Pediatric School Psychology

Series Editor

Paul McCabe, School of Education, Brooklyn College, Brooklyn, NY, USA

The Pediatric School Psychology series presents evidence-based research and practices for prevention, intervention, and treatment of pediatric health issues in school settings. As school psychologists and other educational professionals apply their skills to promote the social and academic success of all students, the information presented in each book in the series facilitates their efforts to understand various health and mental health disorders and target educational delivery to maximize success. Each volume in the series provides analysis by leading experts, who evaluate, synthesize and summarize key research findings and school-related considerations on a specific pediatric disorder. Volume authors critically assess the quality and scholarly design of the extant literature and provide readers with a comprehensive, in depth review of the topic. The information presented in each volume helps scholars and practitioners make informed decisions about identification, evaluation, and treatment of the pediatric health or mental health issue. The overarching goal of the series is to inform and facilitate efforts to enhance the health, mental health, and educational development of students.

More information about this series at http://www.springer.com/series/13561

John S. Carlson · Justin A. Barterian
Editors

School Psychopharmacology

Translating Research into Practice

Springer

Editors
John S. Carlson
School Psychology Program
Michigan State University
East Lansing, MI, USA

Justin A. Barterian
Department of Psychiatry
and Behavioral Health
Ohio State University—Wexner
Medical Center
Columbus, OH, USA

ISSN 2524-8278 ISSN 2524-8286 (electronic)
Pediatric School Psychology
ISBN 978-3-030-15540-7 ISBN 978-3-030-15541-4 (eBook)
https://doi.org/10.1007/978-3-030-15541-4

Library of Congress Control Number: 2019935158

This Springer imprint is published by the registered company Springer Nature Switzerland AG.
The registered company address is: Gewerbestrasse 11, 6330 Cham, Switzerland

We dedicate this book to all the school-aged children and their families who struggle with accessing evidence-based mental health treatments. We hope this book can further support the availability of effective treatment approaches that match the complex etiology of psychological/psychiatric disorders. To that end we know that school personnel are important stakeholders in promoting children's academic and developmental success and this book too was written for those heroes who serve our children daily. We hope this book may help to further break down the walls built up around the settings in which children receive mental health care and developmental nurturing.

A special thank you to my wife, Michelle and my children, Alex, Madalyn, and Brady, who supportively allow me to pursue my diverse scientist-scholar-practitioner interests.

John S. Carlson

Thank you to my wife, Alicia, for her continued support and my daughter, Morgan, for the welcome distractions.

Justin A. Barterian

Preface

Students are only eligible for special education services if demonstratable school-related functioning deficits are present. This presents numerous challenges both ethically and professionally when working with interdisciplinary teams regarding diagnostic decision-making for those school-aged children with mental health disorders (e.g., ADHD, social anxiety) who are responding favorably to physician-prescribed psychotropic treatments. If the effects of medication treatment no longer result in significant functioning deficits in the school setting, does this mean that psychotropic medications can prevent a student's need for more resource-intense special education services? If so, does this mean that it might be cost-effective for public school funding to go towards medication consultation by physicians and/or psychotherapy consultations by psychologists with such investments focused on reducing the cost of special education services through prevention efforts?

Siloed approaches to promoting children's developmental functioning and care for when mental health challenges are present are not best practice. Schools, hospitals, physician offices, and community-based mental health centers often work in isolation around a child's mental health needs. The investigative report surrounding the Sandy Hook Elementary School Shootings provides a very clear example of the problems with these current siloed systems of care. Collaboration around integrative mental health treatment is best practice and aligns with the etiological complexity surrounding serious mental health disorders impacting children and adolescents. Mental health providers and systems of care must adapt to better meet the needs of children, families, and school systems serving children with mental health challenges. This is a public health issue. One with significant costs when inadequate siloed care is provided. What will it take to break down silos? How do we better integrate care across these silos, especially for our children and families most in need?

Health Service Psychologist training programs (i.e., clinical, counseling, school) rarely attend to the role of medications when preparing professionals in the area of mental health treatments. Evidence clearly indicates higher rates of psychotropic medication treatment utilization when compared to psychotherapy. Insurance, marketing, pragmatic barriers, misinformation/lack of information surrounding evidence-based treatments, family values, and other social factors play a role in treatment selection. Mental health professionals, especially those working in schools must seek out a balanced knowledge base across psychiatry/psychology and play an active role in disseminating evidence-based biopsychosocial practices to those in need. How do we better expose mental health professionals to all evidence-based mental health practices? What will it take to improve communication and consultation skills across school and community settings?

School Psychopharmacology: Translating Research into Practice was written to address these persistent questions that challenge our work. Chapter contributors from the field of psychology and psychiatry highlight the importance for greater attention on school psychopharmacology across the fields of psychiatry, psychology, and education.

East Lansing, MI, USA John S. Carlson
Columbus, OH, USA Justin A. Barterian

Contents

Editors and Contributors

About the Editors

John S. Carlson, Ph.D. is a professor and director of clinical training of the School Psychology Program within the College of Education at Michigan State University. He is a health service psychologist and licensed psychologist (MI), holds a B.S. in child psychology from the University of Minnesota and his M.A. and Ph.D. in school psychology from the University of Wisconsin-Madison. He completed his predoctoral internship at Primary Children's Medical Center, Department of Psychiatry, in Salt Lake City, UT. In addition to his faculty work at MSU, Dr. Carlson provides mental health consultation to children, families, and schools within his private practice, Child and Adolescent Psychological Services, PLC in East Lansing, MI. Dr. Carlson has authored or coauthored over 80 articles within peer-reviewed journals and chapters within books. He coauthored a book titled *Counseling Students in Levels 2 and 3: A PBIS/RTI Guide* published by Corwin: A Sage Company and a book titled *101 Careers in Education* that he published with his father through Springer Publishing Company. During his tenure at Michigan State University, he has been instrumental in working with interdisciplinary colleagues to propose, secure, direct, and co-direct training and research grants/contracts now totaling over 8 million dollars.

Justin A. Barterian, Ph.D. is a clinical assistant professor in the Department of Psychiatry and Behavioral Health at the Ohio State University—Wexner Medical Center. He is a licensed psychologist (OH) and earned his B.S. in psychology from Wayne State University and his M.A. and Ph.D. in school psychology from Michigan State University. Dr. Barterian completed his predoctoral internship at the Milton Hershey School in Hershey, PA. Additionally, he completed a postdoctoral fellowship in the Research Unit in Pediatric Psychopharmacology at the Ohio State University—Wexner Medical Center, where he worked on several clinical trials examining psychosocial and psychopharmacological treatments for children with ADHD and disruptive behavior disorders. Dr. Barterian's research focuses on the efficacy of psychopharmacological, psychosocial, and neurofeedback interventions for school-aged and college-aged students with ADHD, selective mutism, social anxiety, and other mental health difficulties. Additionally, Dr. Barterian provides psychological assessment and cognitive-behavioral treatment services to adolescents and college students with ADHD, learning disorders, and related comorbidities in the outpatient clinic at Harding Hospital.

Contributors

Sally Askar Michigan State University, East Lansing, MI, USA

Justin A. Barterian Department of Psychiatry and Behavioral Health, Ohio State University Wexner Medical Center, Columbus, OH, USA

Nathan J. Blum The Children's Hospital of Philadelphia, Perelman School of Medicine at University of Pennsylvania, Philadelphia, PA, USA

John S. Carlson Michigan State University, East Lansing, MI, USA

Adrianna Crossing Michigan State University, East Lansing, MI, USA

Brian Daniels University of Massachusetts, Boston, Boston, MA, USA

Courtney Darr East Lansing, MI, USA

Kristen E. Dewey The Ohio State University, Columbus, OH, USA

George J. DuPaul Lehigh University, Bethlehem, PA, USA

Sarah Edwards School of Medicine, University of Maryland, Baltimore, MD, USA

Cristan Farmer Pediatrics & Developmental Neuroscience Branch, National Institute of Mental Health, National Institutes of Health, Bethesda, MD, USA

Alexander G. Fiks The Children's Hospital of Philadelphia, Perelman School of Medicine at University of Pennsylvania, Philadelphia, PA, USA

Melanie K. Franklin Lehigh University, Bethlehem, PA, USA

Anisa N. Goforth University of Montana, Missoula, MT, USA

Elizabeth C. Grier Independent Private Practice, Columbia, SC, USA

James P. Guevara The Children's Hospital of Philadelphia, Perelman School of Medicine at University of Pennsylvania, Philadelphia, PA, USA

Danielle Haggerty Michigan State University, East Lansing, MI, USA

Olivia G. Holter University of Montana, Missoula, MT, USA

Rebecca Hommer Pediatrics & Developmental Neuroscience Branch, National Institute of Mental Health, National Institutes of Health, Bethesda, MD, USA

Sharon A. Hoover School of Medicine, University of Maryland, Baltimore, MD, USA

Elizabeth H. Jeffords Independent Private Practice, Columbia, SC, USA

Heather Joseph School of Medicine, University of Pittsburgh, Pittsburgh, PA, USA

Alicia R. Khan University of Maryland, Baltimore County, Baltimore, MD, USA

Shabana Khan School of Medicine, University of Pittsburgh, Pittsburgh, PA, USA

Rachel Korest Michigan State University, East Lansing, MI, USA

Katherine Krive Michigan State University, East Lansing, MI, USA

Thomas Kubiszyn University of Houston, Houston, TX, USA

Jill Leon Pediatrics & Developmental Neuroscience Branch, National Institute of Mental Health, National Institutes of Health, Bethesda, MD, USA

Alyse Ley Michigan State University, East Lansing, MI, USA

Jed Magen Michigan State University, East Lansing, MI, USA

Jennifer A. Mautone The Children's Hospital of Philadelphia, Perelman School of Medicine at University of Pennsylvania, Philadelphia, PA, USA

Cristin McDermott School of Medicine, University of Pittsburgh, Pittsburgh, PA, USA

Allison Meinert University of Houston, Houston, TX, USA

Zachary B. Millman University of Maryland, Baltimore County, Baltimore, MD, USA

Sarah S. Mire University of Houston, Houston, TX, USA

Andy V. Pham Florida International University, Miami, FL, USA

Thomas J. Power The Children's Hospital of Philadelphia, Perelman School of Medicine at University of Pennsylvania, Philadelphia, PA, USA

Christina Sakai Floating Hospital for Children at Tufts Medical Center, Boston, MA, USA

Jason Schiffman University of Maryland, Baltimore County, Baltimore, MD, USA

Monique Simpson School of Medicine, University of Pittsburgh, Pittsburgh, PA, USA

Allison Siroky Michigan State University, East Lansing, MI, USA

Brian Smith Michigan State University, East Lansing, MI, USA

Youeun Song School of Medicine, University of Pittsburgh, Pittsburgh, PA, USA

Robert J. Volpe Northeastern University, Boston, MA, USA

Courtney Walker School of Medicine, University of Pittsburgh, Pittsburgh, PA, USA

Heidi J. Wehring School of Medicine, University of Maryland, Baltimore, MD, USA

Justina Yohannan Michigan State University, East Lansing, MI, USA

Chapter 1
Introduction to School Psychopharmacology

John S. Carlson

Introduction

Promoting the academic and social success of school-aged children requires a tiered approach to mental health service delivery and an accurate picture of how families currently access mental health services to address their child's emotional, behavioral, and social needs. Mental health service utilization research, as well as the latest understanding of evidence-based care for serious mental health disorders, clearly demonstrates the importance of implementing multimodal treatments (e.g., parent/teacher interventions, cognitive behavioral therapy, psychostimulants/antidepressants) that match the biopsychosocial needs of youth with psychiatric diagnoses. According to prevalence estimates derived from a recent national survey of over 50,000 households with children in the United States, most prevalent in school-aged youth (ages 3–17) are psychiatric diagnoses related to behavior/conduct problems (7.4%, approximately 4.4 million children), anxiety (7.1%, approximately 4.1 million), and depression (3.2%, approximately 1.9 million children; Ghandour, Sherman, Vladutiu, Ali, Lynch, Bitsko, & Blumberg, 2019). Providing evidence-based mental health care to this substantial group of children and adolescents requires a seamless coordination of services across educational and health service sectors (e.g., school, clinic, community mental health center) to address the complex needs associated with these psychiatric diagnoses.

School psychopharmacology is the study of psychotropic medications (see Table 1.1 for the most commonly prescribed classes; Sultan et al., 2018) within the school-aged population with special attention given to the impact of these medications on school-related functioning (Carlson, 2001). This area of study has relevance to a number of stakeholders across multiple contexts (e.g., school, home, community) including school administrators, teachers, parents, children, psychologists, and

J. S. Carlson (✉)
Michigan State University, East Lansing, MI, USA
e-mail: carlsoj@msu.edu

J. S. Carlson and J. A. Barterian (eds.), *School Psychopharmacology*,
Pediatric School Psychology, https://doi.org/10.1007/978-3-030-15541-4_1

Table 1.1 Medication classes commonly used to treat child and adolescent mental health disorders

Class of psychotropic medication (specific example)	Potential target behaviors	Possible side effects
Antidepressants		
Selective serotonin reuptake inhibitors (SSRIs) (citalopram, escitalopram, and fluoxetine)	• Obsessive thoughts • Compulsive behaviors • Depressive symptoms	• Drowsiness • Stomach upset • Headache
Serotonin and norepinephrine reuptake inhibitors (SNRIs) (venlafaxine, and duloxetine)	• Depressive symptoms • Anxiety symptoms • Panic attacks	• Dizziness • Headache • Insomnia
Antipsychotics Atypical antipsychotics (aripiprazole, olanzapine, quetiapine, and risperidone)	• Schizophrenia symptoms • Mood regulation	• Hypotension • Motor impairments • Memory difficulties
Typical antipsychotics (haloperidol)	• Psychotic symptoms • Autism-irritability	• Sedation • Weight gain
Stimulants and other ADHD medications (methylphenidate, dexmethylphenidate, lisdexamfetamine atomoxetine, and guanfacine)	• Inattention • Hyperactivity • Impulsivity	• Diminished appetite • Weight loss • Sleep difficulties

Note Source: Sultan et al. (2018)

physicians. Given that schools are often the only or primary source of mental health treatment for children and adolescents (Power, Eiraldi, Clarke, & Mazzuca, 2005; Simon, Pastor, Reuben, Huang, & Goldstrom, 2015), translating school psychopharmacology research into practice is especially important. The purpose of this edited book is to provide an efficient and effective overview of psychopharmacology related to school-related learning and behavior, school contexts, and school-aged populations.

School Psychopharmacology: *Translating Research into Practice* contributes to the child psychopharmacology literature via its focus on legal, ethical, and professional issues related to the use of psychotropic medications in school-aged populations. Following a review of legal, ethical, and professional considerations, this book uniquely opens with a set of case study examples from the educational setting to highlight those situations, where a physician consultation may be warranted following failure to respond to psychosocial treatments being implemented in the school, home, and community settings. A review of effective medications for youth presenting with externalizing disorders (e.g., conduct problems, hyperactivity), internalizing disorders (e.g., depression, anxiety), autism spectrum disorder, psychosis, and mood dysregulation are presented. Special attention is given to the side effects of psychotropic medication and the importance of balancing treatment decisions within a comprehensive cost–benefit analysis. Considerations for the use of psychotropic medications when working with young children and diverse populations are then reviewed. Implications for service sector coordination and ideas for how to engage in practical medication evaluations specific to the school context are examined. The book concludes with a look back at the case studies presented initially, for which a cost–benefit analysis would warrant treatment of a child's school-related dysfunction with a psychotropic medication(s). Within each case study, a data-based approach to evaluating the medication outcomes in the school setting is offered. Implications of prescription practices on the roles and responsibilities of school personnel are highlighted throughout this book. In sum, this edited book brings together experts from across the fields of school psychology, clinical psychology, and child psychiatry to be the only edited book currently published that is focused on child psychopharmacology with specific attention to the school setting.

Arguments Against and for Psychotropic Medications

Psychotropic medication use in school-aged populations is especially controversial and this controversy has only grown in intensity as the number of children prescribed medications has increased over the past 20–30 years. Estimates derived from a national database from 2008 indicated more than 7 million children (0–18 years) were prescribed psychotropic medications (Sultan et al., 2018). Given increased rates of psychotropic prescriptions since 2008, it is reasonable to assume more than 8 million children (approximately 16%) in the United States (US) were prescribed psychotropic medications in 2018. To provide context, this number appears to be slightly more than the total number (6.7 million; 13%) of children and youth (ages 3–21) reported as receiving special education services in the US during the 2015–2016 school year (National Center for Education Statistics, 2018).

Arguments against and for the use of psychotropic medications in children and adolescents are well documented (Carlson & Crossing, 2019). Examples of arguments against use include (a) a mismatch between the child's needs and treatment due to insufficient problem identification/analysis (e.g., differential diagnosis), (b) psychosocial treatments work and they must be utilized first, when possible, (c) the need to do no harm as some medications result in problematic side effects and long-term impacts are largely unknown, (d) the need to do good and the need to teach skills and competencies associated with promoting positive social–emotional functioning and development, and (e) nonadherence to medication treatment and the challenges associated with children and adolescents taking medications as prescribed. Important ethical issues too are at play within school psychopharmacology given issues of assent and consent related to treatment decisions. Specific examples of arguments for use include (a) the evidence-base behind the short-term impact of medications on numerous psychological disorders, (b) the insufficiency of psychosocial interventions in improving dysfunction, (c) the need to do no harm and reduce potentially harmful behaviors (e.g., suicidal or aggressive behaviors), (d) the need to do good and the possibility that some medications may lead to improved developmental outcomes, and (e) the positive safety-efficacy profile of psychotropic medications approved by the Food and Drug Administration (FDA) when taken as prescribed. This mix of reasons against and for psychotropic medication treatment use may result in confusion and uncertainty especially for how caregivers should best address school-aged youth's mental health dysfunction. This becomes even more difficult when emotional and behavioral symptoms fail to respond as expected to effectively implemented, evidence-based psychosocial interventions. Such persistent, intractable, and impactful symptoms may leave parents, teachers, and children themselves at a loss for how to reduce psychological distress and its resulting consequences including how this distress may impact later development.

Impaired social, emotional, or behavioral functioning within the school setting is often the target of psychological consultations with medical personnel. Psychotropic medications are one treatment approach along the continuum of mental health services provided to school-aged children, usually reserved for a very narrow subset of cases according to treatment guidelines found in psychology, pediatrics, psychiatry, and primary care (e.g., American Academy of Pediatrics, 2011). Many parents are unwilling to consider or follow through on a psychotropic treatment approach for their child, while others do so cautiously. Schools can play an important role in documenting the failure of Tier 2 (i.e., strategic interventions) and Tier 3 (i.e., tertiary interventions) psychosocial interventions. Providing parents with clear data about how children may be failing to demonstrate improvements in school-related functioning is paramount to data-based decision making around evidence-based mental health care. In addition, school personnel in coordination with physicians can help to gather the data necessary to help parents support or refute their difficult decision to initiate a trial of psychotropic medication to target school-based improvements in social–emotional, behavioral, and/or academic functioning.

Trends in Mental Healthcare Utilization

A national increase in inpatient hospitalization for suicide, suicidal ideation, and self-injury in children and adolescents (104% increase between 2006 and 2011), and especially in youth 10–14 years of age (151%), demonstrates a pressing need to address serious mental health issues impacting school-aged youth in the United States (Torio, Encinosa, Berdahl, McCormick, & Simpson, 2015). Youth with severe mental health impairment have been persistently undertreated as demonstrated by a recent study examining trends in mental health care (Olfson, Druss, & Marcus, 2015). Based on an analysis of trends in outpatient use of mental health services by persons 6–17 years of age in the United States, the percentage of youth receiving any type of outpatient mental health service was 13.3% in 2010–2012. For this same period of time, youth who were defined as having a severe mental health impairment were receiving outpatient mental health services at relatively low rates. Only one in four (26.1%, up from 16.1% from 1996 to 1998) children and adolescents with serious mental health needs were reported to be receiving outpatient psychotherapy services. Only one in three (31.8%, up from 17.7% from 1996 to 1998) were reported to be treated with psychotropic medication within outpatient mental health care services. Specifically, stimulants (22.6%), antidepressants (13.4%), and antipsychotic (7.5%) classes were reported as most frequently utilized within this 2010–2012 sample of children and adolescent presenting with serious mental health concerns. In sum, only about half of children and adolescents with significant mental health needs are being treated within outpatient mental health settings and the majority are being treated by primary care physicians (35%) or psychiatrists (26%; Anderson, Chen, Perrin, & Van Cleave, 2015).

While healthcare utilization by caregivers of children and adolescents with serious mental health impairment appears to be increasing over the past 20 years, mental health care utilization within the general population of households including children who have been diagnosed with a psychiatric disorder, paints a slightly different picture. A study of national trends in mental health care utilization related to any childhood-onset mental health disorder (see Table 1.2; Olfson & Marcus, 2010) indicates an infrequent use of psychotherapy as a standalone treatment (8.5%) within outpatient mental health services. More frequently, psychotherapy is being utilized in combination with psychotropic medication (33.4%). Even more frequently, children and adolescents with mental health concerns are being treated with psychotropic medication used alone (58.1%). This is especially true for school-aged children diagnosed with Attention Deficit Hyperactivity Disorder who are predominately prescribed medications by their primary care physician and at rates even higher than psychiatrists (73.7% vs. 61.4%; Anderson et al., 2015). Issues of treatment utilization are especially important to consider in the context of cost to families. Out-of-pocket costs for professional behavioral health services are approximately $100 a year more than similar costs for physician behavior health services (Walter, Yuan, & Cabral, 2017).

Trends in outpatient mental healthcare utilization for children and adolescents with a diagnosed psychiatric condition appears to indicate that utilization of psychotherapy, alone or in combination with psychotropic medication is declining, whereas treatments that rely only on psychotropic medications appear to be increasing across time. In a general population sample (N = 53,622) of households in the United States, substantially higher growth across time can be seen for psychotropic medication use when compared to psychotherapy (see Table 1.3).

A substantial percentage of school-aged youth with severe mental health impairments or diagnosed psychiatric conditions are not being treated within the healthcare system. Instead, educational systems of care are often left to attend to these unmet mental health care needs (Power et al., 2005). Moreover, when families are accessing mental health care for their children and adolescents with mental health challenges, use of psychotropic medications are most frequently employed when compared to

Table 1.2 Trends in outpatient mental health care utilization for childhood-onset mental health disorders

Service Utilization, Type	1998 (%)	2007 (%)	Difference 1998–2007 (%)
Psychotherapy, alone	13.1	8.5	−4.6
Psychotherapy, with psychotropic medication	40.7	33.4	−7.3
Psychotropic medication, alone	46.2	58.1	+11.9

Note Includes DSM codes 299, 312–315, 317–319, 307, except 307.2 and 307.8
Source Olfson and Marcus (2010) (N = 605)

Table 1.3 Trends in use of psychotropic medications and psychotherapy by school-aged youth (6–17 years)

Treatment, Type	1996–1998 (%)	2003–2005 (%)	2010–2012 (%)	15-year trend (%)
Psychotropic medication	**5.5**	**7.0**	**8.9**	**+3.4**
Stimulants	4.0	4.9	6.6	+2.6
Antidepressants	1.5	2.5	2.6	+1.1
Antipsychotics	0.2	0.9	1.2	+1.0
Psychotherapy	**4.2**	**5.0**	**6.0**	**+1.8**

Note Source: Olfson et al. (2015) (N = 53,622)

psychotherapy approaches. Schools and behavior within schools are substantially impacted by these trends in psychotropic medication use in school-aged populations (Simon et al., 2015) and support the need for greater attention to translating research into practice in school psychopharmacology.

Implications of Prescription Trends on Schools and Training

Increases in prescriptions of psychotropic medications in school-aged populations have led to increased involvement of school personnel within medication treatment-related roles (Carlson, Demaray, & Hunter-Oehmke, 2006; Shahidullah & Carlson, 2014). Rates of psychotropic medication, especially atypical antipsychotics which present with worrisome side effect profiles, have increased substantially in recent years (Olfson et al., 2015). At the same time, evidence-based psychosocial interventions are failing to be implemented as expected in both school (e.g., Hicks, Shahidullah, Carlson, & Palejwala, 2014) and community-based (Bruns et al., 2016) settings due to numerous systemic barriers. Given these challenges, mental health professionals working in schools must have a firm understanding of how psychotropic medications fit into a comprehensive psychological service delivery model now more than ever. Numerous publications and resources have been targeted to school personnel related to child psychopharmacology (e.g., Carlson, Brinkman, Majewicz-Hefley, 2006; Carlson, Kruer, Ogg, Mathiason, & Magen, 2007; Carlson & Shahidullah, 2014; Carlson, Thaler, & Hirsch, 2005; DuPaul & Carlson, 2005, Kubiszyn, Carlson, & DeHay, 2005) but the need for resources like Lloyd and colleagues (2016) describing effective service sector coordination to more effectively connect physicians, school personnel, and families is now more important than ever given increased trends in psychotropic medication treatment approaches for childhood-onset mental health disorders.

More than 20 years ago, the American Psychological Association (1995) called for an additional focus on training psychologists in psychopharmacology. A specific set of guidelines was developed to assist in the training of psychologists in evidence-based psychopharmacological interventions. Yet, even the most basic education related to psychotropic medication remains missing from many university training programs (Shahidullah & Carlson, 2014), leaving many school-based mental health professionals unprepared to coordinate services and monitor outcomes of school-aged youth treated with psychotropic medications. It is our hope that this edited book will be one of many resources that can help to (a) improve basic educational training related to evidence-based psychopharmacological interventions (in combination with psychosocial approaches) in school-aged populations and (b) increase service sector coordination of services for youth presenting with mental health disorders that are not responsive to evidence-based psychosocial interventions. Toward this goal, a brief review of each of the chapters found in this edited book is presented.

Chapter 2 (DuPaul & Franklin, 2019) addresses the legal, ethical, and professional issues related to the use of psychoactive medications in school-aged populations. Specific attention is given the implications of these issues for the roles and responsibilities of school personnel when working with families and physicians around medication treatment decisions.

Chapter 3 highlights a series of case studies for disorders impacting school-aged youth that commonly are prescribed psychopharmacological treatments. Within each case study [Attention Deficit Hyperactivity Disorder (Askar, 2019); Conduct Disorder (Haggerty, 2019); Depression (Yohannan, 2019); Social Anxiety Disorder (Darr, 2019); Autism Spectrum Disorder (Siroky, 2019); Psychosis (Korest, 2019); Bipolar Disorder (Crossing, 2019)], readers are provided a general case overview including impacted school functioning, targeted school-based intervention goals/behaviors, a description of a failed evidence-based psychosocial treatment approach implemented in the classroom, and rationale for the need for more intensive services including a medical consultation. The purpose of each case study is to provide readers with a sense of the social, emotional, behavioral, and developmental costs associated with each child's current behavioral functioning within the school and home settings.

Chapter 4 (Joseph, Walker, McDermott, Song, Simpson, & Khan, 2019) reviews the evidence for the use of psychotropic medications, including stimulants, atypical antipsychotics, and antihypertensives, to treat externalizing disorders, such as attention deficit hyperactivity disorder, oppositional defiant disorder, and conduct disorder, in children and adolescents. Both the intended and side effects of medication treatments (e.g., stimulants, non-stimulants, antipsychotics, mood stabilizers) commonly used to treat these externalizing disorders are reviewed. Professional guidelines for the treatment of externalizing disorders in school-aged populations are presented.

Chapter 5 (Smith, Ley, Krive, & Magen, 2019) reviews the evidence for the use of psychotropic medications, including selective serotonin reuptake inhibitors, tricyclic antidepressants, and anxiolytics to treat depression and anxiety (e.g., generalized anxiety disorder, social anxiety disorder, obsessive–compulsive disorder) in children and adolescents. The intended and side effects of medication treatments commonly used to treat internalizing disorders in school-aged youth are described. Professional guidelines for the treatment of anxiety and depression are presented.

Chapter 6 (Farmer, Leon, & Hommer, 2019) reviews the evidence for the use of a variety of psychotropic medications, such as antidepressants, atypical antipsychotics, and stimulants, to treat the symptoms of autism spectrum disorder (i.e., irritability, inattention, hyperactivity, sleep problems, restricted and repetitive behaviors, social communication problems) in children and adolescents. The intended and side effects of medications commonly used to treat symptoms of autism spectrum disorder are described. Professional guidelines for the treatment of autism spectrum disorder in school-aged children are discussed.

Chapter 7 (Millman, Wehring, Khan, Edwards, Hoover, & Schiffman, 2019) reviews the evidence for the use psychotropic medications such as mood stabilizers, typical antipsychotics, and atypical antipsychotics for the treatment of psychosis in school-aged youth. Both the intended and side effects of medication treatments (i.e., first-generation antipsychotics, second-generation antipsychotics) commonly used to treat psychotic symptoms are reviewed. In addition, the impact of using adjunctive psychosocial interventions in combination with psychotropic medication treatment for psychosis is presented. The chapter concludes with implications for school personnel and the importance of interprofessional collaboration when working with youth presenting with psychosis.

Chapter 8 (Grier, Jeffords, & Dewey, 2019) reviews the evidence for the use psychotropic medications such as mood stabilizers, typical antipsychotics, and atypical antipsychotics for the treatment of mood dysregulation disorders in children and adolescents. Both the intended and side effects of medication treatments (mood stabilizers, antipsychotics, anticonvulsants, antidepressants, stimulants) commonly used to treat mood dysregulation are reviewed. The chapter concludes with implications for school personnel and the importance of interprofessional collaboration when working with youth presenting with mood dysregulation.

Chapter 9 (Kubiszyn, Mire, & Meinert, 2019) highlights the commonly experienced side effects of psychotropic medication use in school-aged children. In addition, less common but life-threatening side effects are discussed with specific attention to the implications of prescriptions carrying "black-box" warnings. To help guide the thought processes that undergird risk–benefit analysis, a framework for stakeholder's (e.g., prescribers, parents, school professionals) communications is provided.

Chapter 10 (Barterian, 2019) discusses the special considerations associated with the use of psychotropic medications in young children. Emphasis is placed on the importance of a thorough cost-to-benefit analysis prior to and during psychiatric treatment. The paucity of available efficacy data in young children and the unique short- and long-term side effect concerns are reviewed.

Chapter 11 (Goforth, Pham, & Holter, 2019) highlights the importance and need to be sensitive to the cultural context of a child and her family when considering treatment plans that involve psychotropic medications. Special considerations are provided for how school personnel can create an open and clear pattern of communication with diverse families who choose to medicate their children. A brief primer on cultural psychiatry and the integration of clinical services with school support are presented. Recommendations for school personnel when providing mental health services to diverse children and families, with a focus on psychopharmacological treatment for children are reviewed.

Chapter 12 (Power, Mautone, Blum, Fiks, & Guevara, 2019) highlights the importance of linking school personnel with treatment providers in the community. An overview of integrated behavioral health and the benefits to care coordination to school-aged youth experiencing social, emotional, and behavioral challenges is presented. The role of school psychologists in IBH contexts is reviewed. Limitations of current models of integrated care, future directions for research, and implications for training and practice are discussed.

Chapter 13 (Volpe, Daniels, & Sakai, 2019) presents an overview of assessment and medication-monitoring procedures that can be completed in the school setting to collect information on symptom severity/improvement, adverse events, and educational outcomes associated with psychopharmacological treatment. Commonly encountered systemic barriers to these procedures and solutions to these challenges are presented.

Chapter 14 highlights case studies involving psychotropic medication treatment approaches to improve school functioning. Within each case study [Attention Deficit Hyperactivity Disorder (Askar, 2019); Conduct Disorder (Haggerty, 2019); Depression (Yohannan, 2019); Social Anxiety Disorder (Darr, 2019); Autism Spectrum Disorder (Siroky, 2019); Psychosis (Korest, 2019); Bipolar Disorder (Crossing, 2019)], readers are provided a general case overview of the child's treatment plan, targeted goals/behaviors, an overview of a classroom-based medication evaluation plan, and an overview of treatment response communicated back to the child's family/physician. The purpose of each case study is to provide readers with a sense of how to measure the impact of psychotropic medication on a child's current behavioral functioning within the school and home settings.

References

American Academy of Pediatrics. (2011). ADHD: Clinical practice guideline for the diagnosis, evaluation, and treatment of attention-deficit/hyperactivity disorder in children and adolescents. *Pediatrics, 128,* 1007–1022.

American Psychological Association. (1995). *Final report of the BEA working group to develop a Level 1 curriculum for psychopharmacology education and training.* Washington, DC: Author.

Anderson, L. E., Chen, M. L., Perrin, J. M., & Van Cleave, J. (2015). Outpatient visits and medication prescribing for US children with mental health conditions. *Pediatrics, 136,* e1178–e1185.

Bruns, E. J., Kerns, S. E. U., Pullmann, M. D., Hensley, S. W., Lutterman, T., & Hoagwood, K. E. (2016). Research, data, and evidence-based treatment use in state behavioral health systems, 2001–2012. *Psychiatric Services, 67,* 496–503.

Carlson, J. S. (2001). Empirical support for training in school psychopharmacology. *Trainers' Forum: Periodical of the Trainers of School Psychologists, 20,* 6–11.

Carlson, J. S., & Crossing, A. E. (2019). Arguments for and against the use of psychotropic medication within school-aged populations. In M. Burns (Ed.), *Introduction to school psychology: Controversies and current practices.* Oxford: Oxford University Press.

Carlson, J. S., & Shahidullah, J. D. (2014). Best practices in assessing the effects of psychotropic medications on student performance. In P. L. Harrison & A. Thomas (Eds.), *Best practices in school psychology: Systems-level services* (pp. 361–374). Bethesda, MD: National Association of School Psychologists.

Carlson, J. S., Thaler, C. L., & Hirsch, A. J. (2005). Psychotropic medication consultation in schools: An ethical and legal dilemma for school psychologists. *Journal of Applied School Psychology, 22,* 29–41.

Carlson, J. S., Brinkman, T., & Majewicz-Hefley, A. (2006). Promoting an understanding of medication treatment outcomes for school-aged children diagnosed with autism. *The California School Psychologist, 11,* 33–42.

Carlson, J. S., Demaray, M. K., & Hunter-Oehmke, S. (2006). A survey of school psychologists' knowledge and training in child psychopharmacology. *Psychology in the Schools, 43,* 623–633.

Carlson, J. S., Kruer, J. L., Ogg, J. A., Mathiason, J. B., & Magen, J. (2007). Methylphenidate, atomoxetine, and caffeine: A primer for school psychologists. *Journal of Applied School Psychology, 24,* 127–146.

DuPaul, G., & Carlson, J. S. (2005). Child psychopharmacology: How school psychologists can contribute to effective outcomes. *School Psychology Quarterly, 20,* 206–221.

Ghandour, R. M., Sherman, L. J., Vladutiu, C. J., Ali, M. M., Lynch, S. E., Bitsko, R. H., & Blumberg, S. J. (2019). Prevalence and treatment of depression, anxiety, and conduct problems in US children. *The Journal of Pediatrics, e3,* 256–267. https://doi.org/10.1016/j.jpeds.2018.09.021.

Hicks, T. B., Shahidullah, J. D., Carlson, J. S., & Palejwala, M. (2014). Nationally Certified School Psychologists' use and reported barriers to using evidence-based interventions in schools: The influence of graduate program training and education. *School Psychology Quarterly, 29,* 469–487. https://doi.org/10.1037/spq0000059.

Kubiszyn, T., Carlson, J. S., & DeHay, T. (2005). Pediatric psychopharmacology: An update on internalizing disorders. *School Psychology Quarterly, 20,* 135–154.

Lloyd, B. P., Torelli, J. N., & Symons, F. J. (2016). Issues in integrating psychotropic and intensive behavioral interventions for students with emotional and behavioral challenges. *Journal of Emotional and Behavioral Disorders, 24,* 148–158.

National Center for Education Statistics. (2018). *Children and youth with disabilities.* Retrieved November 29, 2018, from https://nces.ed.gov/programs/coe/indicator_cgg.asp.

Olfson, M., & Marcus, S. C. (2010). National trends in outpatient psychotherapy. *American Journal of Psychiatry, 167,* 1456–1463.

Olfson, M., Druss, B. G., & Marcus, S. C. (2015). Trends in mental health care among children and adolescents. *The New England Journal of Medicine, 372,* 2029–2038.

Power, T. J., Eiraldi, R. B., Clarke, A. T., & Mazzuca, L. B. (2005). Improving mental health service utilization for children and adolescents. *School Psychology Quarterly, 2005,* 187–205.

Shahidullah, J. D., & Carlson, J. S. (2014). Survey of Nationally Certified School Psychologists' roles and training in psychopharmacology. *Psychology in the Schools, 51,* 705–721. https://doi.org/10.1002/pits.21776.

Simon, A. E., Pastor, P. N., Reuben, C. A., Huang, L. N., & Goldstrom, I. D. (2015). Use of mental health services by children ages six to 11 with emotional and behavioral difficulties. *Psychiatric Services, 66,* 930–937. https://doi.org/10.1089/cap.2017.0077.

Sultan, R. S., Correll, C. U., Schoenbaum, M., King, M., Walkup, J. T., & Olfson, M. (2018). National patterns of commonly prescribed psychotropic medications to young people. *Journal of Child and Adolescent Psychopharmacology, 28,* 158–165.

Torio, C. M., Encinosa, W., Berdahl, T., McCormick, M. C., & Simpson, L. A. (2015). Annual report on health care for children and youth in the United States: National estimates of cost, utilization and expenditures for children with mental health conditions. *Academic Pediatrics, 15,* 19–35.

Walter, A. W., Yuan, Y., & Cabral, H. J. (2017). Mental health services utilization and expenditures among children enrolled in employer-sponsored health plans. *Pediatrics, 139,* S127–S135.

Chapter 2
Legal, Ethical, and Professional Issues Related to Use of Psychotropic Medications in School-Aged Populations

George J. DuPaul and Melanie K. Franklin

Introduction

Psychologists and related school professionals (e.g., school nurse, special educator) play a critically important role in the psychopharmacological treatment of child and adolescent disorders. This is due, in large part, to the exponential increase in the use of pharmacological interventions and multimodal protocols (i.e., combined medication and psychosocial strategies) for treating a growing number of mental disorders (Olfson, He, & Merikangas, 2013; Ryan, Katsiyannis, & Ellis, 2015; Visser et al., 2014). In addition, a plethora of empirical studies show clear effects, both positive and negative, of psychotropic medications on child cognitive, behavioral, social, and emotional functioning (Brown et al., 2008). Because untreated disorders (e.g., ADHD) can negatively impact school performance, there is increased use of pharmacotherapy to ameliorate deleterious symptoms (e.g., Nyarko et al., 2017). Psychologists are in a great position to collect data that will inform medication-related decisions including evaluation of whether pharmacotherapy is warranted and, if so, what medication and/or dosage will optimize outcomes. School psychologists are particularly well positioned for this evaluation role given their access to direct measures of child functioning on an ongoing basis.

Given the important involvement of psychologists and school professionals in psychopharmacological treatment, the purpose of this chapter is to address legal, ethical, and professional issues related to the use of psychoactive medications in the school-aged population. Specific attention will be given to the implications of these issues for the roles and responsibilities of school personnel when working with families and physicians around medication treatment decisions. First, we provide an overview of legal and ethical issues that should be considered in the context of psychopharmacological treatment in school settings. Next, a variety of roles and

G. J. DuPaul (✉) · M. K. Franklin
Lehigh University, Bethlehem, PA, USA
e-mail: gjd3@lehigh.edu

J. S. Carlson and J. A. Barterian (eds.), *School Psychopharmacology*, Pediatric School Psychology, https://doi.org/10.1007/978-3-030-15541-4_2

responsibilities are described for school psychologists. Third, the implications of legal, ethical, and professional issues for school personnel are discussed. The chapter concludes with a list of readings and websites that may be helpful for readers seeking more information on this topic.

Overview of Legal and Ethical Issues

Over the past 50 years, psychotropic medication use for children and adolescents has greatly increased as a form of treatment and symptom management (DuPaul & Carlson, 2005; Mazur-Mosiewicz, Pierson, & McIntosh, 2009; Steinhausen, 2015). Despite the rise in psychopharmacological interventions, however, there is a dearth of research and knowledge on the use of these medications in the pediatric population (Koelch, Schnoor, & Fegert, 2008). Although certain risks accompany the use of psychopharmacological treatments, the emerging research supports that for many disorders, best-practice treatment includes a combination of psychotherapy and psychopharmacology (Arnold, Hodgkins, Caci, Kahle, & Young, 2015). The limited state of research (aside from treatment of attention deficit/hyperactivity disorder [ADHD] with stimulant medication) combined with the historically controversial practice of utilizing psychopharmacological treatments in children warrants close consideration of legal and ethical issues relevant to pharmacotherapy (Koelch et al., 2008; Ryan, Katsiyannis, Losinski, Reid, & Ellis, 2014).

Practitioners face a variety of ethical and legal challenges with the use of psychotropic interventions. Despite the burgeoning supportive research on this type of treatment, the lack of clear information on the immediate (e.g., insomnia, appetite reduction) and long-term (e.g., impacts on fertility, concomitant alcohol use) adverse side effects of psychotropic medications for children and adolescents leaves room for subjective decision-making and potentially deleterious outcomes (Koelch et al., 2008). The state of knowledge on the safety and efficacy of psychotropic drugs is also dependent on the age of the patient. In general, there are less comprehensive medication treatment standards for younger children, making use riskier in younger populations. Alternatively, given that psychotropic medication may lead to significant symptom reduction and improvement in behavioral functioning, the advantages of this treatment for certain individuals may far outweigh the risks (Brown et al., 2008).

Complications in psychotropic medication use lend themselves to controversial ethical decisions involving indicated dose, over/underdosing, and improper use for the purposes of enhancement. Additionally, legal issues such as off-label use, health insurance coverage, and liability for adverse side effects can further challenge practitioners in their treatment planning (Gutheil, 2012). For the pediatric population, in particular, practitioners must balance best-practice treatment with legal and ethical standards in order to maximize the safety and positive long-term outcomes for the children and adolescents under their care. When utilizing psychotropic interventions, medical and mental health practitioners face different obstacles (e.g., inadequate health insurance coverage, lack of knowledge, and limited patient contact) that may interfere with best-practice care. A team-based approach to treatment planning and evaluation can be an effective way to overcome some of the challenges and subjectivity inherent to this type of practice through data-based decisions and monitoring of the safety and progress of children and adolescents (DuPaul & Carlson, 2005; Mazur-Mosiewicz et al., 2009; Roberts, Floress, & Ellis, 2009; Ryan et al., 2014). Involving important stakeholders such as physicians, children, families, schools, and other allied health professionals is important to best support children's treatment plans and maintain the safety of children in school settings and beyond.

Challenges for Physicians

Traditionally, medical decisions involving prescription of psychotropic medications have fallen under the purview of physicians (Ball, Kratochwill, Johnson, & Freuhling, 2009). Children's infrequent contact with their physicians, limited opportunity for physicians to directly assess functioning in home and school settings, and sporadic communication with healthcare professionals typically precludes a comprehensive understanding of the utility and safety of pharmacotherapy for each individual child. Treatment decisions should be individually determined based on evidence-based practice and cost–benefit analysis (Gutheil, 2012). Best-practice treatment for one child may differ from that of another child, depending on the specific needs and circumstances. Practitioners have a duty to weigh the possible risks and benefits of each type of treatment to determine the optimal care plan for each child. This individualized approach, however, often leaves room for subjective decision-making that can potentially compromise the legal and ethical practice of various treatment modalities. To overcome these obstacles, it is particularly important for practitioners to take great care in understanding and explaining all possible treatment options as well as monitoring the effects of treatment in order to maintain best-practice procedures (Gutheil, 2012).

Physicians face certain pressures and barriers to treatment that may compromise the safety and utility of psychotropic medication use in children and adolescents (Gutheil, 2012). For example, pressures from insurance companies and managed care organizations may limit the physician from choosing the optimal first-choice medication in favor of less expensive or insurance-covered medications. Additionally, due to clinical schedule constraints, physicians may have insufficient time to spend with their patients to develop important relationships and/or gain a comprehensive understanding of patients' reactions to treatments. Other pressures may include limited information on polypharmacy, professional inertia, inducements from drug companies and other stakeholders, professional coding restrictions, and infrequent patient visits.

As with all treatments, many psychotropic medications are associated with possible risks (Hilt et al., 2014). Physicians are faced with the challenge of finding the optimal dosage of the most appropriate medication that will lead to maximal benefits with minimal adverse side effects (Gutheil, 2012; Rappaport, Kulick, & Phelps, 2013). Further compounding these decisions are considerations of age in the context of ethical use of medication (Spetie & Arnold, 2007). In the pediatric population, it is paramount to consider developmental differences in symptom presentation to accurately determine the need for psychopharmacological treatment; both over- and under-use of medication can have extremely detrimental side effects to the short- and long-term outcomes of patients. Stark differences in the pediatric population due to factors such as age, comorbidities, developmental progress, and parental involvement can also limit the efficacy and safety of specific treatments. The limited research literature on psychotropic medication use in the pediatric population leaves room for error in practice and threatens the safety of this population (e.g., Bramness, Engeland, & Furu, 2007).

Particularly because physicians have limited interaction with their patients, to best address these challenges and maximize the safety and efficacy of psychotropic medication interventions, physicians should collaborate with other health-based practitioners to corroborate and support their medical decision-making (DuPaul & Carlson, 2005; Rappaport, Kulick, & Phelps, 2013). Although the decision to medicate a patient may originate in the physician's office, the practicalities of medication use occur in a child's functional settings (e.g., school, home), thus necessitating the involvement of other practitioners and systems in psychotropic medication management (Power & Bradley-Klug, 2012).

One primary functional setting for children is the school. Although school personnel cannot make prescriptive determinations, they have certain responsibilities to administer and monitor the effects of medications during the school day (Mazur-Mosiewicz et al., 2009). Schools have frequent access to children and a unique capability and obligation to implement and evaluate certain interventions that can optimize academic and other areas of functioning (DuPaul & Carlson, 2005; Roberts et al., 2009). Given the frequency of pediatric medication use, mandated legal responsibilities, and the unique position of the school to instigate change, it is imperative for school-based practitioners to be trained in and knowledgeable about psychotropic agents as well as to be involved in a child's treatment plan (DuPaul & Carlson, 2005; Mazur-Mosiewicz et al., 2009; Roberts et al., 2009; Ryan et al., 2014).

School Involvement

Data from the 2011–2012 National Health Survey estimated that approximately 7.5% of children between the ages of 6–17 had taken medication, within the past 6 months of the survey, for emotional or behavioral difficulties (Howie, Pastor, & Lukacs, 2014). Because children spend a large portion of their time in the school setting, as the use of psychotropic medication for children and adolescents increases, so does school involvement (Nyarko et al., 2017; Roberts et al., 2009). Schools are faced with considerable responsibility in medication administration and management that is dictated by both federal and state standards. Although legal obligations stipulate school responsibility, the gray area of the law combined with external challenges (e.g., practitioner training, resources) can create complicated ethical considerations surrounding psychotropic medication use. School-based actions must comply with both legal and ethical standards in order to best support students, families, and external practitioners.

School-Based Legislation

Specific legal standards provide protections to ensure that all students have access to a free and appropriate education (FAPE) whether or not they are taking medication (Section 504 of the Rehabilitation Act of 1973, 2000). According to the Individuals with Disabilities Education Act (IDEA, 2004) and Section 504 of the Rehabilitation Act of 1973 (2000), if students require medication during the school day to access an appropriate education, schools are unable to selectively deny the administration of psychoactive prescriptions or to delegate administrative responsibilities to parents. Rather, schools are legally required to dispense medications during school hours.

Conversely, for students who are not taking medications, schools with federal funding cannot require parents to obtain prescriptions for their children as a prerequisite for gaining access to educational services (e.g., attending school, receiving an evaluation of need for special education support, and receiving special education services; IDEA, 2004; Jacob & Hartshorne, 2007). Further, the determination of impairment under Sect. 504 must be made "without regard to the ameliorative effects of measures such as medication" (U.S. Department of Education, 2016). Although all states with federal funding are bound to these standards, state laws further clarify and expound upon federal legislation to provide state-specific standards for the schools' role in medication involvement (e.g., standards for drug administration responsibilities, involvement of school nurse versus unlicensed individuals; Mazur-Mosiewicz et al., 2009; Ryan et al., 2014). Legislation surrounding school involvement with psychotropic medication places tremendous pressure on school personnel to handle and control substances about which they may have very little training or knowledge. Perhaps due, in part, to the potential discrepancy between training and expected practice, legal standards necessitate the need for trained individuals within the school system to take a role in medication management. To address challenges that arise due to inconsistencies in legal policies, it is of utmost importance to establish clear and consistent state guidelines that address administration procedures, training of personnel, documentation requirements, storage requirements, monitoring procedures, and psychotropic medications to increase the safety of psychotropic medication usage within the school system (Ryan et al., 2014).

Another important aspect of federal legislation concerns parent and child rights under the Family Educational Rights and Privacy Act (FERPA; U.S. Department of Health and Human Services, 2015) and the Health Insurance Portability and Accountability Act (HIPAA; U.S. Department of Health and Human Services, 2014). Both of these pieces of legislation limit the accessibility and disclosure rights of personal information and thereby protect the privacy of children in school and medical settings. FERPA requires schools to obtain consent before disclosing certain personally identifiable information (e.g., health records, transcripts) from a student's educational records (U.S. Department of Health and Human Services, 2015). The HIPAA Privacy Rule also protects personal health information by preventing different organizations (e.g., hospitals, pediatrician offices) from disclosing certain information to outside parties without formal consent (U.S. Department of Health and Human Services, 2014). Although these Acts are of paramount importance to the protection of children and their families, the information sharing restrictions can also limit communication between important stakeholders (e.g., physicians, schools) and interfere with comprehensive care.

Challenges for School Psychologists

Like physicians, school-based practitioners face their own unique legal and ethical challenges when working with children in the school setting (Mazur-Mosiewicz et al., 2009). Allied mental health professionals have training in treatment evaluation and data-based decision-making as well as frequent contact with children in important functional settings (Mazur-Mosiewicz et al., 2009; Roberts et al., 2009). Particularly, due to concerns with the limited knowledge base on standards for pediatric psychotropic agent usage, the involvement of school practitioners in decisions about and evaluations of psychopharmacological treatment may help to increase the safety, effectiveness, and ethical practice of psychopharmacological interventions (DuPaul & Carlson, 2005; Roberts et al., 2009). Because of their training in treatment implementation and evaluation, evidence-based decision-making, data collection, and location within the school environment, school psychologists in particular, are in an ideal position to support physicians in psychotropic pediatric treatment (DuPaul & Carlson, 2005; Mazur-Mosiewicz et al., 2009). Despite these qualifications, however, school psychologists often have insufficient training in clinical psychopharmacology, leading to a plethora of legal and ethical challenges.

In spite of the critical role of school psychologists in medication management, the main governing body for school psychologists; the National Association of School Psychologists (NASP) has no standards for medication training, and the American Psychological Association (APA), another important governing organization for psychologists, only advises general standards that are not specific to school psychology (Roberts et al., 2009). A primary legal and ethical responsibility of all health-based practitioners is to practice only within the bounds of their competence, yet many school psychology graduate programs do not provide the requisite training in this area. Most school psychologists obtain limited to no education in psychopharmacology during their academic training and acquire most of their information from workshops and related readings (Mazur-Mosiewicz et al., 2009). Both NASP and APA, however, have standards for training school psychologists in data-based decision-making and accountability, home–school collaboration, legal and ethical practice, and professional development which are all important aspects of best-practice and acquiring new competencies (Roberts et al., 2009). Although it is possible to gain external training in psychopharmacological interventions, the lack of standards for academic training creates a deficit in practice that can have negative legal and ethical implications for school psychologists and the children that they serve.

Even though school psychologists frequently recommend and implement behavioral interventions, school psychologists typically are not allowed to prescribe or initiate pharmaceutical interventions (Ball et al., 2009; Roberts et al., 2009). As part of informed consent, however, school psychologists have an ethical responsibility to discuss empirically supported treatments with children and their families (DuPaul & Carlson, 2005; Roberts et al., 2009). Empirically supported treatments often include a combination of psychosocial and psychopharmacological interventions (Arnold et al., 2015; Baweja et al., 2016). Failing to provide comprehensive information on various treatment options (e.g., psychotropic agents) could constitute a violation of ethical practice. These dual roles force school psychologists to walk a fine line in their joint responsibilities to communicate various treatment options (e.g., medication) to families and also to avoid prescriptive recommendations that could result in legal turmoil (Ball et al., 2009). Further complicating this responsibility are the limited standards put in place for training in clinical psychopharmacological interventions. School psychologists are expected to communicate about and monitor these interventions in school children, but might have a very limited knowledge base on the use and effects of psychotropic agents.

Just as with psychosocial interventions, school psychologists have the responsibility to help evaluate and implement best-practice care for students in the school system. Depending on children's specific needs and care plan, this responsibility may extend to include a role in psychotropic medication management. Some of these responsibilities include monitoring behavioral, social–emotional, and academic outcomes; coordinating with intervention teams; facilitating communication between various stakeholders (e.g., school personnel, families, physicians); creating a comprehensive plan of therapeutic interventions; and interfacing with physicians (Lloyd, Torelli, & Symons, 2016). School psychologists need to monitor the effectiveness of treatments and also assist in evaluating the risks and benefits of different treatment options to provide comprehensive and ethical practice.

The role of the school psychologist necessitates communication about treatment options that they may have limited knowledge about; implementation of treatments that are initiated by outside practitioners; and evaluation of children's reactions to various interventions. In order to fulfill these obligations in an ethical manner, school psychologists must be given the skills to build competency in pharmacological interventions. Currently, legal and ethical standards to provide services surrounding psychotropic medication use conflict with the limited training standards of school psychologists in this domain, creating a potential deficit in practice and the care of children. To help resolve some of these legal and ethical concerns, dictating specific

Table 2.1 Psychopharmacological treatment of children and adolescents: possible roles for school psychologists

1. Diagnostic decision-making and determining the need for medication
2. Consulting with physicians and families to assess medication effects on academic, social, and behavioral functioning in school settings
3. Assisting physicians and families to determine the optimal dosage of medication for enhancing academic, social, and behavioral outcomes
4. Assessing and supporting adherence with prescribed pharmacological regimens
5. Facilitating integration of medical, psychosocial, and educational interventions in support of individual students

training standards to better prepare school psychologists for the realities of the school system (e.g., trends toward increasing psychotropic use) will help to maintain the safety and efficacy of treatments and provide support to physicians and families in optimizing outcomes for children and adolescents.

Professional Roles and Responsibilities

School psychologists have several critically important roles and responsibilities related to the psychopharmacological treatment of children and adolescents (see Table 2.1). These roles include (a) diagnostic decision-making and determining need for medication; (b) consulting with physicians and families to assess medication effects; (c) assisting physicians and families to determine the optimal dosage of medication: (d) assessing and supporting adherence with prescribed regimens; and (e) facilitating integration of interventions.

Psychologists can provide valuable information to assist families and physicians in determining whether medication is necessary for a child or adolescent. This information is chiefly gathered in the context of a comprehensive evaluation of a student's psychological, behavioral and educational functioning. Stated differently, diagnostic assessment activities typically conducted by psychologists working with the school-aged population will provide data regarding the nature of children's difficulties, severity and chronicity of symptomatic behaviors, and the impact of symptoms on student functioning across multiple domains. In addition, if data are gathered in the context of a multi-tier system of behavioral support, then psychologists should be able to determine the degree to which students respond to Tier 1 and 2 interventions. A lack of response to Tier 1 and 2 interventions could indicate the need to implement a more intensive treatment such as psychotropic medication. In this context, decisions could be made through linking assessment data to treatment options, assessing the need for medication beyond psychosocial and educational interventions, and selecting the least intrusive options as first-line strategies. In addition, psychologists can assist physicians in selecting medications that are empirically supported for treating specific disorders in school-aged populations.

One of the most important roles for school psychologists is to provide data to assist physicians in evaluating the effects of medication. Specifically, behavioral assessment methods can be used to monitor medication effects on academic (e.g., curriculum-based measurement [CBM] probes), social (e.g., self- and teacher-report), and behavioral (e.g., teacher and parent behavior rating scales) functioning. Data can be collected across medication dosage conditions including a non-medication assessment phase (e.g., baseline or placebo, if available). Psychologists can collaborate with others (i.e., school nurse, family, physician) to coordinate findings and the latter can be communicated in a concise, timely fashion to facilitate treatment decisions. In addition, school psychologists can advocate with school and health care professionals for practices that integrate care across settings and help facilitate integration by setting up communication mechanisms (e.g., protected electronic communications) that are compliant with FERPA and HIPAA standards.

Several important features should be included in a medication evaluation (Power, DuPaul, Shapiro, & Kazak, 2003). First, the medication trial should be designed through consultation between school professionals and the prescribing physician. Specific timelines, procedures, and measures should be identified and agreed upon a priori. In addition, areas of functioning (e.g., academic, behavioral, and social) should be prioritized in terms of desired medication outcomes. Brief, objective, psychometrically sound measures (e.g., behavior rating scales, direct observations) are highly desirable given the need for short-term, continuous monitoring of medication effects. In addition to the desired outcomes, possible adverse side effects should be identified and measured. Data for the monitoring protocol should be collected across treatment phases, perhaps in the context of a single-subject research design (for details, see Volpe, Heick, & Gureasko-Moore, 2005 and Chap. 13 of this book). Both outcome and adverse side effect data can then be summarized in a graph or table to facilitate interpretation. Finally, psychologists can collaborate with physicians to reach conclusions about medication treatment and clearly communicate findings and recommendations to parents.

As part of the medication monitoring process, psychologists may also assist physicians in determining optimal dosage; which is defined as the lowest dosage associated with clinically significant improvement with minimal adverse side effects (see Power et al., 2003). Typically, this is accomplished by identifying and monitoring one or two primary outcomes that are deemed to be of highest priority. Although decisions about the dosage associated with the greatest improvement are inherently subjective to some degree, psychologists can advocate for the use of data to inform dosage recommendations.

Findings from three national surveys indicate that the majority of school psychologists have assisted physicians with medication monitoring, although respondents also reported that this activity comprised less than 5% of their workload. Gureasko-Moore, DuPaul, and Power (2005) surveyed 438 National Association of School Psychologists (NASP) members and found approximately 55% of respondents had been involved in medication monitoring for students with ADHD at least once in a given school year. Psychologists reported using teacher and parent behavior ratings, direct observations, and work samples for this purpose. Similarly, Carlson, Demaray, and

Hunter-Oehmke (2006) surveyed 320 practicing NASP members with 62% reporting having worked with physicians and families to evaluate medication effects. Respondents indicated that nearly 25% of their cases involved students who were being treated with one or more medications. Most recently, Shahidullah and Carlson (2014) collected survey data from 817 randomly selected nationally certified school psychologists with an excellent 72% usable response rate. A minority of respondents reported providing direct services such as monitoring behavioral response (28%) or side effects (23%) to psychotropic treatment, and developing medication treatment goals from assessment data (14%). Alternatively, school psychologists were much more likely to report providing indirect services such as behavior management consultation to teachers of students receiving pharmacotherapy (96%), implementing adjunctive psychosocial treatment (87%), and providing assessment data to physicians (84%). School psychologists from all survey samples reported having had very little in the way of training in child psychopharmacology; for example, less than 20% of respondents reported receiving formal coursework in this area during their graduate studies (Gureasko-Moore et al., 2005).

Another very important role for psychologists in the context of pharmacotherapy is to assess and support adherence with prescribed medication regimens. Adherence is defined as the extent to which an individual's behavior, in this case taking medication, coincides with medical advice (i.e., prescription) (Haynes, 1979). As such, medication adherence can vary along a continuum ranging from never taking medication as prescribed to always taking medication as prescribed. Unfortunately, low adherence with pharmacotherapy is common (Osterberg & Blaschke, 2005) and medications for chronic diseases are taken as prescribed only about 50% of the time (Peterson, Takiya, & Finley, 2003). Adherence can be assessed in several ways (e.g., drug assays, pill counts, patient reports) and psychologists can contribute by collecting relevant data such as how often students take medication at school as prescribed. In addition, psychologists can help support adherence by implementing educational strategies (e.g., written instructions plus modeling and behavioral rehearsal), behavioral procedures (e.g., prompting adherent behaviors), and/or multicomponent interventions (e.g., education plus self-management) (Rapoff, 2010).

A final important role for psychologists in the medication management of school-aged populations is to collaborate with physicians, school personnel, and other professionals engaged in treatment to determine the sequence of interventions as well as how multimodal strategies can be integrated. Although sequencing of treatments may be determined, in part, by response to intervention protocols (e.g., implement and assess Tier 2 behavioral strategies before adopting more intensive Tier 3 strategies), because medication falls outside the school purview it is important to consider whether pharmacotherapy should precede psychosocial and educational treatment or vice versa. For example, initiating treatment for attention deficit hyperactivity disorder (ADHD) with behavioral parent training has been found superior to beginning intervention with psychostimulant medication in terms of child outcomes and parent engagement with intervention (Pelham et al., 2016) as well as with respect to cost-effectiveness (Page et al., 2016). In addition, multimodal or combined treatment protocols may optimize outcomes at lower dosages for each treatment. For example, Fabiano et al. (2007) examined the interactive effects of four dosages of methylphenidate (including placebo) and three levels of intensity of behavior modification in an analog classroom setting for children with ADHD. Within-group analyses indicated that the combination of the lowest medication dosage and lowest intensity behavioral strategy led to academic and behavior outcomes analogous to those obtained with the highest dosage of medication or the most intensive behavioral intervention alone. Thus, the combination of medication and psychosocial treatment may lessen concerns regarding adverse side effects typically associated with higher medication dosages and resistance to behavioral interventions that require more teacher time or classroom resources.

Implications for School Personnel

School professionals, particularly school psychologists, are mandated to practice within the bounds of their training. However, to increase the safety of and compliance with school-based legal mandates surrounding psychotropic agents, school psychologist's formal training must be expanded to include education on medication-based interventions. Standardized training dictated by the governing bodies of school psychologists (i.e., NASP, APA) should incorporate mandated courses on pediatric pharmacological interventions so that school psychologists can appropriately and ethically support physicians, fulfill their role within the school, and most importantly, increase the safety and effectiveness of psychotropic agent use with children.

Another main barrier to legal and ethical practice surrounding psychopharmacological interventions is the deficit in communication between school-based and external practitioners. By utilizing the unique strengths of each stakeholder (e.g., families, physicians, school psychologists) involved in a child's care, it is possible to maximize child outcomes across all settings. For this reason, it is of paramount importance to set up systems of open communication between the school and outside practitioners and to provide education to school-based workers and physicians to emphasize the importance of a team-based approach to care. Additionally, this proactive communication between systems can be helpful in setting up guidelines of collaboration that will comply with legal and ethical standards. Further, to increase competencies of practitioners involved in pediatric care, reciprocal efforts to enhance knowledge and training about school and health-based issues should be emphasized.

In general, there is a great need for more research evaluating the safety and efficacy of psychopharmacological interventions to help guide practitioners. More conclusive and detailed information on the short- and long-term effects (both positive and negative) of medications can help reduce the subjectivity in treatment decisions and maximize outcomes for children. Utilizing data-based monitoring techniques in the school system can help to provide evidence surrounding the use of these treatments to further bolster the understanding of these interventions in functional settings. With more information about these treatments, the challenges between law and ethics may be assuaged, enhancing the quality of care for the pediatric population and their families.

Because of their unique role within the school system and relevant training, school psychologists are in an ideal position to serve as liaisons between important stakeholders. Streamlining care will promote best-practice care and optimize outcomes for children in the school setting and beyond. By accounting for the current deficits in practice and understanding of psychotropic interventions, the monitoring and implementation of these interventions can be enhanced to provide more ethical and effective treatment.

Summary

School psychologists can play a variety of important roles with respect to pharmacotherapy including assisting physicians in determining the need for medication treatment, monitoring effects of psychotropic drugs, determining the dosage that optimizes school functioning while not leading to adverse side effects, promoting child and parent adherence with medication prescriptions, and working with a treatment team to determine the best sequence and/or combination of interventions to address students' emotional and behavioral difficulties. There are a variety of important ethical and legal tenets that should be considered when school professionals are engaged in these medication treatment support roles. In particular, the ethical requirement to practice within the parameters of one's training has important relevance given the limited instruction that school professionals typically receive regarding pharmacotherapy procedures and principles. Clearly, greater attention to medication-related issues in preservice training is necessary given the growing use of psychotropic drugs in the pediatric population. Chief among legal considerations are requirements to protect sensitive medical and educational information. Psychologists, school professionals, and physicians should collaborate to proactively design communication and intervention assessment procedures that adhere to legal standards while insuring comprehensive treatment support for students with emotional and behavioral disorders.

List of Readings

Giles, L. L., & Martini, D. R. (2016). Challenges and promises of pediatric psychopharmacology. *Academic Pediatrics*, *16*, 508–518.

This article provides a summary of evidence-based psychopharmacological interventions for pediatric medical conditions. The authors describe the efficacy, safety, and clinical use of different drug types (e.g., stimulants, antidepressants) which help guide pediatric health providers in treatment decisions.

Rappaport, N., Kulick, D., & Phelps, L. (2013). Psychotropic medications: An update for school psychologists. *Psychology in the Schools, 50*, 589–600.

This review focuses on the utilization of medication for pediatric depression, anxiety, and bipolar disorder. This article provides information that will aid school psychologists and other practitioners in communicating with physicians and caregivers. A summary of treatment options as well as clear, detailed tables about common drug types and adverse side effects are included.

Ryan, J. B., Katsiyannis, A., Losinski, M., Reid, R., & Ellis, C. (2014). Review of state medication policies/guidelines regarding psychotropic medications in public schools. *Journal of Child and Family Studies, 23*(4), 704–715.

State procedures regarding school medication policies vary widely. This article provides a review of various state procedures and offers guidance on best practice for establishing state guidelines concerning the use of psychotropic medications in public schools.

List of Websites

Laws and Guidance

https://www2.ed.gov/policy/landing.jhtml

This U.S. Department of Education resource contains links to the text of key pieces of education-related legislation (e.g., IDEA, FERPA) as well as other guiding documents (e.g., Dear Colleague Letters).

http://www.apa.org/pi/disability/dart/legal/

The DisABILITY Resources Toolbox (DART) Toolkit II: Legal Issues, published by the American Psychological Association highlights key pieces of legislation in the context of psychological practice. Summaries of key policies as well as practice suggestions are included in the toolkit.

References

Arnold, L. E., Hodgkins, P., Caci, H., Kahle, J., & Young, S. (2015). Effect of treatment modality on long-term outcomes in attention-deficit/hyperactivity disorder: A systematic review. *PLoS ONE, 10*(2), e0116407.

Ball, C. R., Kratochwill, T. R., Johnston, H. F., & Fruehling, J. J. (2009). Limited prescription privileges for psychologists: Review and implications for the practice of psychology in the schools. *Psychology in the Schools, 46*, 836–845.

Baweja, R., Belin, P. J., Humphrey, H. H., Babocsai, L., Pariseau, M. E., Waschbusch, D. A., … Waxmonsky, J. G. (2016). The effectiveness and tolerability of central nervous system stimulants in school-age children with attention-deficit/hyperactivity disorder and disruptive mood dysregulation disorder across home and school. *Journal of Child and Adolescent Psychopharmacology, 26*, 154–163.

Bramness, J. G., Engeland, A., & Furu, K. (2007). Use of antidepressants among children and adolescents–did the warnings lead to fewer prescriptions? *Tidsskrift for den Norske Laegeforening, 127*(20), 2653–2655.

Brown, R. T., Antonuccio, D., DuPaul, G. J., Fristad, M., King, C. A., Leslie, L. K., … Vitiello, B. (2008). *Childhood mental health disorders: Evidence base and contextual factors for psychosocial, psychopharmacological, and combined interventions*. Washington, DC: American Psychological Association.

Carlson, J. S., Demaray, M. K., & Hunter-Oehmke, S. (2006). A survey of school psychologists' knowledge and training in child psychopharmacology. *Psychology in the Schools, 43*, 623–633.

DuPaul, G. J., & Carlson, J. S. (2005). Child psychopharmacology: How school psychologists can contribute to effective outcomes. *School Psychology Quarterly, 20*, 206–221.

Fabiano, G. A., Pelham, W. E. Jr., Gnagy, E. M., Burrows-MacLean, L., Coles, E. K., Chacko, A., … Robb, J. A. (2007). The single and combined effects of multiple intensities of behavior modification and methylphenidate for children with attention deficit hyperactivity disorder in a classroom setting. *School Psychology Review, 36*, 195–216.

Gureasko-Moore, D., DuPaul, G. J., & Power, T. J. (2005). Stimulant treatment for ADHD: Medication monitoring practices of school psychologists. *School Psychology Review, 34*, 232–245.

Gutheil, T.G. (2012). Reflections on ethical issues in psychopharmacology: An American perspective. *International Journal of Law and Psychiatry, 35*, 387–391.

Haynes, R. B. (1979). Introduction. In R. B. Haynes, D. W. Taylor, & D. C. Sackett (Eds.), *Compliance in health care* (pp. 1–7). Baltimore: The Johns Hopkins University Press.

Hilt, R. J., Chaudhari, M., Bell, J. F., Wolf, C., Koprowicz, K., & King, B. H. (2014). Side effects from use of one or more psychiatric medications in a population-based sample of children and adolescents. *Journal of Child and Adolescent Psychopharmacology, 24*, 83–89.

Howie, L. D., Pastor, P. N., & Lukacs, S. (2014). Use of medication prescribed for emotional or behavioral difficulties among children aged 6–17 years in the United States, 2011–2012. *NCHS Data Brief, 148*, 1–8.

Individuals with Disabilities Education Act, 20 U.S.C. § 1400 (2004).

Jacob, S., & Hartshorne, T. S. (2007). *Ethics and law for school psychologists* (5th ed.). Hoboken: Wiley.

Koelch, M., Schnoor, K., & Fegert, J. M. (2008). Ethical issues in psychopharmacology of children and adolescents. *Current Opinion in Psychiatry, 21*, 598–605. https://doi.org/10.1097/YCO.0b013e328314b776.

Lloyd, B. P., Torelli, J. N., & Symons, F. J. (2016). Issues in integrating psychotropic and intensive behavioral interventions for students with emotional and behavioral challenges in schools. *Journal of Emotional and Behavioral Disorders, 24*, 148–158.

Mazur-Mosiewicz, A., Pierson, E. E., & McIntosh, D. E. (2009). Legal issues in school health services and school psychology: Guidelines for the administration of medication. *Psychology in the Schools, 46*, 813–819.

Nyarko, K. A., Grosse, S. D., Danielson, M. L., Holbrook, J. R., Visser, S. N., & Shapira, S. K. (2017). Treated prevalence of attention-deficit/hyperactivity disorder increased from 2009 to 2015 among school-aged children and adolescents in the United States. *Journal of Child and Adolescent Psychopharmacology*. https://doi.org/10.1089/cap.2016.0196. Advance online publication.

Olfson, M., He, J., & Merikangas, K. R. (2013). Psychotropic medication treatment of adolescents: Results from the National Comorbidity Survey-Adolescent Supplement. *Journal of the American Academy of Child and Adolescent Psychiatry, 52*, 378–388.

Osterberg, L., & Blaschke, T. (2005). Adherence to medication. *New England Journal of Medicine, 353*, 487–497.

Page, T. F., Pelham, W. E. III, Fabiano, G. A., Greiner, A. R., Gnagy, E. M., Hart, K. C., … Pelham, W. E. Jr. (2016). Comparative cost analysis of sequential, adaptive, behavioral, pharmacological, and combined treatments for ADHD. *Journal of Clinical Child and Adolescent Psychology, 45,* 416–427. https://doi.org/10.1080/15374416.2015.1055859.

Pelham, W. E. Jr., Fabiano, G. A., Waxmonsky, J. G., Greiner, A. R., Gnagy, E. M., Pelham, W. E. III., … Murphy, S.A. (2016). Treatment sequencing for childhood ADHD: A multiple-randomization study of adaptive medication and behavioral interventions. *Journal of Clinical Child and Adolescent Psychology, 45,* 396–415. https://doi.org/10.1080/15374416.2015.1105138.

Peterson, A. M., Takiya, L., & Finley, R. (2003). Meta-analysis of trials of intervention to promote medication adherence. *American Journal of Health-System Pharmacy, 60,* 657–665.

Power, T. J., & Bradley-Klug, K. L. (2012). *Pediatric school psychology: Conceptualization, applications, and strategies for leadership development.* New York: Routledge.

Power, T. J., DuPaul, G. J., Shapiro, E. S., & Kazak, A. E. (2003). *Promoting children's health: Integrating health, school, family, and community systems.* New York: Guilford.

Rapoff, M. A. (2010). *Adherence to pediatric medical regimens* (2nd ed.). New York: Springer.

Rappaport, N., Kulick, D., & Phelps, L. (2013). Psychotropic medications: An update for school psychologists. *Psychology in the Schools, 50,* 589–600.

Roberts, H. J., Floress, M. T., & Ellis, C. R. (2009). Training school psychologists in psychopharmacology consultation. *Psychology in the Schools, 46,* 827–835.

Ryan, J. B., Katsiyannis, A., Losinski, M., Reid, R., & Ellis, C. (2014). Review of state medication policies/guidelines regarding psychotropic medications in public schools. *Journal of Child and Family Studies, 23,* 704–715.

Ryan, J. B., Katsiyannis, A., & Ellis, C. (2015). Increasing role of medication therapy for managing student behavior. *Beyond Behavior, 24,* 31–37.

Section 504 of the Rehabilitation Act of 1973, 34. C.F.R. Part 104.

Shahidullah, J. D., & Carlson, J. S. (2014). Survey of nationally certified school psychologists' roles and training in psychopharmacology. *Psychology in the Schools, 51,* 705–721. https://doi.org/10.1002/pits.21776.

Spetie, L., & Arnold, L. E. (2007). Ethical issues in child psychopharmacology research and practice: Emphasis on preschoolers. *Psychopharmacology (Berl), 191,* 15–26.

Steinhausen, H. (2015). Recent international trends in psychotropic medication prescriptions for children and adolescents. *European Child and Adolescent Psychiatry, 24,* 635–640.

United States Department of Education, Office for Civil Rights. (2016, July 26). *Dear colleague letter and resource guide on students with ADHD.* Retrieved from https://www2.ed.gov/about/offices/list/ocr/letters/colleague-201607-504-adhd.pdf.

United States Department of Health and Human Services. (2014). *Guidance regarding methods for de-identification of protected health information in accordance with the health insurance portability and accountability act (hipaa) privacy rule.* Washington, DC: US Department of Health and Human Services.

United States Department of Health and Human Services. (2015). *US Department of Education. Joint Guidance on the Application of the Family Educational Rights and Privacy Act (FERPA) and the Health Insurance Portability and Accountability Act of 1996 (HIPAA) to Student Health Records.* Washington, DC: US Department of Health and Human Services.

Visser, S. N., Danielson, M. L., Bitsko, R. H., Holbrook, J. R., Kogan, M. D., Ghandour, R. M., … Blumberg, S. J. (2014). Trends in the parent-report of health care provider-diagnosed and medicated attention-deficit/hyperactivity disorder: United States, 2003–2011. *Journal of the American Academy of Child & Adolescent Psychiatry, 53,* 34–46.

Volpe, R. J., Heick, P. F., & Gureasko-Moore, D. (2005). An agile behavioral model for monitoring the effects of stimulant medication in school settings. *Psychology in the Schools, 42,* 509–523.

Chapter 3
Clinical Case Studies: Failing to Respond to Psychosocial Treatments

Sally Askar, Danielle Haggerty, Justina Yohannan, Courtney Darr, Allison Siroky, Rachel Korest and Adrianna Crossing

The purpose of this chapter is to present a series of cases that highlight those situations when children fail to respond to psychosocial treatment approaches in schools and an emergent need for a psychiatric consultation develops. Case studies (Attention Deficit Hyperactivity Disorder, Conduct Disorder, Depression, Social Anxiety Disorder, Autism Spectrum Disorder, Bipolar Disorder, Psychosis) related to each of the mental health conditions reviewed in this book are presented. Each case study provides an overview of the child's presenting problem, background/case description, targeted goals/behaviors for psychosocial intervention, and rationale for a psychiatric consultation referral. The purpose of each case study is to provide readers with a sense of the social, emotional, behavioral, and developmental costs associated with each child's current behavioral functioning within the school and home settings. The rationale for the importance of implementing evidence-based psychosocial interventions and the resulting need for a psychiatric consultation when children fail to respond to school-based psychosocial interventions is presented for each case.

As a follow-up to each case presented in this chapter, Chap. 14 highlights the results of the psychiatric consultation and information is presented for each child as they are prescribed a trial of an evidence-based psychopharmacological treatment. The rationale for selecting medication to improve each child's mental health functioning in school is presented within a cost–benefit analytic approach. Each case study in Chap. 14 provides an overview of the child's treatment plan, targeted intervention goals/behaviors, a medication evaluation plan, and an overview of the school-based treatment response communicated back to the child's family/physician.

S. Askar (✉) · D. Haggerty · J. Yohannan · A. Siroky · R. Korest · A. Crossing
Michigan State University, East Lansing, MI, USA
e-mail: askarsal@msu.edu

C. Darr
East Lansing, MI, USA
e-mail: courtneyldarr@gmail.com

J. S. Carlson and J. A. Barterian (eds.), *School Psychopharmacology*,
Pediatric School Psychology, https://doi.org/10.1007/978-3-030-15541-4_3

Attention Deficit Hyperactivity Disorder

Sally Askar

Presenting Problem

Jim is a 10-year old in the fourth grade. His teacher reports numerous behavioral problems in the classroom that are impacting his academic performance. His symptoms include fidgeting, inattention, talking excessively to his peers, disorganization, and difficulties with self-regulation.

Background

Jim lives with his mom, dad, older brother, and younger sister. He resides in a rural area and his family struggles, financially. Jim's father has been chronically unemployed since Jim was 5 years old and Jim's mother works night shifts at a local hospital as a nurse aide. Jim's 16-year-old brother was diagnosed with ADHD when he was 12 years old and is currently taking Ritalin, a stimulant medication. Jim's younger sister has no history of mental health issues and is a model student according to her first-grade teacher. Jim's father was diagnosed with ADHD when he was 17 years old. He continues to struggle with symptoms of inattention, which negatively impacted his job performance when he was employed. Jim's mother reported smoking cigarettes since she was 18 years old and reported smoking during the first trimester when pregnant with Jim. It is noteworthy that Jim was a preterm baby (4 weeks) and underweight at birth. Jim's parents shared that he was an active toddler and that his behavior began to create problems while in preschool as he was not able to sit still during large group activities. In second grade, Jim's parents shared that he increasingly began to show difficulty focusing and maintaining his attention when completing seat work. Further, they indicated he had trouble socializing in the neighborhood, difficulty sitting still at the kitchen table, and being unable to watch television shows from start to finish.

Case Description

For the past 6 months, Jim's teacher has been noticing an increased difficulty in his ability to pay attention in class. He is making careless mistakes on his homework assignments resulting in low grades. Jim's teacher reports that he has difficulty in responding appropriately to verbal directions as if he doesn't hear them correctly.

Jim also presents as disorganized and constantly forgetful of where he has left his notebook, pencils, and assignments. Classroom observational data indicate that he is frequently off-task and not able to sit still when compared to his peers. Jim infrequently interacts with classmates and often eats alone in the lunchroom. Jim has consistently underperformed on national reading and math assessments, putting him in a Tier 2 intervention level (i.e., small reading and math groups). Jim's teacher recently recommended he be retained in fourth grade because of his low academic performance. Jim's parents note numerous problems within the home setting as he often fails to follow through with their instructions and he struggles to pay attention when sitting down to do his homework. They also note that Jim does not have many friends in the neighborhood and that he often spends time alone playing video games.

Target Behaviors for Intervention/Goals

1. Increase time on task (Token Economy System)

Since Jim was struggling to maintain his attention within the classroom, the goal of targeting his time on task was to improve both the quality and quantity of his seat work. The goal was for Jim to increase his time on academic tasks to a level consistent with his fourth-grade peers.

2. Increase self-regulatory behavior (Self-Monitoring)

Due to difficulties meeting classroom behavior expectations, Jim's behavioral self-monitoring skills were targeted for intervention. The goal was for Jim to improve his ability to self-observe, reflect, and manage his behavior consistent with his teacher's expectations.

3. Improve social interactions with peers (Social–Emotional Curriculum)

Jim's minimal social interaction with peers was targeted for intervention. The goal was to increase his peer interaction with the hope of providing him additional social support given his academic struggles.

Evidence-Based School Interventions

Token Economy. A token economy system (e.g., use of tokens to reinforce on-task behavior) was developed/implemented in Jim's classroom and at home. This classroom-wide intervention was selected to also benefit other students in the classroom. Jim's teacher used stickers as tokens and school supplies as rewards. Students earned stickers when they were observed being on task during independent work time. When students received 10 stickers they could exchange the stickers for a reward (e.g., pens, erasers, notebooks). When students earned a reward, the number of stickers needed to exchange for a reward was increased. Jim's parents also implemented the intervention (i.e., tokens could be exchanged for video game time) while Jim worked on his homework at the kitchen table.

Self-Monitoring. To assist with self-regulatory behaviors, the school psychologist implemented a self-monitoring intervention with Jim. Self-monitoring is where students observe, record, and reinforce their own behavior. Jim's fidgeting behavior and excessive movement during his teacher's presentation of material were the target behaviors identified for improved self-monitoring. A vibration cue (from a watch) served as the prompt for when Jim was required to observe his own behavior. Jim was taught how to use his self-monitoring form at his desk and a reinforcement menu was developed. Behavioral expectations during class periods (e.g., remaining seated at his desk during teacher instruction) were also clarified and prompted.

Social–Emotional Curriculum. An evidence-based social–emotional curriculum, was implemented in Jim's classroom for 45 minutes every week. This curriculum targeted improvement in social–emotional functioning in all students by teaching topics such as emotion management, friendship skills, and communication skills. This intervention was designed to be implemented as a part of the core instructional program within the classroom to assist Jim and his classmates in promoting and maintaining healthy relationships. Skills taught in the classroom were also monitored and reinforced in the home setting.

Rationale for Psychiatric Consultation

Following 12 weeks of implementing a classroom-wide token economy, a self-monitoring intervention directly with Jim, and the social–emotional curriculum, his target behaviors failed to respond as expected. His inability to earn rewards and reinforce his own appropriate behavior created new concerns related to his sense of self. Negative self-talk and his frustration with schoolwork grew. His ability to complete his seatwork worsened and his grades showed further deterioration. A couple of negative interactions with peers (e.g., verbal altercations) emerged. At home, Jim's parents reported increased challenges while completing his homework. They also reported an increased level of stress related to their interactions with him. Jim's parents and teacher also reported Jim beginning to exhibit aggressive behavior and overt defiance toward them when given directions or a task to complete. Jim's increasing externalizing behaviors were particularly worrisome to his parents. A psychiatric consultation was recommended to help address the dysfunction associated with Jim's inattention, hyperactivity, impulsivity, and aggression.

Conduct Disorder

Danielle Haggerty

Presenting Problem

Brian is a 15-year old in the tenth grade who exhibits increasingly aggressive behaviors. He is often truant from school. Brian was recently suspended for 3 days for fighting with another boy in the hallway. He is at-risk for school expulsion and/or juvenile detention.

Background

Brian was born to a teenage mother and father. His father was sentenced to prison for armed robbery. Brian's mother raised him on her own and works two jobs to support them. The family struggles to meet monthly bill obligations. During first grade, Brian was diagnosed with a specific learning disability in reading fluency and oral expression. He had few friends in elementary school and socialized with peers infrequently in the classroom. When Brian did interact with peers, he often was verbally and physically aggressive toward them. When disciplined by his teachers, Brian would often tantrum or try leaving the classroom. He was often sent home by the school because of his aggressive behavior. Due to increased behavioral problems at school, Brian's mother sought parent training sessions from a community-based mental health center during late elementary school. Brian's mother enrolled in the intervention, however, she had to drop out after 3 weeks due to conflicts with her work schedule. Brian's mother currently reports considerable challenges at home with respect to managing her son's behavior as he often fails to follow her household rules (i.e., comes home after his curfew, has friends over when she is at work, doesn't clean up after himself). Brian is known to associate in the community with delinquent peers, who have dropped out of school. Brian's mom worries that he has begun to engage in substance use while out with these friends.

Case Description

Brian has a long history of academic struggles, specifically in reading and oral expression. He has received special education services in these areas since third grade. A review of records and teacher interviews indicates that Brian's behavior has become significantly more aggressive since starting middle school, as he initiates fights at school and curses at teachers unapologetically. His grades currently range from Fs (math, science) to Cs (Digital Media, Spanish). Brian is frequently truant from school and shows limited academic progress. He is at-risk for not graduating on time and must take summer school classes to catch up. During his freshman year, Brian had numerous unexcused absences and often stayed at home, sick, with excused absences. Not only is his attendance a concern, but Brian's behavior within the classroom has become particularly problematic for his math and science teachers. They report Brian is overtly defiant with their requests, he won't engage in seat work, he rarely turns in homework, and that he is disruptive to the learning environment. Other students within these two classes have complained repeatedly about being verbally harassed by Brian despite changes in seating. School personnel are feeling frustrated in managing his behavior and worry his behavior will get worse if additional intervention is not implemented quickly.

Target Behaviors for Intervention

1. Decrease aggressive behavior (Multisystemic Therapy)

Brian's aggressive behavior is evident at school and within the community. Coordination of interventions across home/school was undertaken to reduce his aggressive behavior. The goal was for Brian to completely stop his physical aggression toward other students at school.

2. Improve compliance with requests (Parent/Teacher Management Training)

Brian's lack of compliance with adults across the home/school settings resulted in the implementation of an evidence-based parent/teacher classroom management program. The goal was to increase Brian's compliance with requests to better meet home/school expectations.

3. Increase school attendance (Check and Connect)

Brian's unexcused absences are putting him at-risk for juvenile justice involvement and additional school failure. The goal was to improve Brian's school attendance through regular check-ins with the school psychologist.

Evidence-Based School Interventions

Multisystemic Therapy (MST). Within MST, conduct problems are believed to be influenced and maintained by a reciprocal interaction between an individual and others (i.e., peers, adults). A social worker in the district worked daily with Brian to address his aggressive behavior in school. His mother also attended these meetings during the first hour of the school day and was responsible for driving him to school to ensure his attendance. Brian's school counselor and his resource room teacher were regularly included in these meetings with the goal of promoting an increase in responsible behavior. Brian was taught a set of techniques to control his anger (e.g., label his feelings, relax, verbalize) and he worked on developing appropriate peer relationships within the school building.

Parent/Teacher Management Training (P/TMT). Brian's mother and homeroom teacher were provided an evidence-based, self-administered behavior management program. The goal of that treatment was to replace negative parenting and teaching methods with positive strategies. Brian's mother and homeroom teacher were taught to encourage Brian's anger control and social skills, set limits, monitor activities, develop plans for achievement, and show positive regard within their interactions with him. Brian's teacher was intentional about praising appropriate behavior within the classroom. Brian's mother checked his grades regularly. She also added time in the evenings and on weekends to engage positively (e.g., play cards, watch a show) with him.

Check and Connect. The school psychologist developed a rapport with Brian individually and then also with his mom/him. They set specific behavior goals for improving his attendance. Then a check (examine progress toward attendance goals) and connect (regular/brief meetings after school) intervention was implemented with the goal of increasing Brian's school attendance. As a part of the intervention, Brian was responsible for monitoring his attendance, his grades, and his behavior toward others. The school psychologist helped Brian and his mom apply the skills they were practicing to other settings.

Rationale for Psychiatric Consultation

After 6 weeks of implementing these three evidence-based psychosocial interventions, Brian's interactions with his teachers showed small signs of improvement. In addition, his attendance improved dramatically, largely the result of his mother's commitment to getting him to school each morning. However, additional conduct problems emerged. Brian and a peer were suspended from school after being caught drinking in the school bathroom during lunch. When confronted by the assistant principal, Brian became aggressive and ran from the school. Later that same day Brian was caught stealing food from a local store. Brian was suspended from school for five days and he has a court appearance next week for the shoplifting incident. Most concerning to his mom was Brian's lack of remorse for his actions and his report that everybody was out to get him in trouble. She wondered if his increased paranoia could be due to substance use. A psychiatric consultation was recommended to more effectively address the increased dysfunction associated with Brian's conduct problems at school, at home, and within the community.

Depression

Justina Yohannan

Presenting Problem

Chris is a 13-year old in eighth grade whose grades have declined recently. His teachers reported increased irritability and isolation from his peers. His mom stated that he recently dropped out of the wrestling club and that he appears sad and is more withdrawn at home.

Background

Chris is an only child. His father works as a lawyer and his mother works as a nurse. Chris's mother indicated a family history for alcoholism, anxiety, and depression in both sets of grandparents. In addition, her husband's sister had attempted suicide in college and is currently taking medication for depression. Chris met his developmental milestones and appeared to be a typically developing preschooler. While in elementary school, he struggled to make friends and was reported by teachers to be "a quiet child". Chris's mother noted he rarely has friends over from school and refuses to accept invitations to his classmates' birthday parties. In kindergarten and first grade, he would even "throw temper tantrums" to avoid going. Chris's academic performance is consistent with peers and typically in the A-B range until recently. Last year in the seventh grade, Chris frequently complained about headaches. He often "snapped" at classmates when frustrated. The transition from elementary to middle school was particularly challenging for Chris. His mother stated that the stress associated with the increased expectations of the middle school curriculum was tough on Chris. Some days this stress resulted in his inability to sleep at night and a reduced appetite. By the end of seventh grade, Chris appeared to "adjust well to the demands of middle school" and his teachers reported that he performed well, academically.

Case Description

About 4 weeks ago, both Chris's teachers and parents noted a change in his behaviors. Chris's teachers stated that Chris "has gotten really lazy recently" and that he isn't doing work in class or the homework assignments. His math teacher reported that Chris stares into space during class and does not pay attention during instruction. Chris only turned in one (partially completed) out of the five math homework assignments expected of him within the past week. His other teachers noted similar behaviors. Furthermore, Chris would skip class multiple times a week and go to the office complaining of headaches. The teachers also noted that he started losing his temper more frequently with very little provocation, and that he rarely talked to his friends during lunch and between classes. Chris's parents shared that they were also concerned with his recent behaviors including his decision to drop out of his wrestling club. Chris frequently comes home from school exhausted and when asked to do his chores, he stated that he "didn't have the energy." Chris's mother reported that he looked sad at home. Although he had a close relationship with his parents, he significantly reduced his interactions with them and frequently spent time alone in his room.

Target Behaviors for Intervention

1. Increase work completion (Self-Monitoring)

Since Chris was only turning in 20% of his homework assignments, the goal of targeting this behavior was to improve work completion. Within 8 weeks, the goal was for Chris to turn in 60% of completed homework assignments.

2. Increase appropriate responses to frustration (Cognitive Behavioral Therapy)

Due to inappropriate interactions with peers and other adults, the goal was for Chris to learn appropriate coping skills and use them regularly when he was feeling upset. Chris's teachers recorded his outbursts and noted if they decreased over time.

3. Increase peer interactions (Behavioral Activation/Activity Planning)

Due to parental concerns regarding Chris's avoidance of previously preferred activities and his limited interactions with peers, the goal was for Chris to take part in at least one desired club before, during, or after school.

Evidence-Based School Interventions

Self-Monitoring. The first target behavior addressed was work completion. To address this, a self-monitoring tool aimed at his homework completion was created by the school social worker and taught to Chris. Both the quality and quantity of his work were targeted. Chris recorded when he turned in his completed homework assignment and the grades received. He monitored his progress toward predetermined goals and reinforced himself when those goals were met. As goals were met, they were refined to reflect an increased rate of homework completion. His teachers were also made aware of these goals and provided a reliability check of his self-recording.

Cognitive Behavioral Therapy. The second behavior targeted for intervention was Chris's inappropriate behaviors that resulted from his low frustration tolerance, poor self-regulation, and high level of irritability. To address these difficulties, cognitive behavioral therapy (CBT) techniques were implemented by the school psychologist. This intervention focused on improving his reactions to frustration, developing more effecting problem-solving skills, and creating more positive thoughts and feelings about himself. He met once a week for 8 weeks to learn how to challenge his own negative thoughts, to learn and practice new coping skills, and to improve his interpersonal interactions with peers and adults.

Behavioral Activation/Activity Planning. The final behavior addressed was Chris's avoidance of previously preferred activities (e.g., dropping out of the wrestling club). It is believed that activities that are planned and scheduled in advance are more likely to be completed by those showing signs of depression. To address concerns about his increased isolation and avoidance, the school counselor met with Chris once a week for eight weeks to plan, initiate, and engage in preferred activities that were hypothesized to improve his mood. The counselor worked with Chris to monitor his thoughts and feelings about his involvement in these activities.

Rationale for Psychiatric Consult

The three evidence-based school interventions were not found to be effective in addressing Chris's target behaviors. Chris completed the self-monitoring tool as instructed but did not consistently turn in his homework. He only received a reward during the first week of intervention. Chris also refused to participate fully in cognitive behavioral therapy and behavioral activation planning. He commonly stated "What's the point? This isn't going to fix anything." School personnel struggled to develop rapport and Chris's irritable mood seemed to get in the way of his willingness to fully engage. Chris's teachers noticed increased withdrawal and one of his friends reported to the social worker that Chris recently said that he wished there was a way to "make all of his sadness go away." With the lack of success with the school-based interventions and a worsening of symptoms, a psychiatric consultation was recommended to address Chris's persistent withdrawal, depressed mood, and irritability.

Social Anxiety Disorder

Courtney Darr

Presenting Problem

Kate is a 16-year old in eleventh grade. Her teachers raised concerns regarding her lack of class participation and school avoidance. Her parents expressed concerns regarding her difficulties with developing positive peer relationships, frequent somatic complaints, and issues with school attendance.

Background

Kate is the youngest of three children. According to her parents, Kate had a high level of needs as an infant. She wanted to be constantly near her parents and was frequently fussy. There is a family history of anxiety and depression. Specifically, her mother was diagnosed with generalized anxiety disorder ten years ago. Her oldest brother (a college senior) has struggled with depression. During preschool and kindergarten, Kate had a particularly difficult time separating from her parents. When her father dropped her off to school each morning, Kate would frequently cry and complain. On a few occasions, Kate's parents kept her home instead of taking her to school due to more severe tantrums. She was described as "shy" throughout elementary and middle school. She preferred to play with one or two close friends and infrequently participated in large group activities. During middle school, Kate would frequently "freeze" if called on by a teacher in class. She frequently complained of headaches and stomachaches. Academically, she often received one of the top grades within her classes. During high school, Kate has grown increasingly more withdrawn and socially avoidant. She struggles to form new friendships and describes herself as "awkward around new people." Kate rarely accepts invitations to social events. She often tells her parents "people at school don't like me." Her grades in several of her classes have dropped from As to Cs in the past few months.

Case Description

Now in her junior year of high school, Kate is increasingly struggling with social anxiety and avoidant behavior. Her best friend from her neighborhood recently moved to another state and Kate's peer interactions have declined considerably. She often sits by herself during lunch and walks home by herself after school. Kate's English teacher recently raised concerns regarding her "unusually long bathroom breaks" during his class, which requires frequent group activities and discussion. Kate continues to complain of stomachaches, particularly the night before oral presentations or class exams. As a result, she has missed 14 school days in the past 3 months. Most recently, Kate missed 4 consecutive school days during the week of an oral presentation. Kate's visit to the school office has also increased recently. Three times this past week she has visited the office to call her parents to pick her up from school due to her stomachaches and headaches. At home, Kate is having difficulties falling asleep at night. Most nights she only gets three to four hours of sleep. Her parents too are concerned with an increase in tearfulness and isolation.

Target Behaviors for Intervention/Goals

1. Decrease anxious thoughts and feelings (Cognitive Behavioral Therapy)

Kate's school counselor implemented an evidence-based anxiety intervention to help her develop coping skills/relaxation strategies to reduce social anxiety and accurately identify situations that induce anxiety.

2. Increase class participation (Self-Monitoring)

A self-monitoring plan with increasing weekly goals was developed to have Kate report on how many times she participated in class. Teachers were also asked to record the length of her bathroom breaks to determine if they decreased over time.

3. Increase school attendance (Parent Psychoeducation)

Given Kate's historical issues with attendance, the school psychologist set an attendance goal of 80% for each month. Kate was also expected to reduce the number of times she called home from the school office to one call per week.

Evidence-Based School Interventions

Cognitive Behavioral Therapy. Cognitive behavioral therapy (CBT) is an evidence-based intervention for socially anxious youth. To address Kate's anxious thoughts and feelings, she began participating in a group-based CBT intervention at school. She and three other girls in the group were taught how to identify anxious thoughts/feelings and to engage in relaxation training exercises. Social skills training and identification/alteration of distorted cognitions were also taught . Exposure-based tasks and assignments for practice outside of the group were assigned. Processing these assignments within the group and group practice and modeling helped to reinforce the strategies. The intervention was implemented once a week over 16 weeks, with progress monitored weekly.

Self-Monitoring. Self-monitoring is an evidence-based intervention used to increase and modify behavior. With planning and structure provided by the school counselor, Kate recorded (1) whether she attended each class, (2) how many times she raised her hand during class, and (3) how many times she verbally participated. At the end of each day, if Kate met her individual goals she rewarded herself from the reinforcement menu she created. Kate received a larger reward on Fridays if she achieved her goal during four out of the five school days. Goals were set in consultation with her counselor and increased slightly each week.

Parent Psychoeducation. Training parents on anxiety disorders and treatment techniques is a common feature of evidence-based anxiety interventions. Kate's parents participated in three parent psychoeducation sessions with the school counselor. The counselor used instructional materials to teach Kate's parents about anxiety, the role they may be inadvertently playing in reinforcing Kate's anxiety, and how to help Kate apply the skills learned in her group-based intervention to both home and community settings. Special attention was given to how to address Kate's headaches and stomachaches and resulting school refusal.

Rationale for Psychiatric Consult

After 16 weeks of intervention, it was determined that the evidence-based school interventions were not sufficiently addressing Kate's social anxiety. During Kate's last two group sessions, she refused to participate stating that the session activities "won't make people like me more" and that "everything was fine." During Kate's self-monitoring intervention, she met her early goals (e.g., "raise my hand during one class period during the day") but did not achieve her goals during later weeks. She frequently "forgot" to check out at the end of the day with the school counselor to turn in her self-monitoring sheet. Her grades continued to be well below expectations. Last week, Kate's father overheard her talking on the phone to her older brother about drinking alcohol at a classmate's party she was "forced to go to by Mom." She said that she wanted to "feel more confident" and "forget how other people don't like me." In consultation with their family physician, a psychiatric consultation sought by her parents to address her persistent cognitive distortions, somatic complaints, avoidance of social situations, and poor coping strategies.

Autism Spectrum Disorder

Allison Siroky

Presenting Problem

Danny is a 12-year old in the seventh grade. He has received special education services as a student with ASD since second grade, though he spends almost all day in general education classes. Danny's teachers are concerned about his growing obsession with current events. This has led to frequent class disruptions and a recent physical altercation with a peer.

Background

Danny lives at home with his mom and two older sisters. His parents divorced when he was 3 and his father lives out of state. Danny's developmental and medical history is noteworthy for social and language delays. At age 2, Danny regularly played alongside his older siblings, though he rarely chose to participate in their pretend play. Danny "always had a hard time making and keeping friends" and he "hardly speaks to his siblings or close family." His kindergarten teacher occasionally noted concerns about sharing, transitioning, and fidgeting in his seat. At that time, Danny exhibited frequent tantrums during transitions at home (i.e., before going to school, when asked to help with chores) and an increase in aggressive behaviors (e.g., pinching, grabbing) toward his siblings. Unsure of whether these behaviors were due to underlying anxiety, attention difficulties, or oppositionality, he was assessed by a developmental/behavioral pediatrician. A comprehensive diagnostic assessment resulted in an ASD diagnosis. Impairments in social communication and responsiveness were most prominent. Danny's excessive interest in collecting and reading books also met clinical significance around restricted interests. Danny's cognitive profile indicated above-average cognitive abilities for peers his age. During the past 3 years, Danny has met with a speech-language pathologist for 1 hour every 2 weeks to work on his social communication skills. Improvements in his classroom behavior and peer interactions were noted in the past 2 years.

Case Description

Although Danny has responded well to his current school-based supports, his civics teacher recently noticed an excessive desire to check and recheck news websites during class. When unable to access these websites, Danny would rock back and forth while verbally repeating details about the news stories he read. Other teachers reported similar behaviors, noting that he often disrupted instruction and students' learning. A review of Danny's grades indicated a recent decline in academic performance. He stopped completing in-class assignments and instead would read the news or, when unable to do so, sit in his seat rocking back and forth. This persistent pattern of behaviors led to a referral to the school's problem-solving team. The school psychologist collected initial data via teacher interviews and direct observations of Danny in the classroom. In one observation during Danny's English class, a classmate attempted to engage in discussing a recent news story with Danny. When this classmate shared conflicting information about this event, Danny began to shout and grabbed the student's wrist. When the classmate tried to pull away, Danny would not let go until his teacher redirected him to his seat. A brief conversation with Danny's mother confirmed that he has shown increased interest in the news and current events, though she reported no incidents of aggression at home.

Target Behaviors for Intervention/Goals

1. Communicate appropriately within his classes (Social Scripts)

Danny is frequently speaking out of turn (i.e., without raising his hand, while the teacher is speaking) in class. The goal of implementing a social scripts intervention was to increase the frequency he was contributing appropriately (i.e., waiting until called) to classroom discussion.

2. Increase self-management strategies (Self-Monitoring)

A self-monitoring program was implemented to help Danny decrease the frequency of his engagement in repetitive, stereotyped behaviors (e.g., rocking in his seat). Replacement behaviors (e.g., writing questions down, tapping his foot) were taught, then monitored and reinforced by Danny.

3. Decrease aggressive behavior (Video Self-Modeling)

Danny occasionally displays aggressive behavior (i.e., shouting, grabbing peer's wrist) when his ideas and beliefs are challenged. Danny was taught adaptive social communication skills to use when faced with peer conflict or when others disagreed with him.

Evidence-Based School Interventions

Social Scripts. To decrease the frequency of Danny's inappropriate requests during class, the school psychologist developed a social script to help Danny practice contributing appropriately in class discussions. The script described a specific example of students in a junior high classroom, focusing on one student who wants to ask questions about the lesson. The script describes the students' thought process as they ultimately chose to raise their hand. A visual cue was placed on Danny's planner showing him sitting in his desk with his hand raised. The school psychologist met with Danny daily to review the social script and practice making appropriate requests. The school psychologist also met with Danny's teachers weekly to review expectations and to gather data about his behaviors over time.

Self-Monitoring. A self-management intervention was implemented to support Danny's awareness and regulation of his repetitive, stereotyped behaviors. The school psychologist worked with Danny to identify what it looks and feels like when he begins to rock in his seat and when he starts to describe a news story aloud. Danny and his teachers selected a behavioral cue to remind Danny to check his seat behavior. Danny was taught to use a blank notebook to write down questions to then be checked by his teachers during individual seat work. Access to news/screen time was contingent on his engagement in these self-monitoring techniques.

Video Self-Modeling. A video self-modeling procedure was implemented to help Danny observe and practice appropriate social communication skills when others disagreed with him. The school psychologist worked with Danny to develop a script for responding to disagreements. Danny and a familiar peer practiced and recorded this scripted conversation in various school contexts. Danny reviewed these video clips three times per week and practiced a similar conversation at least one time per week with a novel peer. When he independently provided the correct response during practice conversations, Danny earned 5 minutes to talk about the news with his resource room teacher.

Rationale for Psychiatric Consultation

After nine weeks of school-based psychosocial interventions to address three target behaviors, Danny continued to struggle with managing repetitive, stereotyped behaviors that were disruptive to the classroom learning process. Since the start of these interventions, Danny displayed two more instances of aggressive behavior toward one classmate and one teacher. Due to Danny's limited behavioral improvements, as well as the potential risk of harm to other classmates or school personnel, the school psychologist called a meeting with Danny's mom and teachers. Given his prior history of successfully responding to other school-based supports, Danny's mom decided to consult with a local psychiatrist to discuss medication options for underlying anxiety and/or irritability, which were believed to be functionally related to Danny's recent problematic behaviors at school.

Psychosis

Rachel Korest

Presenting Problem

April is a 15-year old in the tenth grade. Her teachers report low rates of homework completion, a decline in her grades, expression of frequent worries about peer and teacher rejection. April's parents too are concerned especially about her peer and school avoidance, decreased appetite, and increased fatigue at home.

Background

April is an only child. Her mom was born in Mexico and her dad was born in the United States. April's mom has a history of postpartum depression but has no other history of mental health issues. Her family history is noteworthy for Schizophrenia as April's aunt received that diagnosis while in her first year of college. There is no history of mental health issues on April's father side. April's mom works part-time as a Spanish tutor, while April's dad works locally in sales. When April was younger, she had some difficulties making new friends. Sleep issues were noted as occurring nightly and April would often have temper tantrums when she did not get her way. She would frequently complain of stomach aches during school and would have to come home. After taking her to her doctor, it was found that she did not have any gastrointestinal issues. April's parents indicated they believed at the time these symptoms were the result of her age and symptoms of separation anxiety. April's mother reported specific concerns about April's difficulties with rejection during elementary and middle school, specifically when April's friends canceled plans or when they didn't invite her over to play. April's mom remembered a time when April cried for hours because her friend could not come over due to a family conflict. April stated she was worried her friend did not like her and that it was not fair that her friend's parents would not let her come over.

Case Description

During the past 2 weeks, April has shown increased agitation with her friends and family as well as a loss of interest in attending school. Additionally, she presents with increased fatigue, an inability to concentrate, and a decreased appetite. This past week, April stopped showing up for three of her classes. April's teachers reported that she has been displaying atypical behavior in the classes she is attending and that they have observed her sitting alone in the library during the classes she was skipping. In math, her teacher stated she has been sitting away from her friends and resting her head on her desk during most of the class period. In addition, her homework completion and grades have plummeted in recent days. April's parents shared they too have become quite concerned about her behavior at home over the past two weeks. April has appeared agitated, sleeping sporadically throughout the day, and spending a lot of time in her room alone. Additionally, her parents shared she has stopped showering and practicing daily hygiene habits. When April's parents asked April why she has been skipping class, she replied that her friends were making plans to embarrass her in front of her classmates and that her teachers were constantly talking about her behind her back.

Target Behaviors for Intervention/Goals

1. Increase class attendance (Check and Connect)

Class attendance has been an issue for April, especially as it relates to impacting her course grades. The goal was for April to attend every class for at least 4 out of 5 days of the school week. She could skip one class of her choosing each week and sit in the library instead.

2. Engage in daily hygiene habits and improve her social skills (Social Skills Training)

Given the current difficulties in her interactions with her peers, increasing the number of positive connections (i.e., initiating social contacts, engaging positively with others) with her friends were targeted in addition to improving her personal hygiene (i.e., brush her hair/teeth, shower).

3. Distorted thinking (Cognitive Behavioral Therapy)

The severity of April's cognitive distortions and her overall challenges at school were significant enough to the school psychologist who implemented daily 30-minute individual counseling sessions. The goal of these sessions was to reduce her agitation and distorted thinking related to her peers.

Evidence-Based School Interventions

Check and Connect. A check and connect intervention was initiated by April's school counselor to provide her with additional support in increasing her class attendance and overall school performance. At the beginning and end of each school day, April and her school counselor met briefly to discuss her progress. April's teachers monitored her attendance and recorded their observations of her classroom behavior on a daily report card that April was to bring home each day. April's parents were responsible for getting their daughter to school on time and they made notes on the card about her sleeping habits. April's goal was to attend all her classes for at least 4 out of 5 days. April identified the weekly rewards she worked toward. This included being able to take a friend to lunch off campus and being able to go to the library during her study period.

Social Skills Training. To work on self-care and more positive peer interactions, the school social worker implemented a social skills training program with April. This program offered opportunities for modeling, role play, and practicing targeted social behaviors (i.e., complimenting others, social initiation, active listening skills). Once a week, April selected a friend each day to join in on the social skills training to assist with practicing the skills taught. The social worker also provided counseling on the importance of practicing good hygiene. April was asked to self-monitor and report on her hygienic behavior (e.g., showering, brushing her hair/teeth) and her parents were asked to reinforce and support those behaviors at home.

Cognitive Behavioral Therapy. Cognitive behavioral therapy was undertaken via daily 30-minute sessions with the school psychologist. Sessions initially addressed April's distorted thoughts, specifically her belief that her friends were plotting to embarrass her and that her teachers were talking about her behind her back. Strategies were also taught to help address April's hostility and anger towards her family and friends. Homework related to thought stopping and problem-solving were assigned. Improvements were measured through monitoring April's ability to competently carry out the skills taught and the completeness of her ability to record other's reactions to her behavior. Her mother and father were consulted weekly to assist and support April's efforts at home to implement what she was learning at school.

Rationale for Psychiatric Consultation

A 4-week trial of school-based psychosocial interventions and cognitive behavioral therapy techniques resulted in minimal improvement. In the past 2 weeks, April has been increasingly paranoid, telling the school psychologist that she has been meeting with her friends each week to "keep her enemies closer." April's teachers have reported that while she is attending class she leaves for long periods during class under the guise that she needs to use the bathroom. Yesterday, one of April's friends noticed that she had numerous cuts on her forearm that she attempted to cover by wearing a long-sleeve shirt. Alarmed, this friend confided in the school social worker that she believed April had been deliberately cutting herself. School personnel, in collaboration with the family and their physician, referred April for an emergency psychiatric consultation.

Bipolar Disorder

Adrianna Crossing

Presenting Problem

Dylan is a 14-year old in the ninth grade. His teachers report that he has been particularly defiant and disrespectful in recent weeks. Dylan's parents reported to his homeroom teacher that he has been atypically irritable with family members and not acting like himself.

Background

Dylan lives at home with his mom, dad, and two older brothers who live outside the home. Dylan's mother experienced severe postpartum depression following his birth. She was unable to return to work for almost a year and was effectively treated by her doctor. Depression runs in her family and her younger brother committed suicide in college. A review of school records indicated that Dylan struggled with inattention, hyperactivity, and impulsivity in elementary school. Despite school recommendations, Dylan's parents chose not to seek a consultation with his pediatrician regarding these behaviors and potential medication treatments until late in the sixth grade, when Dylan was diagnosed with ADHD. His parents secured school- and community-based psychosocial treatment supports. After a significant decline in grades and a series of outbursts at home and school, Dylan's pediatrician started a trial of psychostimulants in the middle of seventh grade. Treatment onset coincided with increased behavioral problems. He began to act more impulsively and often talked incessantly with peers during class time. Stimulant treatment was discontinued. Dylan has been taking atomoxetine (i.e., non-stimulant) since that time. His grades have recently declined from a high B average to low Cs. His irritability and moodiness reportedly vary from month to month. According to his parents, his peer relationships are volatile as he often makes his friends angry with his words and actions.

Case Description

Since the start of ninth grade, Dylan has shown a high level of disrespect to others in the classroom. He frequently talks out of turn, talks with those around him incessantly, and is noncompliant with requests for seatwork. At home, his parents too have seen an increase in his defiant behavior. He plays video games well into the night and they are concerned with how his limited sleep is impacting his behavior. Dylan's father reported that they have had several arguments in the past week after he woke up to find Dylan still playing video games at 3 a.m. on three different occasions. Concerned about this new habit cutting into his sleep, his father checked in with his homeroom teacher who indicated that he has been coming to school each morning during the past week with an energy drink. She noted that he is being more noncompliant and irritable. She agreed that his getting more sleep may improve his behavior and mood. Yesterday, Dylan's foreign language teacher submitted a behavior referral for insulting and disobeying her when she presented a pop quiz to the class. In a resulting child study meeting the school social worker, school psychologist, behavioral interventionist, and Dylan's homeroom teacher decided on an intensive regimen of psychosocial interventions to support his behavior.

Target Behaviors for Intervention/Goals

1. Improve homework completion and respect toward his teachers (Check and Connect)

Since Dylan is frequently disrupting classroom learning (i.e., distracting peers, showing disrespect toward teachers) and in turn not completing his seatwork, the goal was to increase appropriate academic behaviors in the classroom.

2. Increase compliance with teacher/parent requests (Conjoint Behavioral Consultation)

Dylan's parents and foreign language teacher are reporting significant challenges in managing his behavior. A focus on improving his compliance with adult's requests was implemented via an increased focus on rewarding him for displaying desired behaviors (i.e., differential reinforcement) across home/school settings.

3. Improve peer relations (Social Skills Training)

Dylan is frequently disrupting classroom learning by conversing with peers and his inability to filter his comments is threatening his friendships. Social skills training targeted his impaired social interactions with peers both in and out of the classroom.

Evidence-Based School Interventions

Check and Connect. The school psychologist developed rapport with Dylan through brief daily meetings. Together, they set specific academic behavior goals. Then a check (examine progress toward goals) and connect (meetings after school) intervention was implemented. As a part of the intervention, Dylan was responsible for monitoring his attendance, his homework completion, showing respect for his teachers, and his grades. The school psychologist helped Dylan and his mom apply the skills they were practicing across settings. At the end of each day, they met to assess how he performed on his outlined goals. Meeting his daily goal resulted in a predefined reward.

Conjoint Behavioral Consultation. To increase Dylan's compliance with adult requests, his foreign language and homeroom teachers along with his parents met conjointly once a week with the school social worker to implement a differential reinforcement plan as a part of behavioral consultation. Meetings focused on problem identification, problem analysis, treatment implementation, and treatment evaluation. By focusing on verbal reinforcement of his compliant behavior, the goal was to increase the frequency that Dylan was complying with adult requests and more generally meeting behavioral expectations at home/school.

Social Skills Training. Since the beginning of the school year, Dylan had become increasingly combative with peers, including those in his close group of friends. During the planning meeting for Dylan's interventions, the school psychologist and his social worker felt that he would benefit from an intervention plan that specifically targeted prosocial behavior. Once a week, Dylan met with the school counselor for social skills training involving psychoeducation, social skills modeling, and practice. During these meetings, they set 3 social behavior goals for each week, including eating lunch with his friends, playing video games with his friends or siblings, and working to stop and think prior to communicating his thoughts and feelings with friends.

Rationale for Psychiatric Consultation

After 7 weeks, Dylan showed limited progress with two of his three interventions. He rarely met his behavioral goals and he complied infrequently with adults' requests and remained disruptive and distracting to peers during classwork activities. According to his school counselor, Dylan's relationships with his peers appeared to improve. However, yesterday the counselor noticed marks on Dylan's wrist and communicated his concerns about self-harm to his parents and other school staff. Dylan admitted to self-injurious behavior, but insisted it was an isolated impulsive reaction that resulted from a series of negative interactions with one of his female friends. The school psychologist administered several behavioral rating scales and conducted a structured behavioral health interview which resulted in Dylan's endorsement of a clinically significant level of depressive and impulsive symptoms, along with some worrying indicators related to suicidal ideation. An immediate psychiatric consultation was arranged after his parents communicated these concerns to his primary care physician who was currently managing his medication treatment.

Chapter 4
Effective Medications for Treating Externalizing Disorders

Heather Joseph, Courtney Walker, Cristin McDermott, Youeun Song, Monique Simpson and Shabana Khan

Introduction

Externalizing disorders are psychiatric disorders characterized by behaviors disruptive to the individual's environment (e.g., home, classroom). The most frequent externalizing disorders diagnosed in childhood include attention-deficit hyperactivity disorder (ADHD), oppositional defiant disorder (ODD), and conduct disorder (CD). These disorders often coexist and are frequently comorbid with mood, anxiety, and substance use disorders. Contrary to ADHD, ODD, and CD, intermittent explosive disorder (IED) is an externalizing disorder that typically peaks in the third decade of life (Coccaro, Schmidt, Samuels, & Nestadt, 2004). Thus, despite having a mean age of onset of 15 years, it is more commonly recognized and treated in adults (Kessler et al., 2006).

ADHD is one of the most prevalent psychiatric disorders in childhood, with an estimated childhood prevalence of 5%, followed by ODD and CD each with a prevalence of 3% (American Psychiatric Association, 2013; Canino, Polanczyk, Bauermeister, Rohde, & Frick, 2010). Children with ADHD are more likely than the general population to have ODD (25–50%) and CD (25%) (American Psychiatric Association, 2013). Internalizing disorders are common among children with ADHD, major depressive disorder (12–50%) and anxiety disorders (25–50%), and these children tend to experience greater impairment, younger age of onset, and increased risk of suicidality than children with MDD alone (Daviss, 2008; Costello, Egger, & Angold, 2004).

Although hyperactivity may be the first recognized symptom of ADHD, as early as toddlerhood, it is most often diagnosed in grade school when inattentive symptoms become more prominent and thus impair academic performance. Research has demonstrated that children with ADHD frequently have difficulties in accuracy and

H. Joseph · C. Walker · C. McDermott · Y. Song · M. Simpson · S. Khan (✉)
School of Medicine, University of Pittsburgh, Pittsburgh, PA, USA
e-mail: khans@upmc.edu

J. S. Carlson and J. A. Barterian (eds.), *School Psychopharmacology*,
Pediatric School Psychology, https://doi.org/10.1007/978-3-030-15541-4_4

efficiency of work completion (Barkley, 2014). Even though children with ADHD are six times more likely to have accessed educational services than those without ADHD, children with ADHD are still three times less likely to finish high school and six times less likely to attend higher education (Erskine et al., 2016). The significant impact on the U.S. educational system and the academic performance of children with externalizing disorders makes their identification and treatment of importance.

Attention-Deficit/Hyperactivity Disorder (ADHD)

Psychopharmacological Treatment of ADHD

Behavioral interventions may be sufficient for cases of ADHD with mild impairment and used in conjunction with medications as a part of a comprehensive treatment plan for patients. A landmark study in ADHD, the Multimodal Treatment of ADHD (MTA), found that while medications were highly effective for the core symptoms of ADHD, behavioral interventions provided additional benefits for overall positive functioning and achievement (Jensen, 1999). However, behavioral treatment alone does not always result in a significant improvement of symptoms. Therefore, psychopharmacological intervention is often necessary.

Efficacy and Effectiveness

Stimulants

Stimulant medications are highly efficacious in the treatment of ADHD, and trials in children and adults have shown that 65–75% of subjects with ADHD are stimulant responders (Greenhill, Pliszka, & Dulcan, 2002). In fact, the effect size of stimulant treatment relative to placebo is one of the largest effect sizes for any psychotropic medication (Pliszka & AACAP Work Group on Quality Issues, 2007). Stimulant medications are thought to exert their effect by enhancing synaptic levels of norepinephrine and dopamine in parts of the brain that are associated with attention, motivation, and reward (Volkow et al., 2012). The two classes of stimulants, methylphenidate (MPH) and amphetamine salts, are equally efficacious in the treatment of ADHD (Pliszka & AACAP Work Group on Quality Issues, 2007). There are short-acting (immediate release, IR) and long-acting (sustained, SR; extended release, XR) formulations available for both MPH and amphetamine salts; all formulations are equally efficacious. In general, short-acting formulations require more frequent dosing (two or three times daily), whereas long-acting formulations are typically once daily dosing. The long-acting formulations are used most often due to convenience and increased treatment adherence. Initial response rates to stimulants, if both classes of stimulants are tried, may be as high as 85% (Pliszka & AACAP Work Group on Quality Issues, 2007). As of yet, there does not exist a way to predict which stimulant will produce the best response in a given individual.

While rates of stimulant use continue to grow in the United States (Zuvekas & Vitiello, 2012), most evidence suggests either appropriate prescribing or under-treatment of ADHD, despite public concern regarding overdiagnosis of ADHD and overprescribing of stimulants (Connor, 2011). In a national sample, only one-third of adolescents with ADHD received stimulants and only 48% of patients with ADHD had received any treatment over the previous 12 months, suggesting underdiagnosis and undertreatment of the illness (Merikangas et al., 2010). Studies have also demonstrated gender and ethnic differences in the pharmacologic treatment of ADHD, suggesting that these discrepancies are greater for patients who are minorities or female. Males are more likely to be diagnosed and treated than females and white males are more likely to be diagnosed and treated than Hispanic or African American males (Zuvekas, 2012).

Contraindications

Appetite suppression is one of the more common side effects of stimulant medications. Given this risk, stimulants should be used with caution in those who have failure to thrive or those who are very underweight. Routine monitoring of height, weight, and BMI should be done throughout the course of treatment to monitor growth trajectory. Non-stimulants are preferred if there is a concern for an eating disorder.

Stimulants are contraindicated in the context of active mania or psychosis as they may exacerbate these symptoms. Though stimulants are not absolutely contraindicated in patients with bipolar disorder or comorbid substance use, non-stimulants are generally first-line medications in these populations. Stimulants should not be used in patients with comorbid psychotic disorders.

Non-stimulant medications are preferred in patients with structural cardiac lesions. If stimulants are necessary due to significant or distressing behavioral symptoms, providers should collaborate closely with a pediatric cardiologist. Relative contraindications also exist. For patients with specific cardiac risk factors (Table 4.1), an electrocardiogram (ECG) and pediatric cardiology consult should be obtained prior to initiating stimulant medication. Importantly, however, routine cardiac evaluation prior to the use of stimulant medications in healthy individuals (no cardiac history) is unnecessary. Nonetheless, the FDA recommends that patients treated with ADHD medications, be periodically monitored for changes in heart rate and blood pressure.

Table 4.1 Risk factors for cardiovascular disease/side effects

History of severe palpitations, fainting, seizures, exercise intolerance (not accounted for by obesity)
Family history of sudden or unexplained death at a young age (<35 years)
Postoperative Tetralogy of Fallot, coronary artery anomalies, subaortic stenosis
Chest pain, arrhythmias, hypertension or syncope[a]

[a]These may be signs of a condition called hypertrophic cardiomyopathy, which is associated with sudden cardiac death

Non-stimulants

Non-stimulant medications are also helpful in the treatment of ADHD, particularly when stimulant medications have been tried and are not well tolerated. Non-stimulant medications may also be used in conjunction with stimulants to target residual symptoms of ADHD not fully responsive to stimulant monotherapy. Non-stimulant medications are preferred in children who may have a contraindication to receiving stimulants.

Atomoxetine is a noradrenergic reuptake inhibitor that has been shown to be superior to placebo in the treatment of ADHD (Pliszka & AACAP Work Group on Quality Issues, 2007). In general, this medication has little effect on appetite and sleep, as compared to stimulants and may also prove beneficial in the setting of ADHD with comorbid anxiety (Pliszka & AACAP Work Group on Quality Issues, 2007). It is often used in the setting of patients with comorbid substance use as there is little abuse potential compared to stimulant medications. Unlike stimulants however, it may take up to 12 weeks for patients to see full treatment effects and, although no deaths from suicide have been reported, the FDA mandates that a blackbox warning for suicidal ideation be included for this medication (Bushe & Savill, 2014).

Other medications that are FDA-approved for the treatment of ADHD, include long-acting alpha-agonists such as guanfacine and clonidine. Alpha-agonists are often used for patients with comorbid conditions such as tics or aggression and can improve some side effects of stimulants, such as insomnia (Pliszka & AACAP Work Group on Quality Issues, 2007). Alpha-agonists have been shown to have a small to moderate effect size for the treatment of ADHD (Pliszka & AACAP Work Group on Quality Issues, 2007). Clinical consensus suggests that alpha-agonists are more successful in treating the hyperactive and impulsive symptoms of ADHD as opposed to the inattentive symptoms (Pliszka & AACAP Work Group on Quality Issues, 2007). They are generally well tolerated and the common side effect of sedation can be advantageous in patients with sleep disturbance. Due to their effect on blood pressure, they may cause dizziness and increase the risk of falls and syncope. Thus, patients should be advised to stay hydrated to avoid low blood pressure.

Tricyclic antidepressants (TCAs), though not FDA-approved for the treatment of ADHD, have been shown to be effective in studies of both children and adults with ADHD. TCAs require a baseline ECG and frequent monitoring of plasma levels, and may have unpleasant side effects making them undesirable to patients. TCAs are contraindicated in children with cardiac conduction abnormalities, as they can prolong the QTc interval and in rare cases, lead to torsades de pointes. TCAs can also activate psychotic symptoms in those with a psychotic disorder (Klykylo, Bowers, Weston, & Jackson, 2014). Finally, TCAs should be used with caution in those with seizure disorders, as they may lower the seizure threshold.

Bupropion is sometimes used in the treatment of ADHD due to its effects on dopamine and norepinephrine neurotransmission. It has shown modest efficacy for treatment of ADHD symptoms, though it is contraindicated in patients with current seizure disorders and may exacerbate tics in patients with underlying tic disorders (Pliszka et al., 2006).

Oppositional Defiant Disorder (ODD) and Conduct Disorder (CD)

Psychopharmacological Treatment of ODD and CD

Research demonstrates that medications are only partially effective in the management of oppositional defiant disorder (ODD) and conduct disorder (CD) and that behavioral interventions should be applied prior to a trial of medication (Steiner & Remsing, 2007). Medications are only recommended to target specific symptoms such as aggression, mood lability, and impulsivity as well as specific comorbid disorders. The psychopharmacological treatment of ODD and CD consists of stimulants, other non-stimulant ADHD medications, antidepressants, mood stabilizers, and antipsychotics (Grant & Leppink, 2015; Steiner, 2007). The current literature base focuses mainly on the use of antipsychotics and stimulants in the treatment of ODD and CD due to high rates of comorbidity with ADHD and aggressive behaviors (Grant, 2015). Additionally, lithium is the most studied and frequently prescribed mood stabilizer in the treatment of CD due to an extensive body of research which has shown efficacy in the treatment of behavioral symptoms and aggression (Grant, 2015).

Each class of medication has a different mechanism of action, however, there are similarities between the agents in each individual group. Carbamazepine and valproic acid each bind to voltage-dependent sodium channels, however, at different sites, which leads to an increase in neuronal firing. Valproic acid also increases the level of gamma-aminobutyric acid (GABA) in the brain, however, there is much debate on how this phenomenon occurs (Schachter, 2017). Both groups of antipsychotics, typicals and atypicals, bind to dopamine 2 receptors (D2), however, the atypicals have a decreased binding affinity which has been attributed to producing their less severe side effect profiles (Kapitanyan & Su, 2016). Unfortunately, there is not a firm grasp on how these classes of medications cause anti-aggression effects, however, it has been hypothesized that dopamine plays a role in the development and implementation of aggressive behaviors. It is also theorized that reduced GABA activity can lead to an increase in aggression (Siever, 2008)

Efficacy and Effectiveness

Pharmacologic interventions of ODD have not been sufficiently evaluated and completed studies have notable limitations including small sample size and the presence of comorbid disorders; therefore, no pharmacological interventions are FDA-approved for the treatment of ODD or CD (Turgay, 2009). However, several double-blind placebo-controlled studies have supported the use of medication to improve oppositional behaviors in the context of other diagnoses (Steiner, 2007).

Controlled clinical trials for CD have shown promise in the treatment of aggression and impulsivity with mood stabilizers, antipsychotics, and stimulants. Given limited evidence of clinical effectiveness of these medications in the treatment of ODD and CD, the potential risks of medication use should be carefully considered. As is the case with ODD, it is recommended that comorbid disorders are treated with the appropriate medications before targeted pharmacological treatment of CD symptoms (Steiner, 2007). If a child is nonresponsive to one medication trial, another class of medication should be tried instead of adding additional psychotropic medications to the current regimen (Steiner, 2007).

Stimulants and Non-stimulants

Due to the high comorbidity rate of ADHD and ODD or CD, there have been several studies evaluating the efficacy of stimulant and non-stimulant ADHD medications to treat these disorders. With regards to stimulants, a placebo-controlled parallel study of 84 children and adolescents diagnosed with CD with or without ADHD showed that methylphenidate (MPH) had a short-term positive effect on conduct behaviors (Klein et al., 1997). Another placebo-controlled study of adolescents with the diagnosis of ADHD and CD or ODD showed that methylphenidate was effective in decreasing verbal and physical aggression over placebo (Kaplan, Busner, Kupietz, Wasserman, & Segal, 1990). Additionally, a randomized placebo-controlled study examining the use of a stimulant in addition to parent training in children with the diagnosis of ADHD and ODD or CD showed 70% of participants were much improved on the Clinical Global Impressions-Improvement (CGI-I) along with notable improvement in disruptive behaviors and social competence (Aman et al., 2014).

Two non-stimulant medications studied in this population are atomoxetine and clonidine. The response of atomoxetine in youth with comorbid ADHD and ODD was evaluated in a double-blind placebo-controlled study which showed atomoxetine improved symptoms in both diagnoses although the comorbid group may require higher doses of medication than ADHD youth without comorbid ODD (Newcorn,

Spencer, Biederman, Milton, & Michelson, 2005). Four RCTs were completed with atomoxetine measuring aggression with the primary diagnosis of ADHD and secondary diagnoses including ODD, depression, and generalized anxiety disorder (GAD) demonstrated a small effect size indicating atomoxetine may not be the best medication for the treatment of aggressive behaviors (Pappadopulos et al., 2006). In an RCT comparing clonidine with placebo added to ongoing stimulant therapy for ADHD with comorbid ODD or CD, clonidine in combination with stimulant therapy was effective in improving conduct behaviors on the conduct subclass of the Conner's Behavior Checklist (Hazell & Stuart, 2003). Another RCT was performed with children and adolescents comparing MPH, clonidine, and the combination of MPH with clonidine, which showed no significant difference between the three treatment groups in reducing aggressive behaviors, however, this study has several limitations including no placebo control group and only 8 subjects in each treatment arm (Connor, Barkely, & Davis, 2000).

Antipsychotics

The Treatment Recommendations for the use of Antipsychotics for Aggressive Youth (TRAAY) study recommends the use of an atypical antipsychotic first in the treatment of aggression over typical antipsychotics given reduced likelihood of causing severe side effects such as neuroleptic malignant syndrome, tardive dyskinesia, and cognitive impairment (Pappadopulos et al., 2003). Prior research conducted with typical antipsychotics found haloperidol to be more effective than placebo, however, it was not well tolerated and the results were comparable to lithium in the treatment of aggression in children diagnosed with CD (Campbell et al., 1984).

Regarding atypical antipsychotics, studies have been conducted with risperidone, olanzapine and quetiapine in the treatment of aggression for children and adolescents with OD and CD. Much of this literature has the previously mentioned limitations including small sample sizes, short duration of treatment, and comorbid diagnoses. The majority of research with atypical antipsychotics has been completed with risperidone in the treatment of ODD. Some of these studies were conducted with children that have comorbid intellectual disabilities and ADHD, which may cloud the generalizability to specifically ODD or CD (Buitelaar, Van der Gaag, Cohen-Kettenis, & Melman, 2001). A randomized placebo-controlled trial comparing parent training plus a stimulant with the addition of risperidone or placebo after 3 weeks of stimulant treatment in children with the diagnoses of ADHD and ODD or CD showed a statistically significant decrease in aggression and disruptive behaviors. In addition, 79% of the participants showed a very much improved score on the CGI-I in the group receiving risperidone augmentation over placebo (Aman et al., 2014). Preliminary data from a retrospective study provides support for future studies investigating olanzapine in the treatment of aggression (Masi et al., 2004). A clinical case series was published demonstrating that 5 out of 6 cases of aggressive youth responded to olanzapine; efficacy or safety of the medication cannot be determined from this study (Soderstrom, Rastam, & Gilberg, 2002). Only one randomized controlled trial has been conducted with quetiapine that demonstrated that it might be effective for the treatment of CD. The study enrolled 19 subjects, of which 8 completed the entire trial (Connor, McLaughlin, & Jeffers-Terry, 2008).

It is recommended that atypical antipsychotics are started at low doses and that the dose is increased slowly to an adequate treatment dose for 2 weeks or greater before rendering the medication ineffective. If an initial atypical antipsychotic is ineffective after an adequate trial, then a second atypical should be tried. After failing two atypical antipsychotic trials, it may be reasonable to pursue a mood stabilizer or typical antipsychotic. If a patient has a partial response to an atypical antipsychotic, it would be rational to add a mood stabilizer to the medication regimen. There is limited long-term data on the risk of chronic use of atypical antipsychotics in youth and the use of these medications should be reevaluated after 6 months (Pappadopulos et al., 2003).

Mood Stabilizers

Three mood stabilizers, lithium, valproate, and carbamazepine, have been studied for the treatment of aggression in children and adolescents diagnosed with ODD and CD. Of these medications, lithium has the most data with 3 out of 4 placebo-controlled studies showing positive results (Gérardin, Cohen, Mazet, & Flament, 2002; Malone, Delaney, Luebbert, Cater, & Campbell, 2000; Campbell, 1984; Rifkin et al., 1997). The evidence for the use of valproate and carbamazepine in children and adolescents with ODD or CD and aggression is limited to one placebo-controlled trial each (Donovan et al., 2000; Cueva et al., 1996).

Despite lithium being the most effective mood stabilizer in the treatment of OD and CDD, children and adolescents are frequently deterred from this medication due to the requirement of frequent blood draws for lithium level monitoring, along with side effects of tremors, nausea, vomiting, ataxia, and weight gain (Pappadopulos et al., 2006). Carbamazepine also has potential adverse effects, such as hepatotoxicity and metabolic derangements (Pappadopulos et al., 2006). Valproate requires blood draws for dose monitoring and can be associated with gastrointestinal distress, thrombocytopenia, and hyperammonemia (Schachter, 2017).

Contraindications

There are no absolute contraindications for the medications used in the treatment of oppositional defiant disorder and conduct disorder, however, there are several populations in which we need to closely monitor for side effects or worsening of preexisting conditions, such as children with a diagnosis of a cardiac arrhythmias, obesity, or diabetes mellitus. It is important to obtain baseline laboratory testing prior to starting antipsychotics or mood stabilizers to ensure that the child is an appropriate candidate for these classes of medication and to monitor for side effects.

It is also crucial to take into consideration if an adolescent is of child bearing age when choosing medication due to the risk of birth defects associated with mood stabilizers, especially valproic acid (Schachter, 2017).

Intermittent Explosive Disorder (IED)

Psychopharmacological Treatment of Intermittent Explosive Disorder (IED)

Patients with intermittent explosive disorder (IED) who are either resistant or refractory to behavioral treatment may be referred to a psychiatrist for medication management. Medications used may include antidepressants, mood stabilizers, and antipsychotic medications. These medications can be used alone or in combination. The mechanism of anti-aggression effect of these medications is not well understood. Research has implicated several neurobiological deficits associated with impulsive aggression involving dysregulation of neurotransmitters including serotonin, dopamine, noradrenaline, glutamate, and GABA (Siever, 2008).

Efficacy and Effectiveness

There are currently no medications approved by the FDA to treat IED and no studies conducted in children or adolescents with IED to demonstrate efficacy of medication. However, children and adolescents with IED are sometimes treated with medications that have demonstrated some efficacy in treating aggressive behaviors in adults.

Antidepressants

Selective Serotonin Reuptake Inhibitors (SSRIs) are antidepressants commonly prescribed for the treatment of depression and anxiety in children and adolescents. Several studies have demonstrated some benefit of using SSRI in adults with IED or aggression. Fluoxetine has been the most studied, but other SSRIs are reasonable options. A 12-week double-blind, randomized controlled trial was conducted with 100 adults with IED and impulsive aggressive behavior comparing fluoxetine and placebo. Moderate to large improvement occurred in significantly more patients who received fluoxetine than placebo (66 vs. 29%). Fluoxetine's effect on impulsive aggressive behavior in these subjects was most pronounced on measures of verbal aggression and aggression against objects. A significant effect was not seen on aggression against others or self (Coccaro, Lee, & Kavoussi, 2009).

Mood Stabilizers and Antiepileptic Drugs (AEDs)

A12-week randomized controlled trial comparing lithium with placebo in 59 adult inmates with chronic impulsive aggressive behavior found that aggression decreased significantly more in the individuals receiving lithium (Sheard, Marini, Bridges, & Wagner, 1976). Antiepileptic drugs (AEDs), also known as anticonvulsants, are frequently used in the treatment of seizure disorder and some are used as mood stabilizers. A review of randomized controlled trials found that most of the common AEDs, particularly those that block sodium channels and/or have GABA-related mechanisms of action, are effective in reducing the frequency and intensity of impulsive aggressive outbursts (Stanford, Anderson, Lake, & Baldridge, 2009). This includes phenytoin, carbamazepine, oxcarbazepine, lamotrigine, valproate/divalproex sodium, and topiramate. A systematic review of 14 studies with data from 672 adult participants for four antiepileptic medications (valproate/divalproex, carbamazepine, oxcarbazepine, and phenytoin) concluded that the body of evidence is mixed and insufficient to allow any conclusions to be drawn about the use of antiepileptic medication in the treatment of aggression and associated impulsivity (Huband, Ferriter, Nathan, & Jones, 2010). A meta-analysis of 10 randomized controlled trials of 498 adult participants found evidence of efficacy for carbamazepine/oxcarbamazepine, phenytoin, and lithium; further randomized controlled trials were recommended given the limitations of the studies reviewed (Jones et al., 2011).

Antipsychotics

The efficacy and tolerability of antipsychotics have not been established for intermittent explosive disorder and these drugs are not generally recommended unless they are indicated for a comorbid disorder (e.g., bipolar disorder) that may respond to antipsychotics.

Contraindications

If increased impulsive aggression is a manifestation of mania, an SSRI may exacerbate symptoms. Furthermore, SSRIs have a blackbox warning, indicating that antidepressants may increase the risk of suicidal thinking and behavior in some children and adolescents with major depressive disorder, and close monitoring for suicidal ideation is necessary.

Guidelines

There are several resources that provide algorithms and guidance for the treatment of ADHD. The Texas Children's Medication Algorithm Project is one such evidence-based consensus resource for the treatment of several disorders, including ADHD. This source is continually updated to reflect the ever-expanding body of research in the field. Additionally, given the availability of so many pharmacologic treatments, it is useful for prescribers and non-prescribers alike (Pliszka et al., 2006). Another useful resource is the practice parameter from the American Academy of Child and Adolescent Psychiatry (AACAP) which can be found on their website and outlines evidence-based guidelines for the effective diagnosis and treatment of ADHD (Pliszka & AACAP Work Group on Quality Issues, 2007). The Treatment Recommendations for the use of Antipsychotics for Aggressive Youth (TRAAY) address severe impulsive aggression in children and adolescents with a variety of disorders and include 14 main recommendations for the treatment phases of evaluation, acute treatment, stabilization, and maintenance (Pappadopulos et al., 2003).

Conclusion

Externalizing disorders are prevalent in childhood and include ADHD, ODD, CD, and IED and Table 4.2 provides an overview of medications used to treat these disorders. The most common behavior disorder of childhood is ADHD. There are two classes of medications used to treat ADHD: stimulants and non-stimulant medications. Stimulant medications, including methylphenidate and amphetamine salts, are FDA-approved and highly efficacious for ADHD. A case control, 10-year prospective follow-up study of ADHD youth into young adulthood found evidence that stimulant treatment decreases the risk for subsequent comorbid psychiatric disorders and academic failure (Biederman, Monuteaux, Spencer, Wilens, & Faraone, 2009). Atomoxetine and long-acting alpha-agonists are FDA-approved non-stimulant medications for ADHD. Tricyclic antidepressants and bupropion, though not FDA-approved, have been shown to be effective for ADHD symptoms.

There are no FDA approved medications to treat ODD, CD, and IED. Medications are only partially effective in the management of ODD and CD and behavioral interventions are recommended before a medication trial. Psychopharmacological treatment of ODD, CD, and IED may include stimulants, non-stimulant ADHD medications, antidepressants, mood stabilizers, or antipsychotics.

A thorough diagnostic evaluation is essential to ensure accurate diagnosis and to assess for and address comorbidities. Each individual responds differently to medication and children on medications must be closely monitored by a physician. When assessing the benefits and risks of prescribing a medication, one must consider the severity of the disorder and its impact on a child's functioning at home, school, and social situations. In situations where the disorder results in significant impair-

Table 4.2 Medications used in the treatment of externalizing disorders

Medication (Generic)	Brand name	Mechanism of action	FDA approval state		
			ADHD	ODD/CD	IED
Amphetamine preparations					
Mixed amphetamine salts	Adderall	Blocks NE and DA reuptake and increase release of NE and DA to synapses. Enhances NE and DA actions in various brain regions, may improve concentration, executive function, wakefulness, hyperactivity	Yes, age 3–12	N/A	N/A
	Adderall XR		Yes, 6 years and up		
Dextroamphetamine	Dexedrine		Yes, age 6–16		
Lisdexamfetamine	Vyvanse		Yes, 6 years and up		
Methylphenidate preparations					
Methylphenidate	Methylin	Blocks NE and DA reuptake; enhances NE and DA actions in various brain regions, may improve concentration, executive function, wakefulness, hyperactivity	Yes, age 6–12	N/A	N/A
	Ritalin (short acting)		Yes, age 6–12, and adults		
	Methylin ER		Yes, 6 years and up		
	Concerta (long acting)		Yes, 6 years and up		
	Metadate CD		Yes, age 6–17		
Dexmethylphenidate	Focalin		Yes, age 6–17		
	Focalin XR		Yes, 6 years and up		
Selective norepinephrine reuptake inhibitor					
Atomoxetine	Strattera	Blocks NE reuptake; increases NE and DA in prefrontal cortex	Yes, 6 years and up	No	N/A

(continued)

Table 4.2 (continued)

Medication (Generic)	Brand name	Mechanism of action	FDA approval state		
			ADHD	ODD/CD	IED
Selective norepinephrine and dopamine reuptake inhibitor					
Bupropion	Wellbutrin (IR, SR, XL)	Blocks NE and DA reuptake	No (off label use)	N/A	N/A
Tricyclic antidepressants					
Nortriptyline		Blocks NE and serotonin reuptake	No (off label use)	N/A	N/A
Alpha-2-Agonists					
Clonidine	Kapvay (XR)	Central actions on postsynaptic alpha-2A receptors in prefrontal cortex	Yes, ages 6–17 years	No	N/A
Guanfacine	Tenex Intuniv (XR)		Yes, ages 6–17 years	N/A	N/A
Selective serotonin reuptake inhibitors					
Fluoxetine	Prozac	Blocks serotonin reuptake, thus increasing synaptic concentration of serotonin	N/A	N/A	No
Sertraline	Zoloft				
Citalopram	Celexa				
Escitalopram	Lexapro				
Fluvoxamine	Luvox				
Anti epileptic drugs					
Phenytoin	Dilantin	Sodium channel blocker	N/A	No	No
Carbamazepine, Oxcarbazepine	Tegretol, Trileptal	Sodium channel blocker			

(continued)

Table 4.2 (continued)

Medication (Generic)	Brand name	Mechanism of action	FDA approval state		
			ADHD	ODD/CD	IED
Lamotrigine	Lamictal	Sodium channel blocker			
Topiramate	Topamax	Sodium channel blocker, enhancing GABA function, antagonizing Glutamate receptor			
Valproate/divalproex	Depakote	Sodium channel blocker, enhancing GABA function			
Mood stabilizer					
Lithium	Eskalith	Unknown. May influence serotonin and norepinephrine reuptake and glutamate clearance	N/A	No	No
Antipsychotics					
Olanzapine	Zyprexa	Block D2 receptors	N/A	No	N/A
Quetiapine	Seroquel				
Haloperidol	Haldol				
Risperidone	Risperidal				

Key: *NE* Norepinephrine; *DA* Dopamine, *IR* Immediate Release, *SR* Sustained Release, *XL/XR* Extended Release, *N/A* Not Applicable ment despite adequate behavioral interventions, a trial of medication may allow the child to better function, manage symptoms, and benefit from academic and relation interventions intended to improve functioning across settings.

List of Websites

- http://www.chadd.org/

  This website from Children and Adults with Attention-Deficit/Hyperactivity Disorder (CHADD) provides information for parents and caregivers of children with ADHD.

- http://www.aacap.org/AACAP/Families_and_Youth/Facts_for_Families/FFF-Guide/FFF-Guide-Home.aspx

  The American Academy of Child and Adolescent Psychiatry (AACAP) provides resources online regarding the diagnosis and treatment of externalizing disorders in children and adolescents.

Suggested Readings

- Pliszka, S. R., Crismon, M. L., Hughes, C. W., Conners, K. C., Emslie, G. J., Jensen., P. S., … Lopez, M. (2006). The Texas Children's Medication Algorithm Project: Revision of the Algorithm for Pharmacotherapy of ADHD. *Journal of the American Academy of Child and Adolescent Psychiatry, 45,* 642–657.

  This article presents an evidence-based treatment algorithm for ADHD.

- Pappadopulos, E., MacIntyre, J. C., Crismon, M. L., Findling, R. L., Malone, R. P., Derivan, A., … Felton, C. J. (2003). Treatment recommendations for the use of antipsychotics for aggressive youth (TRAAY). Part II. *Journal of the American Academy of Child & Adolescent Psychiatry*, *42*(2), 145–161.

  This article presents evidence-based treatment recommendations for children exhibiting aggression.

- Pliszka, S., AACAP Work Group on Quality Issues. (2007). Practice parameter for the assessment and treatment of children and adolescents with attention-deficit/hyperactivity disorder. *Journal of the American Academy of Child & Adolescent Psychiatry*, *46*(7), 894–921.

  This article provides evidence-based guidelines for the diagnosis and treatment of ADHD.

References

Aman, M. G., Bukstein, O. G., Gadow, K. D., Arnold, L. E., Molina, B. S., McNamara, N. K., ... Butter, E. M. (2014). What does risperidone add to parent training and stimulant for severe aggression in child attention-deficit/hyperactivity disorder?. *Journal of the American Academy of Child & Adolescent Psychiatry, 53*(1), 47–60.

American Psychiatric Association. (2013). *Diagnostic and statistical manual of mental disorders (DSM-5®)*. American Psychiatric Pub.

Barkley, R. A. (2014). *Attention-deficit hyperactivity disorder: A handbook for diagnosis and treatment*. Guilford Publications.

Biederman, J., Monuteaux, M., Spencer, T., Wilens, T. E., & Faraone, S. V. (2009). Do stimulants have a protective effect on the development of psychiatric disorders in youth with ADHD? A ten-year follow-up study. *Pediatrics, 124*(1), 71–78.

Buitelaar, J. K., Van der Gaag, R. J., Cohen-Kettenis, P., & Melman, C. T. M. (2001). A randomized controlled trial of risperidone in the treatment of aggression in hospitalized adolescents with subaverage cognitive abilities. *Journal of Clinical Psychiatry, 62*(4), 239–248.

Bushe, C. J., & Savill, N. C. (2014). Systematic review of atomoxetine data in childhood and adolescent attention-deficit hyperactivity disorder 2009–2011: focus on clinical efficacy and safety. *Journal of Psychopharmacology, 28*(3), 204–211.

Campbell, M., Small, A. M., Green, W. H., Jennings, S. J., Perry, R., Bennett, W. G., & Anderson, L. (1984). Behavioral efficacy of haloperidol and lithium carbonate: a comparison in hospitalized aggressive children with conduct disorder. *Archives of General Psychiatry, 41*(7), 650–656.

Canino, G., Polanczyk, G., Bauermeister, J. J., Rohde, L. A., & Frick, P. J. (2010). Does the prevalence of CD and ODD vary across cultures? *Social Psychiatry and Psychiatric Epidemiology, 45*(7), 695–704.

Coccaro, E. F., Lee, R. J., & Kavoussi, R. J. (2009). A double-blind, randomized, placebo-controlled trial of fluoxetine in patients with intermittent explosive disorder. *The Journal of Clinical Psychiatry, 70*(5), 653–662.

Coccaro, E. F., Schmidt, C. A., Samuels, J. F., & Nestadt, G. (2004). Lifetime and 1-month prevalence rates of intermittent explosive disorder in a community sample. *The Journal of Clinical Psychiatry*.

Connor, D. F. (2011). Problems of overdiagnosis and overprescribing in ADHD: are they legitimate?. *Psychiatric Times, 28*(8), 14–14.

Connor, D. F., Barkely, R. A., & Davis, H. T. (2000). A pilot study of methylphenidate, clonidine or the combination in ADHD comorbid with aggressive oppositional defiant and conduct disorder. *Clinical Pediatrics, 39*, 15–25.

Connor, D. F., McLaughlin, T. J., & Jeffers-Terry, M. (2008). Randomized controlled pilot study of quetiapine in the treatment of adolescent conduct disorder. *Journal of Child and Adolescent Psychopharmacology, 18*(2), 140–156.

Costello, E. J., Egger, H. L., & Angold, A. (2004). Epidemiology of anxiety disorders. In *Phobic and anxiety disorders in children and adolescents: A clinician's guide to effective psychosocial and pharmacological interventions* (p. 61).

Cueva, J. E., Overall, J. E., Small, A. M., Armenteros, J. L., Perry, R., & Campbell, M. (1996). Carbamazepine in aggressive children with conduct disorder: A double-blind and placebo-controlled study. *Journal of the American Academy of Child and Adolescent Psychiatry, 35*(4), 480–490.

Daviss, W. B. (2008). A review of co-morbid depression in pediatric ADHD: Etiologies, phenomenology, and treatment. *Journal of Child and Adolescent Psychopharmacology, 18*(6), 565–571.

Donovan, S. J., Stewart, J. W., Nunes, E. V., Quitkin, F. M., Parides, M., Daniel, W., et al. (2000). Divaloproex treatment for youth with explosive temper and mood lability: A double-blind, placebo-controlled crossover design. *American Journal of Psychiatry, 157*(5), 818–820.

Erskine, H. E., Norman, R. E., Ferrari, A. J., Chan, G. C., Copeland, W. E., Whiteford, H. A., et al. (2016). Long-term outcomes of attention-deficit/hyperactivity disorder and conduct disorder: a systematic review and meta-analysis. *Journal of the American Academy of Child and Adolescent Psychiatry, 55*(10), 841–850.

Gérardin, P., Cohen, D., Mazet, P., & Flament, M. F. (2002). Drug treatment of conduct disorder in young people. *European Neuropsychopharmacology, 12,* 361–370.

Grant, E. J., & Leppink, E. W. (2015). Choosing a treatment for disruptive, impulse-control and conduct disorders. *Current Psychiatry, 14*(1), 29–36.

Greenhill, L. L., Pliszka, S., & Dulcan, M. K. (2002). Practice parameter for the use of stimulant medications in the treatment of children, adolescents, and adults. *Journal of the American Academy of Child and Adolescent Psychiatry, 41*(2), 26S–49S.

Hazell, P. L., & Stuart, J. E. (2003). A randomized controlled trial of clonidine added to psychostimulant medication for hyperactive and aggressive children. *Journal of the American Academy of Child and Adolescent Psychiatry, 42*(8), 886–894.

Huband, N., Ferriter, M., Nathan, R., & Jones, H. (2010). Antiepileptics for aggression and associated impulsivity. *The Cochrane Library.*

Jensen, P. S. (1999). A 14-month randomized clinical trial of treatment strategies for attention-deficit/hyperactivity disorder. *Archives of General Psychiatry, 56*(12), 1073–1086.

Jones, R. M., Arlidge, J., Gillham, R., Reagu, S., van den Bree, M., & Taylor, P. J. (2011). Efficacy of mood stabilisers in the treatment of impulsive or repetitive aggression: Systematic review and meta-analysis. *The British Journal of Psychiatry, 198*(2), 93–98.

Kaplan, S. L., Busner, J., Kupietz, S., Wasserman, E., & Segal, B. (1990). Effects of methylphenidate on adolescents with aggressive conduct disorder and ADHD: A preliminary report. *Journal of the American Academy of Child and Adolescent Psychiatry, 29*(5), 719–723.

Kapitanyan, R., & Su, M. (2016, May 5) Second generation (atypical) antipsychotic medication poisoning. UpToDate.

Kessler, R. C., Coccaro, E. F., Fava, M., Jaeger, S., Jin, R., & Walters, E. (2006). The prevalence and correlates of DSM-IV intermittent explosive disorder in the National Comorbidity Survey Replication. *Archives of General Psychiatry, 63*(6), 669–678.

Klein, R. G., Abikoff, H., Klass, E., Ganeles, D., Seese, L. M., & Pollack, S. (1997). Clinical efficacy of methylphenidate in conduct disorder with and without attention deficit hyperactivity disorder. *Archives of General Psychiatry, 54,* 1073–1080.

Klykylo, W., Bowers, R., Weston, C., & Jackson, J. (2014). *Green's child and adolescent clinical psychopharmacology* (5th ed., p. 251). Page: Lippincott Williams & Wilkins.

Masi, G., Milone, A., Canepa, G., Millepiedi, S., Mucci, M., & Muratori, F. (2004). Olanzapine treatment in adolescents with severe conduct disorder. *European Psychiatry, 21,* 51–57.

Malone, R. P., Delaney, M. A., Luebbert, J. F., Cater, J., & Campbell, M. (2000). A double-blind placebo-controlled study of lithium in hospitalized aggressive children and adolescents with conduct disorder. *Archives of General Psychiatry, 57,* 649–654.

Merikangas, K. R., He, J. P., Burstein, M., Swanson, S. A., Avenevoli, S., Cui, L., … Swendsen, J. (2010). Lifetime prevalence of mental disorders in US adolescents: Results from the National Comorbidity Survey Replication–Adolescent Supplement (NCS-A). *Journal of the American Academy of Child & Adolescent Psychiatry, 49*(10), 980–989.

Newcorn, J. H., Spencer, T. J., Biederman, J., Milton, D. R., & Michelson, D. (2005). Atomoxetine treatment in children and adolescents with attention-deficit/hyperactivity disorder and comorbid oppositional defiant disorder. *Journal of the American Academy of Child and Adolescent Psychiatry, 44*(3), 240–248.

Pappadopulos, E., MacIntyre, J. C., Crismon, M. L., Findling, R. L., Malone, R. P., Derivan, A., … Felton, C. J. (2003). Treatment recommendations for the use of antipsychotics for aggressive youth (TRAAY). Part II. *Journal of the American Academy of Child & Adolescent Psychiatry, 42*(2), 145–161.

Pappadopulos, E., Woolston, S., Chait, A., Perkins, M., Connor, D. F., & Jensen, P. S. (2006). Pharmacotherapy of aggression in children and adolescents: efficacy and effect size. *Journal of the Canadian Academy of Child and Adolescent Psychiatry, 15*(1), 27–39.

Pliszka, S., AACAP Work Group on Quality Issues. (2007). Practice parameter for the assessment and treatment of children and adolescents with attention-deficit/hyperactivity disorder. *Journal of the American Academy of Child and Adolescent Psychiatry, 46*(7), 894–921.

Pliszka, S. R., Crismon, M. L., Hughes, C. W., Corners, C. K., Emslie, G. J., & Jensen, P. S. (2006). The Texas Children's Medication Algorithm Project: Revision of the algorithm for pharmacotherapy of attention-deficit/hyperactivity disorder. *Journal of the American Academy of Child and Adolescent Psychiatry, 45*(6), 642–657.

Rifkin, A., Karajgi, B., Dicker, R., Perl, E., Boppana, V., Hasan, N., et al. (1997). Lithium treatment of conduct disorder in adolescents. *American Journal of Psychiatry, 154*(4), 554–555.

Schachter, S. (2017, February 27) Antiseizure drugs: mechanism of action, pharmacology and adverse effects. UpToDate.

Sheard, M. H., Marini, J. L., Bridges, C. I., & Wagner, E. (1976). The effect of lithium on impulsive aggressive behavior in man. *American Journal of Psychiatry, 133*(12), 1409–1413.

Siever, L. J. (2008). Neurobiology of aggression and violence. *American Journal of Psychiatry, 165*(4), 429–442.

Soderstrom, H., Rastam, M., & Gilberg, C. (2002). A clinical case series of six extremely aggressive youths treated with olanzapine. *European Child and Adolescent Psychiatry, 11,* 138–141.

Stanford, M. S., Anderson, N. E., Lake, S. L., & Baldridge, R. M. (2009). Pharmacologic treatment of impulsive aggression with antiepileptic drugs. *Current treatment options in neurology, 11*(5), 383–390.

Steiner, H., & Remsing, L. (2007). Practice parameter for the assessment and treatment of children and adolescents with oppositional defiant disorder. *Journal of the American Academy of Child and Adolescent Psychiatry, 46*(1), 126–141.

Turgay, A. (2009). Psychopharmacological treatment of oppositional defiant disorder. *CNS Drugs, 23*(1), 1–17.

Volkow, N. D., Wang, G. J., Tomasi, D., Kollins, S. H., Wigal, T. L., Newcorn, J. H., ... Swanson, J. M. (2012). Methylphenidate-elicited dopamine increases in ventral striatum are associated with long-term symptom improvement in adults with attention deficit hyperactivity disorder. *Journal of Neuroscience, 32*(3), 841–849.

Zuvekas, S. H., & Vitiello, B. (2012). Stimulant medication use in children: A 12-year perspective. *American Journal of Psychiatry, 169*(2), 160–166.

Chapter 5
Effective Medications for Treating Internalizing Disorders

Brian Smith, Alyse Ley, Katherine Krive and Jed Magen

Internalizing disorders, which encompass anxiety and depressive disorders, are a challenge to both diagnose and treat in the school-age population. While the diagnostic criteria for children and adolescents are in most cases identical to those used for adults, children may not be cognitively sophisticated enough to report internal feeling states or may be disinclined to talk with teachers, healthcare professionals, or other adults. Behaviors may also differ between the school and home settings. In developmental terms, adolescents are going through the stage of separation-individuation during which they develop a more complex personality, more sophisticated cognitive abilities and become more independent. As a result, they may not be interested in talking about behaviors or internal feeling states that foster dependency and feel invasive to them. With limited self-report information, it can be difficult to differentiate which disorders are present based on external observations. Internalizing disorders are also uniquely challenging to treat due to a more limited evidence base for efficacy of interventions compared to the adult population and treatment risks unique to the school-age population including incomplete knowledge of potential effects of long-term use on developing brains, more sensitivity to side effects, and possibly increased suicidality.

Anxiety disorders are the most prevalent mental health conditions in youth. The prevalence of anxiety disorders in adolescents may be as high as 1 in 3 (Merikangas et al., 2010). Most anxiety disorders have a median age-of-onset of 11 years (Kessler et al., 2007). While rates of anxiety disorders for prepubescent boys and girls are similar, after puberty the rates for girls are nearly double that of boys for most anxiety disorders aside from possibly OCD (now in a separate chapter in DSM-5) and social anxiety. Prevalence of major depressive disorder is reported to be in the range of 1–2% (some studies reference up to 6%) in children (age 6–12) and 4–8% in adolescents. Males and females are equally affected during childhood. Females

B. Smith · A. Ley · K. Krive · J. Magen (✉)
Michigan State University, East Lansing, MI, USA
e-mail: Jed.Magen@hc.msu.edu

J. S. Carlson and J. A. Barterian (eds.), *School Psychopharmacology*, Pediatric School Psychology, https://doi.org/10.1007/978-3-030-15541-4_5

are doubly affected in adolescence and after puberty, the risk for females increases by a factor of two to four (Birmaher et al., 1996; Whittington et al., 2004; Zhou et al., 2015).

Anxiety disorders in youth are undertreated with only 18% of anxious adolescents receiving help (Merikangas et al., 2011). Unfortunately, significant barriers exist that make recognizing and treating childhood anxiety disorders difficult. They often present chiefly as somatic complaints, decline in school performance, social withdrawal, or behavioral disturbances. Children often do not recognize their fears as excessive and unreasonable. Even children with insight into their anxiety conditions often fail to disclose because of fears of being seen as "not normal." Anxiety can at times be a part of normal maturation, and it can be difficult to know when to reassure as normal or label the presenting complaints as pathologic. Developmentally, there are common childhood fears such as stranger anxiety from 12 to 18 months of age but these age-appropriate fears tend to be temporary and not impairing. Because of these factors, it can be more than a decade, especially in the case of Obsessive-Compulsive Disorder, before anxiety disorders are diagnosed or treated.

Untreated anxiety disorders in adolescents, especially when severe are more likely to worsen and continue into adulthood and are a risk factor for adult depression and substance use. Fifty percent of youth recover from anxiety after 3–4 years of follow-up but are more likely to have developed another mental disorder, primarily another form of anxiety, with those receiving treatment less likely to develop a new anxiety disorder (Last, Perrin, Hersen, & Kazdin, 1996). These children often struggle with a variety of significant mental health burdens. For example, a child who has separation anxiety may become an adolescent with social anxiety or more generalized anxiety. Anxiety disorders also commonly co-occur with other mental health conditions. Common comorbidities include depression, substance use disorders, attention deficit hyperactivity disorder, and learning disabilities (Siegel & Dickstein, 2012).

Children and adolescents with anxiety disorders have significant problems in the school setting. They are at risk for underperforming and withdrawing from school prior to achieving their academic goals (Van Ameringen, Mancini, & Farvolden, 2003). Extreme worry in children and adolescents may manifest as somatic complaints leading to excessive absenteeism or the inability to focus on learning due to these physical symptoms. Anxious children have difficulty concentrating on school demands as they focus on fear or unpleasant thoughts replaying in their minds. A child distracted by worry is unable to attend to academic tasks being presented, often resulting in reduced academic achievement and performance. Social anxiety disorder, the excessive fear of embarrassment or humiliation, limits the ability to ask and answer questions, read aloud, complete oral presentations, engage socially, and form relationships (Connolly & Bernstein, 2007). Students with performance anxiety tend to perform poorly on tests due to distressing thoughts regarding the negative potential outcome of a test (von der Embse, Barterian, & Segool, 2013). Avoidance behaviors that are common to all anxiety disorders often impede learning. Avoiding, sometimes through the refusal of new concepts or tasks is a way of dealing with the anxiety around failure or the inability to focus attention on the task at hand. The relationship between anxiety in school settings and academic performance is well established.

Significant anxiety is correlated with poor reading in early elementary school and math achievement in upper elementary school (Ialongo et al., 1995).

Depression causes significant decreases in functioning and affects social skills, cognition, and overall family functioning (Birmaher et al., 1996; March et al., 2004) Major depressive disorder (MDD) is also problematic because there is considerable comorbidity with other psychiatric disorders, episodes are long, and recurrence is common (Zhou et al., 2015). Approximately 60% of youth with MDD have suicidal ideation and 30% attempt suicide (Brent, Baugher, Bridge, Chen, & Chiapetta, 1999). Other outcomes for youth with depression can include substance abuse, early pregnancy, medical illness, legal issues, and difficulties with academics, work, and psychosocial problems (Fergusson & Woodward, 2002).

Since depressive disorders often reoccur, individuals might have multiple episodes over childhood/adolescence and development can stagnate during the episodes. Cognitive, emotional, and social impacts cannot be underestimated. Pervasive symptoms of depression lead to impairments in relationships, coping skills, and academic performance. A depressive episode not only impacts the child's mood but also affects sleep, appetite, self-worth, enjoyment, energy, and ability to concentrate (APA, 2013). These neurocognitive symptoms of depression make participation in learning difficult. Depressed children may be overwhelmed with negative thoughts, self-deprivation, worthlessness, or suicidal ideation rendering them unable to focus on academics or attend to educational material. Academic underachievement is common during depressive episodes. Given these kinds of difficulties, accommodations in the school setting are extremely important until symptoms resolve. Continued learning difficulties in a child who has been treated for depression may be an indication of continued, low level symptoms (Dulcan, 2015). These children will have difficulty concentrating, problems discerning information, and making decisions leading to drastically reduced ability to perform in the school setting. Students with depression often also suffer from comorbid, anxiety, attention deficit hyperactivity disorder, and substance use disorders (Small et al., 2008). Depressed children and adolescents frequently develop impairment in relationship formation and may gravitate toward unhealthy peer relationships or deviant behavior (Birmaher et al., 2007). Poirier and colleagues (2015) demonstrated that approximately 40% of students enrolled in school services for conduct problems had a comorbid depressive disorder. Given the extreme complexity of neurobiology, genetics, epigenetics, and behavior, psychotropic drug development has proven to be extremely difficult. Although Selective Serotonin Reuptake Inhibitors (SSRIs) and Selective Norepinephrine Reuptake Inhibitors (SNRIs) have largely replaced tricyclic antidepressants, the original tricyclic, imipramine, was developed as an antipsychotic because the chemical structure of tricyclics is similar to that of antipsychotics (Ban, 2006). Nevertheless, when Roland Kuhn in Switzerland gave imipramine to 500 patients at his hospital, rather than an antipsychotic effect he observed that patients who were depressed became less depressed (Ramachandraih, Subramanyam, Bar, Baker, &Yeragani, 2011). Imipramine and other tricyclics became the first commonly prescribed and recognized drugs for major depressive disorder (Mulinari, 2015).

The SSRI story is the only instance of purposeful drug development in psychiatry. Originally, investigators like Arvid Carlsson became interested in directed drug development. The monoamine hypothesis of depression indicated that both norepinephrine and serotonin increases in the synaptic cleft might be involved in the effect of antidepressants. They therefore set out to find compounds that increased serotonin. The result, after other compounds were developed, was fluoxetine, and with the development of this and similar agents, the market for drug treatment of depression mushroomed (Perez-Caballero, Torres-Sanchez, Mico, & Berrocoso, 2014).

Clinical trials for new medications are particularly difficult to conduct in children and adolescents, partly because of deficits in oversight in initial trials. Concern for the ethics of exposing children to medications with unknown effects largely limited such trials. Regulatory agencies have put in place stricter guidelines than for adult trials, with ethical oversight in mind, but also encourage the conduct of these trials as many untested drugs are routinely used in clinical practice (Bavdekar, 2013). There has been no truly new, innovative psychotropic drug developed for internalizing disorders since fluoxetine. New drug development will depend on a much finer grained understanding of both neurobiology and the development of a series of biomarkers for disorders so that we are not dependent only on groupings of symptoms that may or may not represent discrete disorders (Hyman, 2013).

Psychopharmacological and Other Treatment of Internalizing Disorders

Anxiety Disorders Treatment

The first-line treatment for mild to moderate anxiety is psychosocial therapy. Specifically, Cognitive Behavior Therapy (CBT) has the best evidence base for treatment of anxiety disorders for children, adolescents, and adults. Important components of therapy include teaching patients and parents about anxiety (psychoeducation), managing avoidance of feared situations through exposure tasks, relaxation techniques (deep breathing, progressive muscle relaxation, and guided imagery), and cognitive techniques to manage anxious thoughts. Kendall used the "Coping Cat" program in the first randomized, controlled trial of individual cognitive behavior therapy for child anxiety (Kendall, 1994). Additional effective forms of psychotherapy include group cognitive behavior therapy, trauma-focused cognitive behavior therapy (TF-CBT), exposure and response prevention (E/RP) for OCD and Social Effectiveness Training for Children (SET-C) for social anxiety (Beidel, Turner, & Morris, 2000). Working with parents therapeutically is important as parents can greatly influence child anxiety disorders through modeling of fear and anxiety, reinforcing anxious coping behaviors, maintaining avoidance, and overly protective, controlling and critical parenting styles.

Although psychotherapy is recommended as the first-line treatment for mild to moderate anxiety, there is a strong evidence base for pharmacological treatment of anxiety in youth. Medications should be considered for the treatment of moderate to severe anxiety where there is functional impairment and/or significant distress. Medications may also be considered as a first-line treatment, even for mild symptoms, where quality CBT is not available or has not resulted in full remission. There are also cases, as with social anxiety, where pharmacotherapy may be necessary for the child to tolerate and benefit from CBT (Connolly & Bernstein, 2007).

Sertraline, possibly with the greatest evidence base, fluvoxamine, and fluoxetine are superior to placebo in multiple randomized, placebo-controlled trials (Rynn, Siqueland, & Rickels, 2001; Walkup et al., 2008; See Table 5.1 for additional information regarding available medications to treat anxiety and depression in children and adolescents). These SSRIs are typically well tolerated aside from mild gastrointestinal symptoms and insomnia. Paroxetine is effective but not used as often due to concerns regarding tolerability including a discontinuation syndrome with flu-like symptoms and possible increase in suicidal thinking. Although all antidepressants have black box warnings about the risk of suicidality in youth, paroxetine may have a greater risk than other class members for children with depression. However, the risk of treatment-emergent suicidality with SSRIs appears to be nonsignificant in youth taking these medications primarily for anxiety disorders (Strawn, Welge, Wehry, Keeshin, & Rynn, 2015).

Psychotropic medications, including the SSRIs, are prescribed with care in this patient population. The rule for prescribing of medications for anxiety in youth is "start low, go slow." This population may be particularly sensitive to side effects. In general, individuals with anxiety are more sensitive to medication side effects plus youth are more sensitive to side effects than adults. An adequate trial length is 6–8 weeks at an age-appropriate dose although early effects are sometimes seen within the first 1–2 weeks. Medications are often started at approximately half the adult dose, but it is not uncommon for older children and younger adolescents to require adult dosing for full benefit. These disorders can decrease in intensity or abate over time. When a significant reduction in anxiety is maintained for approximately one year, one may consider a medication-free trial during a low-stress period.

While the evidence base supports the use of psychotherapy and medications, especially SSRIs, for anxiety in youth, the most robust treatment options as supported by high quality randomized controlled trials appear to be combination treatments involving both therapy and medication. The Child/Adolescent Anxiety Multimodal Study (CAMS), primarily with children with GAD, found a combination of sertraline and CBT to be more effective than either treatment alone. Both combination and monotherapy approaches were superior to placebo (Walkup et al., 2008). The Obsessive-Compulsive Disorder Treatment Study (POTS) also demonstrated the superiority of a combination of sertraline and exposure therapy/relapse prevention over monotherapies. CBT alone was also superior to placebo (Pediatric OCD Treatment Team, 2004). However, in a trial of TF-CBT plus sertraline versus TF-CBT plus placebo, there was not a significant difference in response, positive for each, between the groups (Cohen, Mannarino, Perel, & Staron, 2007). Although SSRIs are

Table 5.1 Medications used in the treatment of internalizing disorders

Medication (generic)	Brand name	Mechanism of action	FDA approval state	
			Major depression	Anxiety
Selective norepinephrine reuptake inhibitor				
Duloxetine	Cymbalta	Blocks NE reuptake; increases NE and DA in prefrontal cortex	No (off-label use)	Yes, GAD ages 7–17
Selective norepinephrine and dopamine reuptake inhibitor				
Bupropion	Wellbutrin (IR, SR, XL)	Blocks NE and DA reuptake	No (off-label use)	No
Tricyclic antidepressants				
Clomipramine		Blocks serotonin (primary, most serotonergic TCA) and NE reuptake	No	Yes, OCD ages 10–17
Selective serotonin reuptake inhibitors				
Fluoxetine	Prozac	Blocks serotonin reuptake, thus increasing synaptic concentration of serotonin	Yes, ages 8–17	Yes, OCD ages 7–17
Sertraline	Zoloft		No (off-label use)	Yes, OCD ages 6–17
Escitalopram	Lexapro		Yes, ages 12–17	No (off-label use)
Fluvoxamine	Luvox		No	Yes, OCD ages 8–17

Key: *NE*—Norepinephrine; *DA*—Dopamine, *IR*—Immediate Release, *SR*—Sustained Release, *XL*—Extended Release, *OCD*—Obsessive-Compulsive Disorder, *GAD*—Generalized Anxiety Disorder

the first-line medication treatments for anxiety in youth, it is possible that SSRIs are not the most effective pharmacotherapy for all anxiety disorders.

Clomipramine appears to be superior to SSRIs for treatment of OCD (Geller et al., 2003). However, SSRIs remain the first-line medication interventions despite modest effect sizes due to clomipramine's more adverse side effect profile and the necessity of reviewing an electrocardiogram before prescribing this tricyclic antidepressant. It may take 10–12 weeks for substantial benefits to occur during a medication trial for OCD and substantial numbers of patients continue to have very distressing symptoms. Medication augmentation strategies for OCD include adding clomipramine (25–75 mg/day), and adding atypical antipsychotics, especially risperidone in children with tics.

There is also evidence supporting the use of Serotonin–Norepinephrine Reuptake Inhibitors for anxiety disorders in children and adolescents. Venlafaxine extended release has been found to be effective for social anxiety and generalized anxiety disorder in randomized, controlled trials (Rynn et al., 2011). Duloxetine has demonstrated similar efficacy in the treatment of generalized anxiety disorder and is FDA-approved for use in children ages 7–17 for this indication (Taylor, 2015).

While the effect size in trials of medication for PTSD is not as robust as for treatment of other forms of anxiety and medication would likely not be a first-line treatment for this condition, an SSRI such as citalopram can be added if necessary. Antiadrenergic medications such as clonidine to decrease hyperarousal and reexperiencing symptoms, prazosin for trauma nightmares, and possibly antipsychotics such as risperidone or quetiapine can sometimes be used to try to address these kinds of more specific symptoms (Cohen & The AACAP Work Group on Quality Issues, 2010).

Whereas SSRIs and SNRIs may be appropriate and effective for anxiety disorders in youth, more care should be taken with prescribing benzodiazepines in this population. Benzodiazepines can be considered, with caution, for specific anxiety conditions such as specific phobias (for example, fear of flying), prior to medical procedures, situational panic, and eating disorders (often given before a meal as the anxiety-provoking event). However, benzodiazepines are often not more effective than placebo in youth. They also have the potential to make things worse. Paradoxical reactions, including aggression and disinhibition, are often encountered, and benzodiazepines have a significant potential for abuse and dependence, especially in an adolescent population in which the initiation of substance abuse is common (O'Sullivan et al., 2015).

Several psychotropic medications have received FDA approval for the treatment of anxiety in children and adolescents. However, the number of medications, primarily SSRIs, is limited as are the indications, primarily for OCD. In addition to duloxetine for Generalized Anxiety Disorder, the SSRIs fluoxetine, fluvoxamine, and sertraline are FDA-approved for the indication of OCD, starting with youth between the ages of 6 and 8 years old, depending on the medication, through age 17. With limited FDA approval, much of the appropriate use of medications in child psychiatry is "off-label." Position statements by both the American Academy of Pediatrics (AAP) and the American Academy of Child & Adolescent Psychiatry (AACAP) support efficacy of SSRIs for pediatric anxiety. Practice parameters from AACAP recommend CBT for youth with mild to moderate anxiety including OCD and PTSD and consideration of medication approaches, especially in combination with psychotherapy, for more severe symptoms (Cohen & The AACAP Work Group on Quality Issues, 2010; Geller & March, 2012). School accommodations are often necessary to alleviate problems when anxiety affects school performance (AACAP-PP Anxiety). Children can obtain services through the Individuals with Disabilities Education Act (IDEA). Anxious students are eligible for services that help to alleviate barriers to learning caused by their disorders (Dulcan, 2015).

Depressive Disorders Treatment

As with anxiety in youth, CBT is likely the first-line treatment for mild to moderate depression. The risk–benefit ratio for medication treatment of depression in youth is controversial. Efficacy in studies is difficult to demonstrate since the placebo response rate is up to 50%, making it difficult to get large enough study populations and demonstrate medication response is significantly different than placebo. A meta-analysis from 2004, reported that fluoxetine was the only SSRI/SNRI that showed a favorable risk–benefit ratio, with sertraline and paroxetine showing equivocal or weak positive risk/benefit ratios and citalopram and venlafaxine showing negative risk/benefit ratios. A meta-analysis of all data from published and unpublished pharmacological randomized controlled trials for the treatment on MDD in children and adolescents demonstrated that, on average, 61% responded to treatment. Up to 50% of patients respond to placebo, and some young people may benefit from psychoeducation, case management, and support (Whittington et al., 2004).

The major risk concerns for antidepressants include suicidal ideation and other serious adverse events such as hypomania or mania in young people with bipolar disorder (Whittington et al., 2004). There have been persistent questions about suicide risk and antidepressants. The Federal Drug Administration and their British equivalent have each examined all available published and unpublished SSRI trials to look at the risk of suicide. Based on this data, they calculate the risk to be 1–2% for (suicidal ideation). This led to an FDA warning (a "black box" as it is bordered in black) regarding a potential increase in suicidality and precipitated a decline in prescribing SSRIs (Hawton & van Heeringen, 2009; Valluri et al., 2010; Whittington et al., 2004). Subsequent investigations, for example, those utilizing large prescription data sets, do not demonstrate an increased risk for suicide among children and adolescents. While the black box warning is still in effect, the data is still in dispute and the real risk, if any, is not at all clear (Bridge et al., 2007; Hammad, Laughren, & Racoosin, 2006). It is also important to note that the FDA statement of 2004 does not absolutely contraindicate the use of antidepressants in youth, instead warning of potential risks. There are significant negative outcomes and risks from not treating depression and anxiety (Hammad, Laughren, & Racoosin, 2006). Although suicidal thinking related to SSRIs is of concern, this risk should not be overstated and an overall decrease in depressive symptoms, including suicidality, is a more likely outcome, and leads to a more positive prognosis. While most antidepressants carry a 1 in 100 risk of increased suicidal thinking in youth, approximately 2 out of 3 respond positively to antidepressants (Bridge et al., 2007). Given this data, the best course of action when treating a child or adolescent with mild or brief depression may be to attempt psychosocial treatments and monitor response. Children and adolescents with moderate to severe depression, suicidal ideation, or poor social support may need a trial of specific psychotherapy combined with antidepressants (Birmaher, 1996; Bridge et al., 2007).

It is common practice in psychiatry to use off-label medications to treat depression. This is especially true in child psychiatry because of the lack of clinical trials in children due to ethical considerations and stricter standards for IRB approval. Such off-label medications include other SSRIs, Serotonin–Norepinephrine Reuptake Inhibitors (SNRIs), bupropion, and mirtazapine, trazodone with augmenting agents such as lithium, lamotrigine, and the atypical antipsychotics. TCAs and Monoamine Oxidase Inhibitors (MAOIs) are out of favor due to significant side effect profiles and greater lethality in overdose. In addition to nortriptyline, only a few other medications are FDA-approved for treatment of depression in youth. These include the SSRIs escitalopram (for age 12 or greater) and fluoxetine (for age 8 or greater; Medicaid Integrity Group, 2013).

The Treatment of Adolescents with Depression Study (TADS) was a multisite, randomized controlled trial that reinforced previous studies demonstrating combination SSRI and psychotherapy as superior to either treatment modality alone. Four hundred thirty-nine volunteers age 12–17 with MDD at baseline were assigned to fluoxetine, placebo, CBT, or fluoxetine + CBT. CBT is the most studied and empirically approved psychotherapy in this population. In a one-year naturalistic follow-up, results were sustained (March et al., 2004).

Fluoxetine is the only medication to show superiority to placebo in depressed children and preteens. This may be due to the actual effects of the drug or due to study design. There are few trials that have assessed the effectiveness for non-SSRI classes of drugs. Studies have shown that mirtazapine, venlafaxine, and tricyclic antidepressants are no more effective than placebo (March et al., 2004). The Treatment of Resistant Depression in Adolescents (TORDIA) study investigated the efficacy of switching to another mediation when the first SSRI was ineffective. Approximately 50% of adolescents respond to a first SSRI treatment. The method was to switch nonresponding adolescents from an SSRI to a second SSRI, switch to venlafaxine (an SNRI), second SSRI + CBT, or venlafaxine + CBT. The findings showed that when the initial trial of SSRI failed, the second trial of a different SSRI or venlafaxine was effective in 40% of the trial subjects. CBT plus medication was more effective than medications alone (Brent et al., 2008).

Recognition and treatment of child or adolescent depression are imperative to improve functioning, wellbeing and academic success. As outlined in the American Academy of Child and Adolescent Psychiatry (AACAP) Practice Parameters, each phase should include psychoeducation, supportive management, and family and school involvement (Birmaher et al., 2007). Parents should advocate for accommodations for their children in the school setting. Depressed students are eligible for services that enable them to continue to learn under the Individuals with Disabilities Education Act (IDEA) and the Americans with Disabilities Act (Dulcan, 2015). The AACAP Practice Parameters recommend "education, support and case management" for children with brief and or mild depression with minimal functional impairment. Cognitive Behavioral Therapy (CBT) and Interpersonal Therapy (IPT) have both been found to be effective in mild depression. If depression is complicated, moderate to severe, or does not respond to supportive psychotherapy, then CBT or IPT and/or antidepressants are recommended. Severe depressive episodes necessitate antidepressant medication treatment. Selective Serotonin Reuptake Inhibitors (SSRIs) are the most widely studied antidepressants in early onset depression.

SSRIs are well tolerated and have few side effects. Other classes of antidepressants (venlafaxine, bupropion) are less well studied but are also used in the treatment of depression in children and adolescents. Once remission is achieved, medication should be continued for 6–12 months to avoid relapse (Birmaher et al., 2007). As earlier discussed, other mental health conditions commonly co-occur with childhood anxiety and depression. These comorbid conditions can be targets of medications. Pharmacotherapy for these common comorbid disorders, such as ADHD, may also result in reduction in depression and/or anxiety.

Contraindications

Care must be taken to screen for family or individual bipolar disorders before prescribing SSRI's, SNRI's, or any antidepressants. These medications can cause mania or rapid cycling in individuals with untreated bipolar disorder. Bipolar disorders often present first or primarily as depressive episodes, and an antidepressant medication given in the absence of a mood stabilizer can destabilize this condition. Disinhibition, activation, and akathisia (intense subjective feeling of restlessness), all of which may look like mania, are also potential side effects of these serotonergic medications (Southammakosane & Schmitz 2015).

The combination of multiple serotonergic medications, including less known suspects such as metoclopramide and triptans, may be problematic due to the potential for serotonin syndrome. Individuals with epilepsy or eating disorders should not receive the antidepressant bupropion due to the risk of seizures. TCAs should be avoided in youth with known cardiac problems or abnormal electrocardiograms.

Conclusions

The internalizing disorders anxiety and depression are prevalent in youth and have significant impacts on academic outcomes and behavioral/social functioning in the school setting. Anxiety disorders, especially separation anxiety, develop in early childhood. Depression typically begins in later childhood and more often in adolescence. These disorders are both under identified and undertreated. What interventions are most appropriate and effective is still not entirely clear due to limitations in the research literature. However, based on current best information, CBT is the non-pharmacologic intervention with the strongest scientific evidence base for effective treatment of anxiety and depression in youth. Medications, primarily the SSRIs, are often appropriate, safe, and effective interventions for child anxiety and depression, especially internalizing disorders of moderate or greater severity. Fluoxetine has the strongest evidence base for pharmacologic treatment of depression in youth whereas sertraline has the strongest evidence base for pharmacologic treatment of anxiety in youth. Although therapy alone and medication alone are both superior to placebo, the overall most effective interventions for depression and anxiety in youth include combinations of medications and psychotherapy, especially CBT.

Suggested Readings

- Dulcan, M., Ballard, R., Poonan, J., & Sadhu, J. (2018). *Concise guide to child and adolescent psychiatry* (5th ed.). Arlington, VA: American Psychiatric Association Publishing.

  This book provides an overview of psychiatric treatment for mental health disorders in children and adolescents.

- Model School District Policy on Suicide Prevention

  This document developed by several professional organizations provides school professionals with information to prevent, assess, and respond to suicide. The document can be found here: https://afsp.org/wp-content/uploads/2016/01/Model-Policy_FINAL.pdf.

List of Websites

- http://www.aacap.org/AACAP/Families_and_Youth/Facts_for_Families/FFF-Guide/FFF-Guide-Home.aspx

  The AACAP Facts for Families Guide provides information on issue that impact children, teenagers, and families.

- http://www.psychiatry.org/patients-families

  This website from the American Psychiatric Association provides information to parents and families regarding mental health problems in children and adolescents.

- https://adaa.org/living-with-anxiety/children

  This website from the Anxiety and Depression Association of America provides specific information regarding anxiety and depressive disorders in children and adolescents.

References

American Psychiatric Association. (2013). *Diagnostic and statistical manual of mental disorders* (5th ed.). Arlington, VA: American Psychiatric Publishing.

Ban, T. A. (2006). The role of serendipity in drug discovery. *Dialogues in Clinical Neuroscience, 8*(3), 335–344.

Bavdekar, S. B. (2013). Pediatric clinical trials. *Perspectives in Clinical Research, 4*(1), 89–99. https://doi.org/10.4103/2229-3485.106403.

Beidel, D. C., Turner, S. M., & Morris, T. L. (2000). Behavioral treatment of childhood social phobia. *Journal of Consulting and Clinical Psychology, 68*(6), 1072–1080. https://doi.org/10.1037/0022-006X.68.6.1072.

Birmaher, B., Brent, D., & AACAP Work Group on Quality Issues. (2007). Practice parameter for the assessment and treatment of children and adolescents with depressive disorders. *Journal of the American Academy of Child and Adolescent Psychiatry, 46*(11), 1503–1526. https://doi.org/10.1097/chi.0b013e318145ae1c.

Birmaher, B., Ryan, N. D., Williamson, D. E., Brent, D. A., Kaufman, J., Dahl, R. E., ... Nelson, B. (1996). Childhood and adolescent depression: A review of the past 10 years. Part I. *Journal of the American Academy of Child & Adolescent Psychiatry, 35*(11), 1427–1439. https://doi.org/10.1097/00004583-199611000-00011.

Brent, D. A., Baugher, M., Bridge, J., Chen, T., & Chiappetta, L. (1999). Age-and sex-related risk factors for adolescent suicide. *Journal of the American Academy of Child and Adolescent Psychiatry, 38*(12), 1497–1505. https://doi.org/10.1097/00004583-199912000-00010.

Brent, D., Emslie, G., Clarke, G., Wagner, K. D., Asarnow, J. R., Keller, M., ... Birmaher, B. (2008). Switching to another SSRI or to venlafaxine with or without cognitive behavioral therapy for adolescents with SSRI-resistant depression: the TORDIA randomized controlled trial. *JAMA, 299*(8), 901–913.

Bridge, J. A., Iyengar, S., Salary, C. B., Barbe, R. P., Birmaher, B., Pincus, H. A., ... Brent, D. A. (2007). Clinical response and risk for reported suicidal ideation and suicide attempts in pediatric antidepressant treatment: a meta-analysis of randomized controlled trials. *JAMA, 297*(15), 1683–1696. https://doi.org/10.1001/jama.297.15.1683.

Cohen, J., & The AACAP Work Group on Quality Issues. (2010). Practice parameter for the assessment and treatment of children and adolescents with posttraumatic stress disorder. *Journal of the American Academy of Child & Adolescent Psychiatry, 49*, 414–430. https://doi.org/10.1016/j.jaac.2009.12.020.

Cohen, J. A., Mannarino, A. P., Perel, J. M., & Staron, V. (2007). A pilot randomized controlled trial of combined trauma-focused CBT and sertraline for childhood PTSD symptoms. *Journal of the American Academy of Child and Adolescent Psychiatry, 46*(7), 811–819. https://doi.org/10.1097/chi.0b013e3180547105.

Connolly, S. D., & Bernstein, G. A. (2007). Practice parameter for the assessment and treatment of children and adolescents with anxiety disorders. *Journal of the American Academy of Child and Adolescent Psychiatry, 46*(2), 267–283. https://doi.org/10.1097/01.chi.0000246070.23695.06.

Dulcan, M. (Ed.). (2015). *Dulcan's textbook of child and adolescent psychiatry* (2nd ed.). Arlington, VA: American Psychiatric Publishing.

Fergusson, D. M., & Woodward, L. J. (2002). Mental health, educational, and social role outcomes of adolescents with depression. *Archives of General Psychiatry, 59*(3), 225–231. https://doi.org/10.1001/archpsyc.59.3.225.

Geller, D. A., Biederman, J., Stewart, S. E., Mullin, B., Martin, A., Spencer, T., & Faraone, S. V. (2003). Which SSRI? A meta-analysis of pharmacotherapy trials in pediatric obsessive-compulsive disorder. *American Journal of Psychiatry, 160*(11), 1919–1928. https://doi.org/10.1176/appi.ajp.160.11.1919.

Geller, D. A., & March, J. (2012). Practice parameter for the assessment and treatment of children and adolescents with obsessive-compulsive disorder. *Focus, 10*(3), 360–373. https://doi.org/10.1016/j.jaac.2011.09.019.

Hammad, T. A., Laughren, T., & Racoosin, J. (2006). Suicidality in pediatric patients treated with antidepressant drugs. *Archives of General Psychiatry, 63*(3), 332–339. doi:https://doi.org/10.1001/archpsyc.63.3.332.

Hawton, K., & van Heeringen, K. (2009). *Suicide. Lancet, 373*(9672), 1372–1381. https://doi.org/10.1016/S0140-6736(09)60372-X.

Hyman, S. E. (2013, March). Psychiatric drug development: diagnosing a crisis. In *Cerebrum: The Dana forum on brain science* (Vol. 2013). Dana Foundation.

Kendall, P. C. (1994). Treating anxiety disorders in children: Results of a randomized clinical trial. *Journal of Consulting and Clinical Psychology, 62*(1), 100–110. https://doi.org/10.1037/0022-006X.62.1.100.

Kessler, R. C., Angermeyer, M., Anthony, J. C., De Graaf, R. O. N., Demyttenaere, K., Gasquet, I., … Kawakami, N. (2007). Lifetime prevalence and age-of-onset distributions of mental disorders in the world health organization's world mental health survey initiative. *World Psychiatry, 6*(3), 168–176.

Ialongo, et al. (1995). The significance of self-reported anxious symptoms in first grade children: Prediction to anxious symptoms and adaptive functioning in fifth grade. *Journal of Child Psychology Psychiatry, 36*, 427–437.

Last, C. G., Perrin, S., Hersen, M., & Kazdin, A. E. (1996). A prospective study of childhood anxiety disorders. *Journal of the American Academy of Child and Adolescent Psychiatry, 35*(11), 1502–1510. https://doi.org/10.1097/00004583-199611000-00019.

March, J., Silva, S., Petrycki, S., Curry, J., Wells, K., Fairbank, J., … Severe, J. (2004). Fluoxetine, cognitive-behavioral therapy, and their combination for adolescents with depression: Treatment for Adolescents with Depression Study (TADS) randomized controlled trial. *JAMA, 292*(7), 807–820. https://doi.org/10.1001/jama.292.7.807.

Medicaid Integrity Group (2013, August). *Antidepressant medications: Use in pediatric patients.* Retrieved from: https://www.cms.gov/medicare-medicaid-coordination/fraud-prevention/medicaid-integrity-education/pharmacy-education-materials/downloads/ad-pediatric-factsheet.pdf.

Merikangas, K. R., He, J. P., Burstein, M., Swanson, S. A., Avenevoli, S., Cui, L., … Swendsen, J. (2010). Lifetime prevalence of mental disorders in US adolescents: Results from the national comorbidity survey replication–adolescent supplement (NCS-A). *Journal of the American Academy of Child & Adolescent Psychiatry, 49*(10), 980–989. https://doi.org/10.1016/j.jaac.2010.05.017.

Merikangas, K. R., He, J. P., Burstein, M., Swendsen, J., Avenevoli, S., Case, B., … Olfson, M. (2011). Service utilization for lifetime mental disorders in US adolescents: Results of the national comorbidity survey–adolescent supplement (NCS-A). *Journal of the American Academy of Child & Adolescent Psychiatry, 50*(1), 32–45. https://doi.org/10.1016/j.jaac.2010.10.006.

Mulinari, S. (2015). Divergence and convergence of commercial and scientific priorities in drug development: The case of Zelmid, the first SSRI antidepressant. *Social Science and Medicine, 138*, 217–224. https://doi.org/10.1016/j.socscimed.2015.06.020.

O'Sullivan, K., Reulbach, U., Boland, F., Motterlini, N., Kelly, D., Bennett, K., & Fahey, T. (2015). Benzodiazepine prescribing in children under 15 years of age receiving free medical care on the general medical services scheme in Ireland. *BMJ Open, 5*(6), e007070. https://doi.org/10.1136/bmjopen-2014-007070.

Pediatric OCD Treatment Team. (2004). Cognitive-behavior therapy, sertraline, and their combination for children and adolescents with obsessive-compulsive disorder: The pediatric OCD treatment study (POTS) randomized controlled trial. *JAMA, 292*(16), 1969–1976. https://doi.org/10.1001/jama.292.16.1969.

Perez-Caballero, L., Torres-Sanchez, S., Bravo, L., Mico, J. A., & Berrocoso, E. (2014). Fluoxetine: a case history of its discovery and preclinical development. *Expert Opinion on Drug Discovery, 9*(5), 567–578. https://doi.org/10.1517/17460441.2014.907790.

Poirier, M., Déry, M., Toupin, J., Verlaan, P., Lemelin, J. P., & Jagiellowicz, J. (2015). Correlates of conduct problems and depression comorbidity in elementary school boys and girls receiving

special educational services. *Psychology in the Schools, 52*(4), 403–418. https://doi.org/10.1002/pits.21832.
Ramachandraih, C. T., Subramanyam, N., Bar, K. J., Baker, G., & Yeragani, V. K. (2011). Antidepressants: From MAOIs to SSRIs and more. *Indian Journal of Psychiatry, 53*(2), 180–182. https://doi.org/10.4103/0019-5545.82567.
Rynn, M., Puliafico, A., Heleniak, C., Rikhi, P., Ghalib, K., & Vidair, H. (2011). Advances in pharmacotherapy for pediatric anxiety disorders. *Depression and Anxiety, 28*(1), 76–87. https://doi.org/10.1002/da.20769.
Rynn, M. A., Siqueland, L., & Rickels, K. (2001). Placebo-controlled trial of sertraline in the treatment of children with generalized anxiety disorder. *American Journal of Psychiatry, 158*(12), 2008–2014. https://doi.org/10.1176/appi.ajp.158.12.2008.
Siegel, R. S., & Dickstein, D. P. (2012). Anxiety in adolescents: Update on its diagnosis and treatment for primary care providers. *Adolescent Health, Medicine and Therapeutics, 3,* 1–16. https://doi.org/10.2147/AHMT.S7597.
Small, D. M., Simons, A. D., Yovanoff, P., Silva, S. G., Lewis, C. C., Murakami, J. L., & March, J. (2008). Depressed adolescents and comorbid psychiatric disorders: are there differences in the presentation of depression? *Journal of Abnormal Child Psychology, 36*(7), 1015–1028. https://doi.org/10.1007/s10802-008-9237-5.
Southammakosane, C., & Schmitz, K. (2015). Pediatric psychopharmacology for treatment of ADHD, depression, and anxiety. *Pediatrics, 136*(2), 351–359. https://doi.org/10.1542/peds.2014-1581.
Strawn, J. R., Welge, J. A., Wehry, A. M., Keeshin, B., & Rynn, M. A. (2015). Efficacy and tolerability of antidepressants in pediatric anxiety disorders: A systematic review and meta-analysis. *Depression and Anxiety, 32*(3), 149–157. https://doi.org/10.1002/da.22329.
Taylor, A. M. (2015, March). *Pediatric focused safety review: Cymbalta (duloxetine).* Retrieved from https://www.fda.gov/downloads/AdvisoryCommittees/CommitteesMeetingMaterials/PediatricAdvisoryCommittee/UCM438955.pdf.
Valluri, S., Zito, J. M., Safer, D. J., Zuckerman, I. H., Mullins, C. D., & Korelitz, J. J. (2010). Impact of the 2004 food and drug administration pediatric suicidality warning on antidepressant and psychotherapy treatment for new-onset depression. *Medical Care, 48*(11), 947–954. https://doi.org/10.1097/MLR.0b013e3181ef9d2b.
Van Ameringen, M., Mancini, C., & Farvolden, P. (2003). The impact of anxiety disorders on educational achievement. *Journal of Anxiety Disorders, 17*(5), 561–571. https://doi.org/10.1016/S0887-6185(02)00228-1.
von der Embse, N., Barterian, J., & Segool, N. (2013). Test anxiety interventions for children and adolescents: A systematic review of treatment studies from 2000–2010. *Psychology in the Schools, 50*(1), 57–71. https://doi.org/10.1002/pits.21660.
Walkup, J. T., Albano, A. M., Piacentini, J., Birmaher, B., Compton, S. N., Sherrill, J. T., … Iyengar, S. (2008). Cognitive behavioral therapy, sertraline, or a combination in childhood anxiety. *New England Journal of Medicine, 359*(26), 2753–2766. https://doi.org/10.1056/nejmoa0804633.
Whittington, C. J., Kendall, T., Fonagy, P., Cottrell, D., Cotgrove, A., & Boddington, E. (2004). Selective serotonin reuptake inhibitors in childhood depression: Systematic review of published versus unpublished data. *Lancet, 363*(9418), 1341–1345.
Zhou, X., Qin, B., Whittington, C., Cohen, D., Liu, Y., Del Giovane, C., … Xie, P. (2015). Comparative efficacy and tolerability of first-generation and newer-generation antidepressant medications for depressive disorders in children and adolescents: Study protocol for a systematic review and network meta-analysis. *BMJ Open, 5*(9), e007768.

Chapter 6
Effective Medications for Treating Individuals with Autism Spectrum Disorder

Cristan Farmer, Jill Leon and Rebecca Hommer

Introduction

The diagnosis of autism spectrum disorder (ASD) reflects a constellation of impairments, both in the domain of social communication and resulting from restricted/repetitive behaviors. The definition of ASD changed slightly in the transition from DSM-IV-TR to DSM-5 in 2015. Under DSM-IV-TR, individuals may have received diagnoses of Asperger's disorder, autistic disorder, or pervasive developmental disorder-not otherwise specified, which were distinguished by varying degrees and patterns of impairment in three domains (social interaction, communication, and restricted/repetitive behaviors). Although not without controversy, the DSM-5 conceptualizes autism as a single spectrum, with varying degrees of impairment, rather than a conglomeration of distinct but related disorders. In the years since the publication of DSM-5, most data indicate that the majority of children who received a diagnosis under DSM-IV-TR remained eligible for diagnosis under DSM-5 (e.g., Smith, Reichow, & Volkmar, 2015).

As many as one in 68 children is diagnosed with ASD (Centers for Disease Control and Prevention (CDC), 2009). The etiology of ASD is unknown, but it is likely variable, and there is a strong genetic component (Robinson et al., 2016). ASD is about four times more common in males than in females, but in females, a diagnosis of ASD is more likely to be associated with intellectual disability (Bishop, Veenstra-VanderWeele, & Sanders, 2016). The full range of cognitive ability is observed in ASD, though average IQ is observed in only about 20%. Cognitive ability, as well as language skills, are among the most important predictors of a child's long-term outcome. ASD is understood to be a life-long disorder; most individuals diagnosed in childhood will continue to meet diagnostic criteria throughout their lifetime, and those who fall off the spectrum appear to still exhibit persistent subtle difficulties.

C. Farmer (✉) · J. Leon · R. Hommer
Pediatrics & Developmental Neuroscience Branch, National Institute of Mental Health, National Institutes of Health, Bethesda, MD, USA
e-mail: cristan.farmer@nih.gov

J. S. Carlson and J. A. Barterian (eds.), *School Psychopharmacology*,
Pediatric School Psychology, https://doi.org/10.1007/978-3-030-15541-4_6

Still, few rigorous data on adult outcomes of individuals with ASD are available. While the available data are at times conflicting, it is clear that adults with ASD have poorer outcomes than their typically developing peers with respect to mental health and independent living (Howlin & Magiati, 2017).

Given the heterogeneity of individuals diagnosed with ASD, it is unsurprising that a great deal of variability is observed in their academic achievement (Keen, Webster, & Ridley, 2016). As with much of the ASD literature, it is worth highlighting some shortcomings before discussing the data. To date, studies of academic achievement in ASD have been biased towards younger children and those with higher IQ. Some authors propose that this is a function of the different expectations for children enrolled in specialized and inclusive education settings (Keen et al., 2016), but the end result is that we have very little knowledge about the academic achievement of individuals with ASD and low IQ, and whether it differs in meaningful ways from individuals with low IQ and no ASD. The data that do exist suggest that the most important factor in determining academic achievement and academic progress in children with ASD is the student's IQ, though uneven patterns of achievement in specific skill areas are common.

Historically, attempts to identify pharmacologic interventions for the core symptoms of ASD focused on putative differences in neurochemical systems that are known to be affected by commonly used medications. The earliest examples of this were studies demonstrating elevated levels of serotonin in the blood of children with ASD, followed by several decades' worth of research on the effectiveness of medications with serotonergic activity. Differences in cholinergic activity in the brains of individuals with ASD led to interest in relevant medications, and data suggesting alterations in neuropeptide hormone systems have spurred study of oxytocin and vasopressin (McCracken, 2011). Still, the fact remains that there are no empirically supported pharmacologic treatments for ASD. For this reason, pharmacologic interventions for ASD have focused on associated (e.g., irritability, inattention, hyperactivity), rather than core (i.e., social communication impairment, restricted and repetitive behaviors), symptoms of the disorder. Interventions targeting attention problems or challenging behavior may allow the child to more fully benefit from his or her educational environment, and to remain in less restrictive settings. Although it is not the topic of this chapter, it should be noted that a handful of empirically supported behavioral interventions do exist (e.g., applied behavior analysis), though no model is clearly superior.

Psychopharmacological Treatment of ASD

Administrative and medical claims-based data suggest that well over half of children and adolescents with ASD are prescribed psychotropic medications, and 10–15% are prescribed three or more medications (sometimes referred to as "polypharmacy") (Mandell et al., 2008; Spencer et al., 2013). This stands in contrast with the fact that there are no FDA-approved medications for the treatment of the core symptoms of ASD. ASD is commonly associated with challenging behaviors such as inattention, hyperactivity, irritability, aggression, and self-injury. Thus, pharmacologic treatment in children and adolescents with ASD is often targeted towards these associated problem behaviors. In fact, the two medications with ASD-specific indications (the neuroleptics aripiprazole and risperidone) are approved for the treatment of irritability (Ji & Findling, 2015). Psychotropic medication use is more common among older children and adolescents with ASD and for those with comorbidity (Mandell et al., 2008; Spencer et al., 2013). Moreover, the development of evidence-based pharmacotherapy practices in the treatment of children with ASD has been largely informed by clinical practice (e.g., systematically studying medications which appear to alleviate behavioral symptoms in both the ASD and non-ASD populations) rather than neurobiological theory.

The most commonly prescribed drug class in children and adolescents with ASD is the neuroleptics. Postsynaptic blockade of the dopamine D_2 receptor is implicated as the primary mechanism of action of these medications, although to a varying extent medications in this class may also affect serotonergic, histaminic, muscarinic, and alpha-1 receptors. Dopamine plays an important role in the initiation of movement and motor control, as well as in multiple cognitive processes, most notably attention, learning, and reward processing; the relationship between neuroleptic effects on dopaminergic transmission and functional outcomes of decreased irritability and aggression is likely complex and has not yet been clearly delineated. High potency (first generation) antipsychotics show stronger D_2 receptor binding and are more likely to be associated with motoric side effects, while newer (atypical, second/third generation) medications appear to affect other dopamine receptors (D_3 and D_4) as well as other neurotransmitters (e.g., serotonin, glutamate). Risperidone, one of the two neuroleptics approved for use in ASD, shows a high degree of dopaminergic D_2 and serotonergic 5-HT_2 receptor antagonism. Aripiprazole, the other approved medication, also has a high affinity for dopaminergic and serotonergic receptors and, in addition to its antagonistic effects, is a partial agonist of the D_2 receptor. Other classes commonly used to target problem behaviors, and to a lesser extent, core symptoms in ASD, include antidepressants (the primary mechanism of action is usually serotonin-related), mood stabilizers (the mechanism of action varies widely by agent, most have GABAergic activity), stimulants (these increase synaptic dopamine and norepinephrine by promoting release and blocking reuptake), and alpha-adrenergic agonists (these mimic the action of epinephrine and norepinephrine by stimulating alpha-adrenergic receptors). Serotonin influences a number of brain and bodily functions including mood, appetite, sleep, memory, and social behavior; GABA is the primary inhibitory (calming) neurotransmitter of the central nervous system; norephinephrine, the hormone responsible for the "fight or flight" response, is centrally associated with increased alertness and attention. All of these neurotransmitters affect brain and behavioral processes that may be abnormal in ASD, but, as is the case with dopaminergic agents, the relationship between neurotransmitter activity and functional outcomes in the individual remains poorly understood.

In this chapter, we summarize some the available empirical data on the efficacy of these medications for the treatment of individuals with ASD, with our strongest focus necessarily on behaviors associated with ASD, rather than the core symptoms. This is not intended to be an exhaustive review, which can be found elsewhere (e.g., Benvenuto, Battan, Porfirio, & Curatolo, 2013). Instead, we communicate the essential knowledge from the current literature that will be of use to school-based professionals.

Efficacy and Effectiveness of Medications for ASD and Associated Symptoms

Irritability. Medications intended to address challenging behaviors associated with ASD are among the most commonly studied, with target behaviors including irritability, aggression, and hyperactivity. Randomized, double-blind, placebo-controlled trials (RCTs) of risperidone, a second generation antipsychotic, have generally led to moderate-to-large improvements in irritability and aggression (e.g., McCracken et al., 2002). Based on two 8-week RCTs and one open label follow up, in 2006, the FDA-approved risperidone for the treatment of irritability associated with autistic disorder in children ages 5–16 years old. The most commonly reported side effects of risperidone in children with ASD are weight gain and somnolence; extrapyramidal symptoms (movement disorders) have been observed in a small number of children with extended use (Kent, Hough, Singh, Karcher, & Pandina, 2013; Pandina, Bossie, Youssef, Zhu, & Dunbar, 2007), and concerns exist about hormonal and metabolic effects of risperidone and other antipsychotics that may accompany long-term use. To minimize side effects and long-term safety concerns, it is recommended that risperidone be prescribed at the lowest effective dose, and it should be noted that higher doses do not always result in greater efficacy.

Although most studies were designed to evaluate the effectiveness of risperidone for irritability, secondary analyses generated interest in whether risperidone might be effective for the core symptoms of ASD (McDougle et al., 2005). At least one small study demonstrated some improvements in social communication symptoms (Nagaraj, Singhi, & Malhi, 2006), but it is unclear whether these improvements can be disentangled from the improvements observed in problem behaviors. Currently, the predominant opinion is that risperidone is not effective for the core symptoms of ASD, but proximal improvements in problem behaviors may result in distal improvements in other behavioral domains.

Aripiprazole, which also has a clinical indication for irritability in ASD (in ages 6–17 years), has also been the subject of several large-scale RCTs. The two studies used as evidence for the FDA indication provided evidence that aripiprazole was superior to placebo (Marcus et al., 2009; Owen et al., 2009). However, a large relapse prevention study suggested that although maintenance therapy might be effective, once the medication has stopped, there is no effect of previous treatment with aripiprazole on the speed of relapse (Findling et al., 2014). Reported adverse events to aripiprazole are variable, ranging from presyncope and agitation to weight gain, somnolence, vomiting, and extrapyramidal symptoms.

In addition to their antiepileptic properties, for which they are often used in children with ASD and co-occurring seizure disorder, medications like valproate are commonly used in various clinical populations to control problem behaviors. These medications do not appear to be as effective as atypical antipsychotics for problem behaviors, though no direct comparison exists. Small RCTs of valproate and its derivative, divalproex sodium, produced conflicting results (one positive, Hellings et al., 2005; and one negative, Hollander et al., 2010). Other small studies have suggested the efficacy of topiramate (Rezaei et al., 2010), and the lack of efficacy of levetiracetam (Wasserman et al., 2006). Overall, the literature on anticonvulsants for problem behaviors reflects relatively small samples with little suggestion of large effects, and few recent investigations of this class exist (Table 6.1).

Inattention and hyperactivity. Interventions for inattention and hyperactivity in children with ASD are the same as those without ASD. The most popular medication for this purpose, the psychostimulant methylphenidate (and extended-release methylphenidate), have been rigorously evaluated in children with ASD. In the largest study, a Research Units on Pediatric Psychopharmacology (RUPP) Autism Network RCT, evidence was found for a moderate degree of response to methylphenidate, but this was less than what is usually observed in typically developing children (Autism Psychopharmacology, 2005). Further, the rate of adverse events, including irritability, decreased appetite, difficulty falling asleep, and abdominal discomfort, was somewhat higher. The same pattern was observed in a small study of extended-release methylphenidate, wherein moderate effects were tempered by relatively high rates of adverse effects (Pearson et al., 2013). It is noteworthy that in the RUPP study, the primary outcome measure was teacher ratings of hyperactivity; while this is common in studies where ADHD-type symptoms are the target, and other studies may collect school-based ratings as secondary outcomes, studies where other problem behaviors or core symptoms are the targets do not often use teacher ratings as the primary index for efficacy.

Partially owing to concern about the rate of side effects observed with methylphenidate, the norepinephrine reuptake inhibitor atomoxetine has also been studied in ASD. Atomoxetine is considered a second-line treatment for ADHD in children and adolescents without ASD, because while it is superior to placebo, it is less effective than stimulants. RCTs ranging in size from 16 to 128 participants demonstrate improvements in ADHD symptoms in children with ASD (Handen et al., 2015; Harfterkamp et al., 2012). Commonly reported side effects do not differ from those in observed in children and adolescents without ASD, and include decreased appetite, nausea/vomiting, fatigue, and mood swings/irritability. Also of note is the existence of a "black box" warning regarding the potential for suicidal ideation in children and adolescents taking atomoxetine.

Another medication commonly used in typically developing children, guanfacine (anti-hyperintensive), has some empirical support for use in ASD. Two RCTs found moderate-to-large effect sizes of guanfacine relative to placebo on hyperactivity

Table 6.1 Selected studies of medications used to treat irritability in ASD

Drug class	Medication	Publication	n	Study design	Study results
Anticonvulsant	Divalproex sodium	Hollander et al. (2010)	27	12 weeks, R, DB, PBO	Significant improvement in irritability
Antipsychotic	Risperidone	McCracken et al. (2002)	101	8 weeks, R, DB, PBO	Improvement in irritability, but no effect on stereotypy or hyperactivity
Antipsychotic	Risperidone	Shea et al. (2004)	79	8 weeks, R, DB, PBO	Improvements in irritability, inappropriate speech, social withdrawal, and stereotypy
Antipsychotic	Risperidone	Kent et al. (2013)	96	6 weeks, R, DB, PBO	Significant improvements on irritability in high-dose group but not low-dose group
Antipsychotic	Aripiprazole	Marcus et al. (2009)	218	8 weeks, R, DB, PBO, fixed dose	Improvements in stereotypy, irritability, inappropriate speech, and compulsions
Antipsychotic	Aripiprazole	Owen et al. (2009)	98	8 weeks, R, DB, PBO, flexible dose	Improvements in irritability
Antipsychotic	Aripiprazole	Findling et al. (2014)	157	16 weeks, relapse-prevention trial in aripiprazole responders, DB, PBO	No significant difference between aripiprazole and placebo in time to relapse during maintenance phase
Glutamatergic	Amantadine	King et al. (2001)	39	4 weeks, R, DB, PBO	No improvement on parent ratings

R randomized, *DB* double-blind, *PBO* placebo-controlled

Table 6.2 Selected studies of medications used to treat inattention and hyperactivity in ASD

Drug class	Medication	Publication	n	Study design	Study results
Stimulant	Methylphenidate	RUPP (2005)	66	4 weeks, R, PBO, crossover	Significant (but small-to-moderate) effects on hyperactivity
Noradrenaline reuptake inhibitor	Atomoxetine	Harfterkamp et al. (2012)	97	8 weeks, R, DB, PBO	Moderate improvement in ADHD symptoms by teacher and parent rating
Noradrenaline reuptake inhibitor	Atomoxetine	Handen et al. (2015)	128	10 weeks, R, DB, four arms (atomoxetine/placebo plus parent training/none)	Both atomoxetine and parent training alone had significant improvements on parent ADHD ratings, while atomoxetine (with or without parent training) also had improvements in noncompliance
Antihypertensive	Guanfacine-XR	Scahill et al. (2015)	62	8 weeks, R, DB, PBO	Significant improvements in parent ADHD ratings

R randomized, *DB* double-blind, *PBO* placebo-controlled

(Handen, Sahl, & Hardan, 2008; Scahill et al., 2015), with an adverse effect profile consisting of drowsiness, fatigue, and decreased appetite (Table 6.2).

Sleep problems. A variety of sleep problems have been described in ASD; while many are behavioral in nature, differences in sleep architecture (i.e., the amount and relative proportion at each sleep stage, like rapid eye movement sleep) have also been noted (Buckley et al., 2010). Sleep problems are related to daytime impairment, both related to the severity of ASD symptoms and more general externalizing and internalizing problems (Cohen, Conduit, Lockley, Rajaratnam, & Cornish, 2014). Melatonin, used frequently in the general population for the treatment of initial insomnia (especially when due to a circadian rhythm disturbance known as delayed sleep–wake phase cycle disorder), is available over-the-counter and is used with frequency in children with ASD. Only one large-scale RCT has been performed in children with ASD; this study documented a significant improvement in sleep quality (e.g., sleep latency, wake after onset, total sleep time) with the use of cognitive behavioral therapy and/or melatonin compared to placebo, with the largest effect size for the combined intervention (Cortesi, Giannotti, Sebastiani, Panunzi, & Valente, 2012). Although melatonin is the only agent that has been studied in a randomized and controlled fashion, registry data suggests that despite a lack of evidence, in the community setting other medications, most often alpha agonists, but also antihistamines, antidepressants, antipsychotics, benzodiazepines, and sedatives, are used to address sleep issues in children with ASD (Malow et al., 2016).

Restricted and repetitive behaviors. Of the two core symptom domains of ASD, the more successfully treated is restrictive and repetitive behaviors (RRB). Investigators were initially hopeful that antidepressants, the medications of choice in the treatment of obsessive-compulsive disorder and other pediatric anxiety disorders, would also help to mitigate the disruptive nature of RRBs in ASD. While smaller studies had indicated that fluoxetine was possibly effective, the definitive study failed to replicate the positive results (Hollander et al., 2005), and disappointingly, a definitive RCT failed to demonstrate an effect of citalopram on RRBs (King et al., 2009). Other drug classes may be promising but have not yet been evaluated in large-scale trials; for example, small studies suggest that divalproex sodium may be effective at reducing RRB (Hollander et al., 2006), and secondary analyses suggest improvements in RRB with risperidone (McCracken et al., 2002). Still, there is no gold-standard pharmacological treatment of RRB in ASD.

Social Communication. Effective medications for the treatment of social communication impairment, a core symptom domain of ASD, remain elusive. A number of medication classes have been explored; some have been selected on the basis of mechanism of action and relationship to neurochemical differences observed in ASD, but many were selected because they had effects in other symptom domains. Examples of the former include the opioid antagonist naltrexone and the GABAergic arbaclofen. Naltrexone was investigated after scientists observed that opioid-treated research animals exhibited decreased social and increased repetitive behaviors, leading them to hypothesize that ASD might be associated with an overproduction of endogenous opioids. Although small, uncontrolled studies have suggested that naltrexone may be associated with decreases in self-injurious behavior, it has not been associated with improvements in social communication (Eichaar, Maisch, Augusto, & Wehring, 2006; Feldman, Kolmen, & Gonzaga, 1999). Based on the hypothesis that ASD may reflect an imbalance between inhibitory and excitatory neuronal activity, and recent animal studies suggesting that these drugs may impact social behavior in drosophila and mouse models, several studies of GABAergic and glutamatergic medications have also been conducted. A recent large RCT of arbaclofen in youth aged 5–21 years found that although arbaclofen failed to differentiate from placebo on a measure of social withdrawal (the study's primary outcome), a subset of participants showed greater improvements on a separate measure of socialization, suggesting that additional studies may be warranted (Veenstra-VanderWeele et al., 2016). Initial evidence for modest efficacy has also been demonstrated for some cholinergic medications (chosen because they are used in the treatment of dementia), such as galantamine (Niederhofer, Staffen, & Mair, 2002) and for some GABAergic medications, such as bumetanide (Lemonnier et al., 2012). However, other small controlled studies of cholinergic drugs have failed to find benefits of these agents for children with ASD (Arnold et al., 2012; Chez et al., 2003). Similarly, while one small RCT suggested that glutamatergic agents such as N-acetylcysteine (Hardan et al., 2012) may be associated with improvements in irritability, several others (memantine, riluzole, amantadine) have not been found efficacious when used alone, but may contribute added benefit when used in combination with antipsychotic medication (Ji & Findling, 2015).

One medication that has generated considerable excitement in recent years is the hormone oxytocin, postulated to improve social cognition and social behavior. However, this literature is marked by fits and starts, in that pilot studies will suggest efficacy that is not confirmed by subsequent larger RCTs. For example, a blinded crossover pilot study of oxytocin resulted in improvement in emotional recognition in adolescents (Guastella et al., 2010). However, a larger study by the same researchers failed to replicate these findings (Guastella et al., 2015), consistent with another moderately sized study (Dadds et al., 2014). Another study documented modest improvements in a parent-rated scale of social impairment after 5 weeks of treatment with oxytocin (Yatawara, Einfeld, Hickie, Davenport, & Guastella, 2016). Because these studies have generally been performed in older children and adolescents with higher cognitive ability, some data do exist on biomarkers associated with oxytocin. For example, one study documented increased activity in the striatum, nucleus accumbens, left posterior superior temporal sulcus, and left premotor cortex during social judgments after oxytocin administration (Gordon et al., 2013). Activity in these areas was found to decrease during nonsocial judgments. Further study is warranted to fully assess the clinical implications of these findings (Table 6.3).

A second group of medications was considered eligible for evaluation of effect on social communication, because they were already evaluated for some other purpose in ASD. In studies of children with ASD where the target symptom is problem behavior or some other noncore symptom, change in the core symptoms is usually evaluated as a secondary outcome. From these data, some hints at possible efficacy have been obtained. However, as described in the section on irritability, the consensus is that these improvements in social behavior are likely sequelae of improvements in problem behavior, rather than a direct effect of the medication. Although evaluation of stimulants has generally held to this pattern (core symptoms secondary outcomes), at least one study of methylphenidate evaluated social communication as a primary outcome. Unfortunately, although a moderate improvement in social communication was observed, the methylphenidate was not well-tolerated and nearly 20% of participants discontinued due to intolerable side effects (Jahromi et al., 2009).

Table 6.3 Selected studies of medications evaluated for the treatment of social communication impairments in ASD

Drug class	Medication	Publication	n	Study design	Study results
Sulfamyl	Bumetanide	Lemonnier et al. (2012)	60	12 weeks, DB, PBO	Some improvement on a parent-rated measure usually used for screening for autism
Hormonal	Oxytocin	Dadds et al. (2014)	38	4 day, R, DB, PBO	No effect of treatment
Hormonal	Oxytocin	Guastella et al. (2015)	50	8 weeks, DB, PBO	No effect of treatment
Hormonal	Oxytocin	Yatawara et al. (2016)	31	5-week crossover (with 4-week washout, total time 14 weeks), R, DB, PBO	Improvement on a parent-rated measure of social impairment but no improvements in repetitive behavior
GABAergic	Arbaclofen	Veenstra-Vander Weele et al. (2016)	150	12 weeks, DB, PBO	No effect of treatment

R randomized, *DB* double-blind, *PBO* placebo-controlled

Professional Guidelines for the Treatment of ASD

The American Academy of Pediatrics issued a policy statement on the management of children with ASD in 2007, and reaffirmed this statement in 2010 and 2014 (American Academy of Pediatrics, 2017). The American Academy of Child and Adolescent Psychiatry issued an updated practice parameter for the assessment and treatment of children and adolescents with ASD in 2014 (Volkmar et al., 2014). Both documents focus on the need to improve functional outcomes for children with ASD and discuss behavioral interventions as an integral aspect of the approach to treatment. Pharmacologic interventions may be indicated to target specific symptoms in the behavioral domains described above (e.g., aggression, inattention, poor sleep). However, such intervention should be considered when behavioral interventions have failed to yield sufficient improvements, and when possible underlying medical and modifiable environmental factors have been reviewed and addressed (e.g., constipation leading to discomfort and manifest as self-injurious or aggressive behavior). Decisions regarding medications should be made in the context of potential risks and benefits to the child, and may be most effective when implemented in conjunction with ongoing behavioral interventions (Aman et al., 2009; Volkmar et al., 2014).

Contraindications

As hyperactivity and inattention are among the most common co-occurring symptoms in children with ASD, there has been a great deal of interest in the side effect profile of drugs used to treat ADHD. Initially, small studies raised concerns about tolerability, and many parents and practitioners were concerned about the possibility of paradoxical effects. Generally, however, medications deemed effective for specific disorders are assumed to be safe for use in children and adolescents with ASD, and side effect profiles are similar in youth with and without ASD, although rates of adverse effects may be somewhat higher in children with ASD (Ji & Findling, 2015). With or without ASD, medical comorbidities may be associated with specific contraindications to certain medications, and decisions regarding medication management should be made by families in conjunction with their child's physician, after a discussion of the medication's potential risks and benefits, and the specific impact that a medication is likely to have on their child.

Conclusions

Despite the fact that there are no FDA-approved (or effective) pharmacologic interventions for the core symptoms of ASD, over half of children with ASD are prescribed a psychotropic medication. Much of this medication use is explained by symptoms and conditions that frequently co-occur with ASD, including attention and hyperactivity problems, irritability, and aggressive behavior. Two medications, aripiprazole and risperidone, hold FDA indications for the treatment of irritability associated with ASD. While other commonly used medications do not hold ASD-specific FDA indications, there are few data to suggest that pharmacologic treatments for specific disorders should not be effective in children with ASD.

Given that the medications effective for use in ASD target associated symptoms such as hyperactivity, inattention, irritability, and other challenging behaviors, pharmacologic intervention may be most helpful for a child whose challenging behaviors interfere with his or her ability to participate in his or her environment. Psychotropic intervention, along with appropriate behavioral intervention, may allow a child to access and benefit from the social and educational environment, and to remain in the least restrictive environment possible. Thus, one should not expect direct effects of psychotropic intervention on educational outcomes, but rather an enabling of the child to take full advantage of educational opportunities.

However, it is important to recognize that many of the medications commonly used in ASD have side effect profiles that may interfere with educational functioning. While the most medically serious side effects associated with the antipsychotics are rare (i.e., dyskinesias and extrapyramidal symptoms), children commonly experience significant weight gain and sedation. Stimulants may be associated with mood lability and decreased appetite, and antidepressants with gastrointestinal symptoms and weight gain. These side effects may have a detrimental effect on the child's ability to take advantage of educational opportunities, and must be monitored closely by the treating physician. Educators may be a key source of information on these possible side effects, which may be most evident during the day and during periods where attentional effort is required. Unfortunately, few RCTs have included school-based ratings as a primary outcome measure, which is an area ripe for improvement.

In summary, pharmacologic interventions for the core symptoms of ASD remain elusive. Researchers continue to explore the possibility that the core symptoms of the disorder may be successfully treated with pharmacologic intervention, with the most excitement centering on neuropeptides like oxytocin and vasopressin. However, several high-quality studies performed in the past 20 years have confirmed the efficacy and safety of several medications that were previously known to be effective in other populations, resulting in an array of empirically supported choices for pharmacologic intervention on symptoms commonly associated with ASD. These symptoms, most frequently in the domains of challenging behavior, interfere with a child's ability to participate in his or her social and educational environment. Successful treatment, then, may allow for the child to fully benefit from his or her surroundings.

Suggested Readings

- Accordino, R., Kidd, C., Politte, L., Henry, C., & McDougle, C. (2016). Psychopharmacological interventions in autism spectrum disorder. *Expert Opinion on Pharmacotherapy, 17,* 937–952.

  A recent review of psychopharmacological medications for individuals with ASD.

- Hollander, E., Kolevzon, A., & Coyle, J. T. (Eds.). (2011). *Textbook of autism spectrum disorders.* Arlington, VA: American Psychiatric Pub.

  A comprehensive text detailing ASD, including risk factors, etiology, evaluation, and treatment.

- Amaral, D., Geschwind, D., & Dawson, G. (Eds.). (2011). *Autism spectrum disorders.* New York: Oxford University Press.

  A comprehensive text detailing ASD, including risk factors, etiology, evaluation, and treatment.

List of Websites

- https://effectivehealthcare.ahrq.gov/topics/asd-medical/research-2017/

  The Agency for Healthcare Research and Quality website houses a review of medical interventions for ASD.

- https://medlineplus.gov/autismspectrumdisorder.html#cat_78

  The MedLinePlus website is a resource for up-to-date information about ASD.

- http://www.nationalautismcenter.org/national-standards-project/

  The National Autism Center has information provides guidelines about how to make choices between available interventions.

References

Aman, M. G., McDougle, C. J., Scahill, L., Handen, B., Arnold, L. E., Johnson, C., … Wagner, A. (2009). Medication and parent training in children with pervasive developmental disorders and serious behavior problems: Results from a randomized clinical trial. *Journal of the American Academy of Child and Adolescent Psychiatry, 48*(12), 1143–1154.

American Academy of Pediatrics. (2017). Resources for Professionals and Families. Retrieved from https://www.aap.org/en-us/about-the-aap/Committees-Councils-Sections/Council-on-Children-with-Disabilities/Pages/Resources-for-Professionals-and-Families.aspx.

Arnold, L., Aman, M. G., Hollway, J., Hurt, E., Bates, B., Li, X., … Williams, C. (2012). Placebo-controlled pilot trial of mecamylamine for treatment of autism spectrum disorders. *Journal of Child and Adolescent Psychopharmacology, 22*(3), 198–205.

Autism Psychopharmacology. (2005). Randomized, controlled, crossover trial of methylphenidate in pervasive developmental disorders with hyperactivity. *Archives of General Psychiatry, 62*, 1266–1274.

Benvenuto, A., Battan, B., Porfirio, M. C., & Curatolo, P. (2013). Pharmacotherapy of autism spectrum disorders. *Brain and Development, 35*(2), 119–127.

Bishop, S. L., Veenstra-VanderWeele, J., & Sanders, S. J. (2016). Attention finally being paid to girls at risk of autism. *Journal of the American Academy of Child and Adolescent Psychiatry, 55*(3), 159.

Buckley, A. W., Rodriguez, A. J., Jennison, K., Buckley, J., Thurm, A., Sato, S., & Swedo, S. (2010). Rapid eye movement sleep percentage in children with autism compared with children with developmental delay and typical development. *Archives of Pediatrics & Adolescent Medicine, 164*(11), 1032–1037.

Chez, M., Buchanan, T., Becker, M., Kessler, J., Aimonovitch, M., & Mrazek, S. (2003). Donepezil hydrochloride: A double-blind study in autistic children. *Journal of pediatric neurology, 1*(2), 83–88.

Cohen, S., Conduit, R., Lockley, S. W., Rajaratnam, S. M., & Cornish, K. M. (2014). The relationship between sleep and behavior in autism spectrum disorder (ASD): A review. *Journal of Neurodevelopmental Disorders, 6*(1), 44.

Centers for Disease Control and Prevention (CDC). (2009). Autism and developmental disabilities monitoring network surveillance year 2006. Principal investigators. Prevalence of autism spectrum disorders—Autism and developmental disabilities monitoring network, United States, 2006. *MMWR Surveillance Summaries, 58*(10), 1–20.

Cortesi, F., Giannotti, F., Sebastiani, T., Panunzi, S., & Valente, D. (2012). Controlled-release melatonin, singly and combined with cognitive behavioural therapy, for persistent insomnia in children with autism spectrum disorders: A randomized placebo-controlled trial. *Journal of Sleep Research, 21*(6), 700–709.

Dadds, M. R., MacDonald, E., Cauchi, A., Williams, K., Levy, F., & Brennan, J. (2014). Nasal oxytocin for social deficits in childhood autism: A randomized controlled trial. *Journal of Autism and Developmental Disorders, 44*(3), 521–531.

Eichaar, G. M., Maisch, N. M., Augusto, L. M., & Wehring, H. J. (2006). Efficacy and safety of naltrexone use in pediatric patients with autistic disorder. *Annals of Pharmacotherapy, 40*(6), 1086–1095.

Feldman, H. M., Kolmen, B. K., & Gonzaga, A. M. (1999). Naltrexone and communication skills in young children with autism. *Journal of the American Academy of Child and Adolescent Psychiatry, 38*(5), 587–593.

Findling, R. L., Mankoski, R., Timko, K., Lears, K., McCartney, T., McQuade, R. D., ... Sheehan, J. J. (2014). A randomized controlled trial investigating the safety and efficacy of aripiprazole in the long-term maintenance treatment of pediatric patients with irritability associated with autistic disorder. *The Journal of Clinical Psychiatry, 75*(1), 22–30.

Gordon, I., Vander Wyk, B. C., Bennett, R. H., Cordeaux, C., Lucas, M. V., Eilbott, J. A., ... Pelphrey, K. A. (2013). Oxytocin enhances brain function in children with autism. *Proceedings of the National Academy of Sciences, 110*(52), 20953–20958.

Guastella, A. J., Einfeld, S. L., Gray, K. M., Rinehart, N. J., Tonge, B. J., Lambert, T. J., et al. (2010). Intranasal oxytocin improves emotion recognition for youth with autism spectrum disorders. *Biological Psychiatry, 67*(7), 692–694.

Guastella, A. J., Gray, K. M., Rinehart, N. J., Alvares, G. A., Tonge, B. J., Hickie, I. B., ... Einfeld, S. L. (2015). The effects of a course of intranasal oxytocin on social behaviors in youth diagnosed with autism spectrum disorders: A randomized controlled trial. *Journal of Child Psychology and Psychiatry, 56*(4), 444–452.

Handen, B., Aman, M. G., Arnold, L. E., Hyman, S. L., Tumuluru, R. V., Lecavalier, L., ... Buchan-Page, K. A. (2015). Atomoxetine, parent training, and their combination in children with autism spectrum disorder and attention-deficit/hyperactivity disorder. *Journal of the American Academy of Child & Adolescent Psychiatry, 54*(11), 905–915.

Handen, B., Sahl, R., & Hardan, A. Y. (2008). Guanfacine in children with autism and/or intellectual disabilities. *Journal of Developmental and Behavioral Pediatrics, 29*(4), 303–308.

Hardan, A. Y., Fung, L. K., Libove, R. A., Obukhanych, T. V., Nair, S., Herzenberg, L. A., ... Tirouvanziam, R. (2012). A randomized controlled pilot trial of oral N-acetylcysteine in children with autism. *Biological Psychiatry, 71*(11), 956–961.

Harfterkamp, M., van de Loo-Neus, G., Minderaa, R. B., van der Gaag, R.-J., Escobar, R., Schacht, A., ... Hoekstra, P. J. (2012). A randomized double-blind study of atomoxetine versus placebo for attention-deficit/hyperactivity disorder symptoms in children with autism spectrum disorder. *Journal of the American Academy of Child & Adolescent Psychiatry, 51*(7), 733–741.

Hellings, J. A., Weckbaugh, M., Nickel, E. J., Cain, S. E., Zarcone, J. R., Reese, R. M., ... Schroeder, S. R. (2005). A double-blind, placebo-controlled study of valproate for aggression in youth with pervasive developmental disorders. *Journal of Child & Adolescent Psychopharmacology, 15*(4), 682–692.

Hollander, E., Chaplin, W., Soorya, L., Wasserman, S., Novotny, S., Rusoff, J., ... Anagnostou, E. (2010). Divalproex sodium vs placebo for the treatment of irritability in children and adolescents with autism spectrum disorders. *Neuropsychopharmacology, 35*(4), 990–998.

Hollander, E., Phillips, A., Chaplin, W., Zagursky, K., Novotny, S., Wasserman, S., & Iyengar, R. (2005). A placebo controlled crossover trial of liquid fluoxetine on repetitive behaviors in childhood and adolescent autism. *Neuropsychopharmacology, 30*(3), 582–589.

Hollander, E., Soorya, L., Wasserman, S., Esposito, K., Chaplin, W., & Anagnostou, E. (2006). Divalproex sodium vs. placebo in the treatment of repetitive behaviours in autism spectrum disorder. *The International Journal of Neuropsychopharmacology, 9*(2), 209–213.

Howlin, P., & Magiati, I. (2017). Autism spectrum disorder. *Current Opinion in Psychiatry, 30*(2), 69–76.

Jahromi, L. B., Kasari, C. L., McCracken, J. T., Lee, L. S., Aman, M. G., McDougle, C. J., … Vitiello, B. (2009). Positive effects of methylphenidate on social communication and self-regulation in children with pervasive developmental disorders and hyperactivity. *Journal of Autism and Developmental Disorders, 39*(3), 395–404.

Ji, N. Y., & Findling, R. L. (2015). An update on pharmacotherapy for autism spectrum disorder in children and adolescents. *Current Opinion in Psychiatry, 28*(2), 91–101.

Keen, D., Webster, A., & Ridley, G. (2016). How well are children with autism spectrum disorder doing academically at school? *An overview of the literature. Autism, 20*(3), 276–294.

Kent, J. M., Hough, D., Singh, J., Karcher, K., & Pandina, G. (2013). An open-label extension study of the safety and efficacy of risperidone in children and adolescents with autistic disorder. *Journal of Child and Adolescent Psychopharmacology, 23*(10), 676–686.

King, B. H., Wright, D. M., Handen, B. L., Sikich, L., Zimmerman, A. W., McMahon, W., … & Hooper, S. R. (2001). Double-blind, placebo-controlled study of amantadine hydrochloride in the treatment of children with autistic disorder. *Journal of the American Academy of Child & Adolescent Psychiatry, 40*(6), 658–665.

King, B. H., Hollander, E., Sikich, L., McCracken, J. T., Scahill, L., Bregman, J. D., … Ritz, L. (2009). Lack of efficacy of citalopram in children with autism spectrum disorders and high levels of repetitive behavior: citalopram ineffective in children with autism. *Archives of General Psychiatry, 66*(6), 583–590.

Lemonnier, E., Degrez, C., Phelep, M., Tyzio, R., Josse, F., Grandgeorge, M., … Ben-Ari, Y. (2012). A randomised controlled trial of bumetanide in the treatment of autism in children. *Translational Psychiatry, 2,* e202.

Malow, B. A., Katz, T., Reynolds, A. M., Shui, A., Carno, M., Connolly, H. V., … Bennett, A. E. (2016). Sleep difficulties and medications in children with autism spectrum disorders: A registry study. *Pediatrics, 137*(Supplement 2), S98–S104.

Mandell, D. S., Morales, K. H., Marcus, S. C., Stahmer, A. C., Doshi, J., & Polsky, D. E. (2008). Psychotropic medication use among medicaid-enrolled children with autism spectrum disorders. *Pediatrics, 121*(3), e441–e448.

Marcus, R. N., Owen, R., Kamen, L., Manos, G., McQuade, R. D., Carson, W. H., & Aman, M. G. (2009). A placebo-controlled, fixed-dose study of aripiprazole in children and adolescents with irritability associated with autistic disorder. *Journal of the American Academy of Child and Adolescent Psychiatry, 48*(11), 1110–1119.

McCracken, J. T. (2011). Pharmacotherapy for autism spectrum disorders. In D. G. Amaral, G. Dawson, & D. Geschwind (Eds.), *Autism spectrum disorders* (pp. 1309–1322). New York, NY: Oxford University Press.

McCracken, J. T., McGough, J., Shah, B., Cronin, P., Hong, D., Aman, M. G., … Research Units on Pediatric Psychopharmacology Autism, N. (2002). Risperidone in children with autism and serious behavioral problems. *The New England Journal of Medicine, 347*(5), 314–321.

McDougle, C. J., Scahill, L., Aman, M. G., McCracken, J. T., Tierney, E., Davies, M., … Vitiello, B. (2005). Risperidone for the core symptom domains of autism: Results from the study by the autism network of the research units on pediatric psychopharmacology. *The American Journal of Psychiatry, 162*(6), 1142–1148.

Nagaraj, R., Singhi, P., & Malhi, P. (2006). Risperidone in children with autism: Randomized, placebo-controlled. *Double-Blind Study. Journal of child neurology, 21*(6), 450–455.

Niederhofer, H., Staffen, W., & Mair, A. (2002). Galantamine may be effective in treating autistic disorder. *BMJ (Clinical Research Ed.), 325*(7377), 1422.

Owen, R., Sikich, L., Marcus, R. N., Corey-Lisle, P., Manos, G., McQuade, R. D., … Findling, R. L. (2009). Aripiprazole in the treatment of irritability in children and adolescents with autistic disorder. *Pediatrics, 124*(6), 1533–1540.

Pandina, G. J., Bossie, C. A., Youssef, E., Zhu, Y., & Dunbar, F. (2007). Risperidone improves behavioral symptoms in children with autism in a randomized, double-blind, placebo-controlled trial. *Journal of Autism and Developmental Disorders, 37*(2), 367–373.
Pearson, D. A., Santos, C. W., Aman, M. G., Arnold, L. E., Casat, C. D., Mansour, R., ... Jerger, S. W. (2013). Effects of extended release methylphenidate treatment on ratings of attention-deficit/hyperactivity disorder (ADHD) and associated behavior in children with autism spectrum disorders and ADHD symptoms. *Journal of Child and Adolescent Psychopharmacology, 23*(5), 337–351.
Rezaei, V., Mohammadi, M.-R., Ghanizadeh, A., Sahraian, A., Tabrizi, M., Rezazadeh, S.-A., & Akhondzadeh, S. (2010). Double-blind, placebo-controlled trial of risperidone plus topiramate in children with autistic disorder. *Progress in Neuro-Psychopharmacology and Biological Psychiatry, 34*(7), 1269–1272.
Robinson, E. B., St Pourcain, B., Anttila, V., Kosmicki, J. A., Bulik-Sullivan, B., Grove, J., ... Ripke, S. (2016). Genetic risk for autism spectrum disorders and neuropsychiatric variation in the general population. *Nature Genetics, 48*(5), 552–555.
Scahill, L., McCracken, J. T., King, B. H., Rockhill, C., Shah, B., Politte, L., ... McDougle, C. J. (2015). Extended-Release Guanfacine for Hyperactivity in Children With Autism Spectrum Disorder. *The American Journal of Psychiatry, 172*(12), 1197–1206.
Shea, S., Turgay, A., Carroll, A., Schulz, M., Orlik, H., Smith, I., & Dunbar, F. (2004). Risperidone in the treatment of disruptive behavioral symptoms in children with autistic and other pervasive developmental disorders. *Pediatrics, 114*(5), e634–e641.
Smith, I. C., Reichow, B., & Volkmar, F. R. (2015). The effects of DSM-5 criteria on number of individuals diagnosed with autism spectrum disorder: A systematic review. *Journal of Autism and Developmental Disorders, 45*(8), 2541–2552.
Spencer, D., Marshall, J., Post, B., Kulakodlu, M., Newschaffer, C., Dennen, T., ... Jain, A. (2013). Psychotropic medication use and polypharmacy in children with autism spectrum disorders. *Pediatrics, 132*(5), 833–840.
Veenstra-VanderWeele, J., Cook, E. H., King, B. H., Zarevics, P., Cherubini, M., Walton-Bowen, K., ... Carpenter, R. L. (2016). Arbaclofen in children and adolescents with autism spectrum disorder: A randomized, controlled, phase 2 trial. *Neuropsychopharmacology.*
Volkmar, F., Siegel, M., Woodbury-Smith, M., King, B., McCracken, J., & State, M. (2014). Practice parameter for the assessment and treatment of children and adolescents with autism spectrum disorder. *Journal of the American Academy of Child and Adolescent Psychiatry, 53*(2), 237–257.
Wasserman, S., Iyengar, R., Chaplin, W. F., Watner, D., Waldoks, S. E., Anagnostou, E., ... Hollander, E. (2006). Levetiracetam versus placebo in childhood and adolescent autism: A double-blind placebo-controlled study. *International Clinical Psychopharmacology, 21*(6), 363–367.
Yatawara, C. J., Einfeld, S. L., Hickie, I. B., Davenport, T. A., & Guastella, A. J. (2016). The effect of oxytocin nasal spray on social interaction deficits observed in young children with autism: A randomized clinical crossover trial. *Molecular Psychiatry, 21*(9), 1225–1231.

Chapter 7
Effective Medications for Treating Psychosis in School-Aged Youth

Zachary B. Millman, Heidi J. Wehring, Alicia R. Khan, Sarah Edwards, Sharon A. Hoover and Jason Schiffman

Introduction

Psychosis is a psychiatric syndrome characterized by hallucinations (perceptions in the absence of stimulation) and delusions (beliefs held tenaciously despite contradictory evidence). Although schizophrenia is the prototypical psychotic disorder, psychosis is common among several distinct Diagnostic and Statistical Manual of Mental Disorders (DSM) diagnoses, including major depressive disorder, bipolar disorder, and substance-induced mental health conditions. *Primary psychotic disorders* (also referred to as *schizophrenia-spectrum* disorders) are those in which the psychosis is considered to be the core feature; that is, psychotic symptoms are not restricted to periods of mood disturbance (e.g., as in major depressive disorder) or organic brain deterioration (e.g., as in Huntington's disease), and are not the direct physiological consequence of a substance (e.g., as in phencyclidine-induced psychosis). In addition to hallucinations and delusions, primary psychotic disorders often involve disorganized behavior (e.g., communication that is difficult to follow) and negative symptoms (e.g., anhedonia). Examples of DSM-5 (American Psychiatric Association, 2013) psychotic disorders include schizophrenia, schizoaffective disorder, and schizophreniform disorder. Despite the numerous diagnoses in which psychotic symptoms can present, recognition of the shared genetic etiology of psychotic disorders has resulted in a recent, fruitful shift in research away from a focus on specific DSM psychotic disorders and toward transdiagnostic psychosis more broadly. Given this trend, in the present chapter, we discuss psychosis primarily in terms of the broad, transdiagnostic syndrome, and indicate specific psychotic disorders when appropriate.

Z. B. Millman · A. R. Khan · J. Schiffman (✉)
University of Maryland, Baltimore County, Baltimore, MD, USA
e-mail: schiffma@umbc.edu

H. J. Wehring · S. Edwards · S. A. Hoover
School of Medicine, University of Maryland, Baltimore, MD, USA

J. S. Carlson and J. A. Barterian (eds.), *School Psychopharmacology*,
Pediatric School Psychology, https://doi.org/10.1007/978-3-030-15541-4_7

Schizophrenia is the most common psychotic disorder, affecting approximately 1% of the population. Across diagnoses, however, psychosis affects nearly 3.5% of individuals worldwide, suggesting that the most likely psychiatric diagnosis for an individual experiencing psychotic symptoms is not schizophrenia (Perälä et al., 2007). The modal age for onset of a first episode of acute psychosis is between 18 and 25, with men tending to be on the earlier end of the age distribution. Psychosis among youth is far less common. Cases of schizophrenia with clinical onset between 13 and 18 years of age occur in approximately 1 in every 1,000 people, or in 0.1% of the population, while those with onset prior to age 13 occur in approximately 1 in every 10,000 people, or 0.01% of the population (Bo & Haahr, 2016). These "early onset" disorders are considered to be more severe variants of psychosis.

Onset and Course of Psychosis

Although highly heterogeneous across individuals, psychotic disorders can be thought of as progressing through several phases throughout the lifespan. Recovery and stabilization are possible for many people with psychosis regardless of stage of illness, but is often facilitated by treatment in the early course of illness (within the first 3 to 5 years).

The prodromal phase. The prodromal period of psychotic illness involves identifiable and clinically significant symptoms of psychosis at a milder level relative to more severe and impairing diagnostic thresholds. The duration of this phase varies across individuals but tends to begin during adolescence, 2–5 years prior to the acute disorder. Although a nonspecific mix of affective disturbance, anxiety, and social withdrawal is common during this period, the hallmark symptoms of the prodrome are *attenuated symptoms of psychosis*, that is, perceptual abnormalities and unusual thoughts or communication that resemble psychotic symptoms but are insufficiently intense, distressing, or impairing to be considered a formal psychotic disorder. Individuals in this phase often experience symptoms such as confusion about what is real, unfounded, or exaggerated suspiciousness of others, or hearing non-distinct sounds that may resemble voices (APA, 2013).

A prodromal phase is identifiable in the majority of people who eventually develop threshold psychosis, suggesting that for most, rather than appearing abruptly, psychosis develops over time. Early intervention for individuals suspected of experiencing an initial psychosis prodrome has shown some promise in preventing or delaying progression to acute psychosis (Thompson et al., 2015). Although a few randomized trials of antipsychotic medication have been conducted for this "high-risk" population, the general consensus is that the clinical benefits do not outweigh the health risks associated with these medications. Instead, psychosocial interventions involving cognitive behavioral therapy, family psychoeducation, and/or social skills training are recommended as first-line treatments (Addington, Addington, Abidi, Raedler, & Remington, 2017).

The psychotic phase. The transition from the prodromal to the psychotic period is characterized by a loss of insight into the nature of the symptoms and a corresponding decline in functioning. In this phase, the individual's perceptual abnormalities and distorted thought content have become more fully formed and their attributions about the source of these experiences have become more elaborate, interconnected, and delusional. Whereas in the prodromal phase, the unusual thoughts and perceptions are ultimately perceived as not real, in the acute psychotic phase this insight is typically lost. Notably, individuals with psychosis may experience delusional conviction in the reality of some symptoms (e.g., in the belief that the world is coming to an imminent end), but maintain insight into the symptomatic nature of others (e.g., the experience of hearing voices). This varying degree of insight across symptoms is considered a marker of illness severity, with intact insight in any domain suggestive of lesser severity. The psychotic phase of illness and its corresponding increase in social withdrawal, anxiety, and odd behaviors (all of which are more common in cases of early onset) significantly interfere with individuals' ability to function normally in social contexts and schools, and can require hospitalization. Unfortunately, it is typically only during the first acute psychotic episode that an individual's friends, family, or teachers recognize that something is seriously wrong.

Recovery and stabilization in the early course of psychosis. The first episode of psychosis and the 5 years following treatment initiation represent a critical juncture in the long-term course of illness. If further functional decline and symptom worsening occur, it most commonly occurs during this period. Fortunately, rapid intervention and organization of family and community resources can in some cases foster a quicker and more complete recovery, improving the chances that the individual can return to a life resembling their previous level of functioning.

Schizophrenia has historically been considered a chronic, devastating, and lifetime illness. Relatively few studies, however, have actually followed those with the disorder for longer than 10 years. As a result, controversy exists concerning the long-term course of psychotic disorders. The American Psychiatric Association notes that 10–15% of individuals with schizophrenia experience only a single episode, and another 10–15% remain severely and persistently psychotic through much of their lives, leaving the vast majority of people somewhere in between in terms of recovery and functioning (Lehman et al., 2004). Recent evidence, however, suggests that nearly half of clients whose psychosis remits following an initial episode are able to achieve normative levels of functioning with very little or no antipsychotic use (Murray et al., 2016). Although greater proportions of individuals with the illness may recover than previously thought, the majority experience some level of enduring difficulties in social functioning and symptoms.

Impact of Psychosis on School Functioning

Mental health concerns associated with psychosis in school-age children can interfere with individuals' ability to reach their full academic potential, including their ability to earn their high school diploma. Children with psychosis are less likely to complete elementary or high school than peers in the general population or with other mental health concerns (Tempelaar, Termorshuizen, MacCabe, Boks, & Kahn, 2017). Adolescence is an important developmental period normally characterized by significant social and cognitive milestones, and youth who become affected with psychosis during this time suffer an interruption to normative development of these skills. Depression, anxiety, substance use, potentially maladaptive beliefs about the intentions of others, low levels of motivation to participate in social activities, and distracting or disorienting psychotic symptoms may result in loss of friends and bully victimization, difficulty completing schoolwork, or complete inability to attend school, the latter often due to hospitalization. These same behaviors can also negatively impact the student's relationships with teachers and staff, some of whom may feel confused or uncomfortable and shy away from the student. It is important for school personnel to be aware of all of these possibilities, with a particular eye toward the common co-occurrence of psychosis and substance use (Schoeler et al., 2016), and to recognize that substances may be used by individuals to alleviate their symptoms despite the fact that use is ultimately likely to exacerbate the illness.

Psychopharmacological Treatment of Psychosis

Available antipsychotic medications for treating psychosis are listed in Table 7.1. Antipsychotic medications fall into two general classes: first-generation antipsychotics (FGAs) and second-generation antipsychotics (SGAs). In the US, the most prevalent agents used for youth with psychotic disorders are the SGAs (Olfson, King, & Schoenbaum, 2015), also known as atypical antipsychotics. Several SGAs, including aripiprazole, risperidone, olanzapine, quetiapine, paliperidone, and lurasidone all have FDA indication for schizophrenia in youth ages 12–13 through 17. In addition, some of these have indications for non-schizophrenia pediatric diagnoses, including autism, bipolar mania, and Tourette's disorder. Other SGAs without FDA approval for schizophrenia includes asenapine (approved for bipolar disorder in youth ages 10–17) and brexpiprazole, cariprazine, clozapine, and ziprasidone, none of which carry FDA indication for youth under age 18. Although various FGAs carry FDA indications for pediatric psychotic disorders, these agents are far less likely to be used as first-line maintenance medications for psychotic symptoms in youth due to their potential adverse effect profile. FGAs such as chlorpromazine may be more frequently used as an "as needed" or PRN medication for aggression. Other FGAs such as haloperidol may be used for maintenance treatment, since it is available in multiple formulations, including long-acting injection.

Selection of an antipsychotic medication for treatment of psychotic symptoms in youth is generally done based on a combination of clinical, client-specific criteria as well as the evidence base in support of available agents. For example, a greater breadth of clinical trial and pharmacokinetic data are generally available for the medications that have sought and been granted FDA approval for schizophrenia in

Table 7.1 List of second-generation antipsychotics discussed in this chapter or approved by the food and drug administration for use with children

Medication name	FDA approval for children	Psychosis-related indications and corresponding age groups, in years
Aripiprazole	Yes	SZ, 13–17; Mania, 10–17
Asenapine	Yes	Mania, 10–17
Brexpiprazole	No	–
Cariprazine	No	–
Clozapine	No	–
Lurasidone	Yes	SZ, 12–17
Olanzapine	Yes	SZ, 13–17; Mania, 13–17
Paliperidone	Yes	SZ, 12–17
Quetiapine	Yes	SZ, 13–17; Mania, 10–17
Ziprasidone	No	–
Risperidone	Yes	SZ, 13–17; Mania, 10–17

Note SZ = schizophrenia. *Source* https://www.ncbi.nlm.nih.gov/books/NBK84656/

youth specifically (e.g., aripiprazole). Other agents, however, may have an increasing body of evidence for either efficacy or safety without FDA approval. In addition, certain medications, such as clozapine, have shown utility in alleviation of some treatment-resistant symptoms, although FDA approval in school-aged students is unlikely due to a number of factors, including a high risk of adverse effects in youth. Related, in addition to the evidence base for efficacy and safety, differential adverse effect risk profiles of the various agents inform antipsychotic selection.

Prevalence of Prescribing

Antipsychotic use in children and adolescents in 2010 was estimated to be 0.1% for younger children (ages 1–6), 0.8% for older children (ages 7–12), and 1.19% for adolescents (ages 13–18) in a retrospective descriptive analysis using a database including 60% of the US retail pharmacies (Olfson, King, & Schoenbaum, 2015). Since psychotic disorders are rare in school-aged youth, the majority of prescriptions for antipsychotic medications in this age group are assumed to be for purposes other than psychosis. As previously noted, some antipsychotics have FDA indications for youth outside the schizophrenia spectrum, such as Tourette's disorder, mania, and autism. Although there are no FDA indications and less data to support their use, antipsychotics are sometimes also used for management of severe aggression in ADHD, disruptive mood dysregulation, impulse control disorders, or other purposes.

Given the low overall antipsychotic prescription among children and adolescents in the US, combined with the multiple non-schizophrenia-spectrum prescribing purposes of the medications, the prevalence of antipsychotic prescription for psychosis in school-aged youth is likely extremely low. A recent study of linked national health registry data for youth ages 0–18 in Norway found the most common diagnoses for antipsychotic prescriptions were hyperkinetic (i.e., ADHD-related) disorders, autism spectrum disorders, anxiety disorders, and depressive illness (Nesvag et al., 2016). Schizophrenia-like psychotic disorders were diagnosed in 11.1% of the males and 18.2% of the females prescribed antipsychotics in this study. An analysis of 2009 medical and pharmacy claims showed that in the US, the most common diagnosis among antipsychotic-treated children and adolescents was ADHD, although most of the youth under age 18 treated with antipsychotics (57–62%) had no out- or inpatient claim including a mental disorder diagnosis (Olfson, King, & Schoenbaum, 2015). Therefore, although the use of antipsychotics, and particularly the SGAs, continue to increase in youth with mental health disorders, the use of antipsychotics for psychosis in youth accounts for only a small percentage of overall antipsychotic prescriptions.

Mechanism of Action

FGA and SGA medications differ in mechanism of action, but it is important to note that most antipsychotics differ at least slightly in receptor affinity from their class counterparts (i.e., within each class of antipsychotics there are receptor affinity differences). Most approved antipsychotic medications are dopamine type 2 (D2) receptor antagonists, with the exception of three agents with partial agonist activity at D2. Symptoms of psychosis are thought to be related to the mesolimbic dopamine pathway in the brain. Blockade of dopamine in other pathways, however, may also occur, resulting in side effects such as extrapyramidal side effects (EPS), hyperprolactinemia, secondary cognitive symptoms, and secondary negative symptoms. Efficacy of FGA antipsychotics is likely related to blockade of postsynaptic D2 receptors. This blockade is thought to result in decreased dopamine transmission in the mesolimbic and perhaps the mesocortical areas of the brain. FGA antipsychotics also may antagonize other receptors, including D2 receptors in non-mesolimbic/non-mesocortical brain areas, which may lead to adverse events. Other receptor antagonism may include serotonergic, alpha-adrenergic, histaminergic, and muscarinic receptor antagonism, in varying degrees across agents. FGA antipsychotics may be classified by potency: high potency medications such as haloperidol and fluphenazine have greater affinity for D2 receptors and higher risk of EPS, whereas low potency medications such as chlorpromazine may have lower D2 affinity but high affinities for other receptors such as muscarinic, acetylcholine, and adrenergic receptors which can lead to higher degrees of sedation and cardiovascular side effects (Correll, 2010).

SGAs are a diverse group of agents with less risk of acute EPS than FGAs at clinical (i.e., antipsychotic) doses. In addition, they are thought to be less likely to cause secondary (i.e., medication-induced) negative symptoms due to their receptor affinity profiles. Three different mechanisms of action are common among the agents, although not all SGAs have each activity. The first is serotonin type 2 receptor and dopamine receptor antagonism (5HT2-DA antagonism). Here, the serotonergic action is thought to contribute to reduced EPS risk. This mechanism is common to all currently marketed SGAs with indication for treatment of schizophrenia, and by contrast, most FGAs do not have significant 5HT effects at therapeutic doses. The second common mechanism of action is D2 antagonism with faster dissociation/weaker affinity for D2 receptors. FGAs have long receptor occupancy times at D2 receptors, but the lower potency SGAs such as clozapine and quetiapine tend to have faster dissociation and/or weaker affinity to bind to D2 than the higher potency SGAs like paliperidone and risperidone. The third mechanism of action common to SGAs is D2 partial agonism (aripiprazole, brexpiprazole, and cariprazine), thought to provide for reduction of D2 hyperactivity in mesolimbic dopamine neurons of individuals with psychosis, and limiting reduction, or providing for partial agonism, of DA activity in the nigrostriatal system. This third mechanism is thought to contribute to the lower rates of extrapyramidal symptoms associated with SGAs. SGAs may also act as antagonists in alpha-adrenergic, histaminergic, serotonergic, and muscarinic receptors at varying degrees across agents, leading to differential adverse effect profiles (Correll, 2010).

Efficacy and Effectiveness of Antipsychotics for Psychosis in School-Aged Youth

Antipsychotic medications are traditionally tested for efficacy and safety for adults for initial FDA indication and marketing, with later trials examining their use in young people. Although psychosis in youth is generally believed to be consistent in etiology and presentation with that seen in adults, important developmental considerations raise questions about the efficacy and safety of these drugs in younger people. Developmental variability in drug metabolism challenges standardized dosing procedures for youth compared with adults, and animal studies suggest that neural and hormonal development during childhood and adolescence may be adversely affected by antipsychotics (Caccia, 2013). Alternative non-antipsychotic acute treatments for psychosis, however, generally remain unavailable, and antipsychotic medication is considered the first-line treatment for youth with psychotic disorders. Below we review the evidence in support of the efficacy and effectiveness of antipsychotic medication for school-aged youth with psychosis.

Antipsychotic Treatment of Psychosis in the General Psychosis Literature

On average, antipsychotics appear to be effective in reducing psychotic symptoms in adults. In a meta-analysis of 116 randomized trials, Leucht and colleagues (2012) reported that antipsychotics reduced rates of psychotic relapse from 64% in placebo conditions to 27% in the treatment conditions over a 12-month period. Critically, the meta-analytic evidence suggests that antipsychotic drugs are more effective in promoting healthy outcomes among individuals when they are administered earlier in the course of illness (Perkins, Gu, Boteva, & Lieberman, 2005). These findings suggest that school personnel may be the key in improving prognoses of psychosis in youth through early identification and referral.

Antipsychotic Treatment of Psychosis Among Youth

Despite the promise of early intervention, evidence concerning the effects of antipsychotic medications for psychosis in school-aged children is extremely limited. The disorder's low prevalence imposes practical difficulties in conducting a reliable body of research, and the severe nature of symptoms raises ethical concerns with prescribing inactive placebos. Thus, there are only a small number of controlled trials to date, many with notable methodological limitations. Although having changed since, antipsychotic agents marketed prior to pediatric drug development legislation enacted in the late 1990s never received adequate evaluation for children and adolescents. Therefore, relative to SGAs, fewer studies are available concerning the use of older agents for pediatric clients. More studies are now recommended specifically for youth in order to establish safety, efficacy, and dosing parameters for all medications, including antipsychotics, that might be prescribed to school-aged individuals (information available at https://www.fda.gov/Drugs/ResourcesForYou/Consumers/default.htm).

Randomized Controlled Trials of Antipsychotic Treatment for Youth with Psychosis

The small number of head-to-head comparison trials of antipsychotic medication for psychosis in youth makes it difficult to establish superiority, either in efficacy or in safety, among available agents. Recently, a meta-analysis of 12 acute (i.e., 6–12 week) trials examined the safety and efficacy of multiple antipsychotics for youth with schizophrenia-spectrum disorders, including aripiprazole, asenapine, paliperidone, risperidone, quetiapine, olanzapine, molindone, and ziprasidone. Efficacy was comparable among the SGAs aripiprazole, paliperidone, risperidone, quetiapine, olanzapine, and the FGA molindone (no longer available in the US), but appeared mixed for asenapine and possibly inferior for ziprasidone (Pagsberg et al., 2017).

Table 7.2 displays the results of several double-blind, randomized trials of acute treatment for schizophrenia in school-aged youth, either placebo-controlled or active comparator. The trials included in this table suggest that the average participating youth experiences approximately 25% reduction in total psychiatric symptoms after

6–12 weeks of treatment, with positive symptoms appearing more responsive than negative symptoms. Although there appears to be a modest effect of symptom reduction, Table 7.2 also suggests that the average youth undergoing treatment continues to experience significant symptoms of psychosis. Further, as demonstrated in the meta-analysis by Pagsberg and colleagues (2017), no clear advantage is visible between available agents.

There are other randomized trials of antipsychotic treatment for youth with psychosis not included in Table 7.2, but most of these studies have involved particularly small sample sizes (i.e., subgroup n's = 12–21) or have lacked a control condition. Studies of clozapine are particularly notable because clozapine is considered a standard intervention for treatment-resistant schizophrenia in adults. Its efficacy for the condition in youth, however, is less well established. In one small study, Kumra and colleagues (2008) found that clozapine ($n = 18$) outperformed high-dose olanzapine ($n = 21$) in treatment-resistant psychosis in youth. They found that 66% of youth treated with clozapine and 33% of youth treated with high-dose olanzapine made clinically meaningful improvements over the 12-week trial (indicated by a $\geq$30% drop in total symptom scores plus a favorable "clinical global impression" rating). Side effects, however, were notable with insomnia, increased salivation, and nasal congestion common in up to two-thirds of participants.

Side Effects of Antipsychotic Medication

A significant limitation to the safe and effective use of antipsychotics among youth with psychosis is their potential to cause adverse effects. SGAs represented a significant advancement in the history of psychosis treatment due to their tendency to cause fewer extrapyramidal symptoms than the FGAs, although it should be noted that these adverse effects still occur with the newer agents. Extrapyramidal symptoms include *acute* or *early symptoms*, such as acute dyskinesia (brief, involuntary muscle movements), akathisia, acute dystonic reactions (involuntary muscle spasms), and pseudoparkinsonism (postural instability, rigidity, tremor, and slowed involuntary movements), as well as *late* or *tardive symptoms*, such as late-onset tardive dyskinesia (which may be permanent in up to one-third of cases). In addition, neuroleptic malignant syndrome, a very rare but potentially life-threatening condition characterized by mental status change, muscle rigidity, fever, and autonomic dysfunction can result from the use of antipsychotic medication, possibly due to the agents' dopaminergic activity. Table 7.3 summarizes common side effects from randomized trials of antipsychotic treatment for psychosis in youth. All of the randomized trials reviewed reported significant side effects that appear to impact adherence, raising concerns about the tolerability and safety of antipsychotic medications.

Despite side effects, absolute contraindications for any medication are relatively rare. They mostly concern hypersensitivity or allergy to the medication or its components; however, in certain circumstances, client-specific issues may lead to decisions that the risk-to-benefit ratio does not warrant antipsychotic treatment. Labeling for

Table 7.2 Results of randomized controlled trials of antipsychotic medication for treatment of schizophrenia and schizoaffective disorder in youth

Study	Medication condition	Dose (mg/day)	% Δ in total symptoms	% Δ in positive symptoms	% Δ in negative symptoms	% Δ in global functioning
Findling et al. (2008)	Aripiprazole	10	−28.49*	−34.40*	−27.16*	20.67*
	Aripiprazole	30	−30.14*	−34.47*	−26.51	28.26*
	Placebo	–	*−22.32*	*−24.45*	*−21.09*	*20.57*
Savitz, Lane, Nuamah, Gopal, and Hough (2015)	Paliperidone	3–9	−28.57	−29.77	−17.65	24.5
	Aripiprazole	2–15	−29.13	−27.55	−18.59	24.8
Singh, Robb, Vijapurkar, Nuamah, and Hough (2011)	Paliperidone	3	−20.63*	−26.02*	−16.27	30.99*
	Paliperidone	6	−15.20*	−19.83*	−9.40	22.98*
	Paliperidone	12	−17.91*	−23.50*	−15.77	19.75*
	Placebo	–	*−8.39*	*−12.99*	*−7.89*	*10.24*
Sikich et al. (2008)	Molindone + Benzatropine	10–140, + 1	−27.08	−33.84	−23.97	32
	Olanzapine	2.5–20	−26.52	−33.71	−21.20	40
	Risperidone	0.5–6	−22.95	−31.46	−19.69	47
Haas et al. (2009a)	Risperidone	1–3	NR*	−23.77*	−22.41*	43.33*
	Risperidone	4–6	NR*	−25.29*	−20.07*	45.11*
	Placebo	–	*NR*	*−11.19*	*−8.26*	*18.72*
Haas et al. (2009b)	Risperidone	0.15–0.6	13.39	18.05	10.73	18.37
	Risperidone	1.5–6	24.48*	28.68*	22.36*	27.45*
Khrykanovskaya et al. (2009)	Olanzapine	2.5–20	−22.35*	−28.95*	−15.26	22.92*
	Placebo	–	*−9.21*	*−11.89*	*−7.26*	*10.2*
Findling et al. (2015)	Asenapine	2.5	−22.38	NR	NR	21.74
	Asenapine	5	−23.02	NR	NR	25.53*

(continued)

Table 7.2 (continued)

Study	Medication condition	Dose (mg/day)	% Δ in total symptoms	% Δ in positive symptoms	% Δ in negative symptoms	% Δ in global functioning
	Placebo	–	*−17.53*	*NR*	*NR*	*17.39*
Findling, McKenna, Earley, Stankowski, and Pathak (2012)	Quetiapine	400	−28.39*	−36.74	−25	30.05
	Quetiapine	800	−29.32*	−39.24*	−24.07	35.07*
	Placebo	–	*−19.91*	*−26.58*	*−20.52*	*23.66*
Findling et al. (2013)[a]	Ziprasidone mITT	40–160	−26.55	−32.88*	−23.50	23.4
	Placebo mITT	–	*−24.03*	*−27.19*	*−22.57*	*17.39*
	Ziprasidone PP	40–160	−27.35	−33.49*	−25.00	25.53*
	Placebo PP	–	*−22.10*	*−24.20*	*−19.74*	*17.39*
Shaw et al. (2006)	Clozapine	12.5–900	−27.78	−48.89	−48.08*	20
	Olanzapine	5–20	−18.84	−28.89	−26.92	9.62
Kumra et al. (2008)	Clozapine	25–900	−41.09	−56.85	−35.92*	31.05
	Olanzapine	5–30	−35.16	−43.75	19.15	22

Note. Trials varied in duration from 6–12 weeks. Although some studies included an open-label extension, values presented here reflect change at the randomization endpoints. Symptom severity was assessed using the Scale for Assessment of Negative/Positive Symptoms in Shaw et al. (2006), and the Brief Psychiatric Rating Scale in Kumra et al. (2008); otherwise, the Positive and Negative Syndrome Scale was used. Global functioning is reported based on the Child and Adolescent Functional Assessment Scale in Sikich et al. (2008) and the Children's Global Assessment Scale in Haas et al. (2009a); otherwise, it is reported based on the Clinical Global Impression, Severity scale. Asterisks denote a statistically significant difference from placebo; for non-placebo, active comparator studies, asterisks denote statistically significant difference from the comparator. NR = not reported

[a]mITT = modified intent to treat analysis, PP = per protocol analysis

Table 7.3 Select adverse events commonly reported in randomized trials of antipsychotic medication for youth with schizophrenia and schizoaffective disorders

	Incidence during trial period (%)	
Adverse event	Range	Median
Somnolence	5.5–29.7	18.35
Headache	4.4–21.6	10.5
Dizziness	1.9–14.9	7.1
Insomnia	5.1–12.3	9.15
Agitation	0–15	5.5
Tachycardia	0–8.5	5
Fatigue	5–8.8	6.95
Nausea	0–10	5.7
Sedation	2.3–11.3	5.4
Vomiting	0–7.1	4.55
Anxiety	0–8.5	5
Akathisia	1.5–16.8	6.6
Extrapyramidal disorder	0–22	11.4

Note. Figures reflect data from each of the independent trials displayed in Table 7.2, with the exception of Shaw et al. (2006) and Kumra et al. (2008), who reported on effects of clozapine for treatment-resistant schizophrenia. Given that clozapine is rarely used in youth and has a considerable side effect profile, these figures are left out of the table. Additionally, some trials reported only those adverse events occurring in >5% of the sample, or provided insufficient data to extract for this table, and thus this table does not represent a comprehensive view of antipsychotic-induced side effects and their prevalence

FGA medications offers general contraindications such as hypersensitivity, blood disorders, bone marrow disorders or suppression, and CNS depression or brain injury. Certain antipsychotics are contraindicated in persons predisposed to a cardiac condition known as QT interval prolongation, such as long QT syndrome, history of arrhythmias, or combined use with other medications. In general, all antipsychotic medications carry a black box warning for risk of increased mortality. In addition, neuroleptic malignant syndrome, tardive dyskinesia, and metabolic changes (e.g., diabetes, weight gain, and hyperlipidemia), hyperprolactinemia, leukopenia, orthostatic hypotension and syncope, seizures, potential for motor or cognitive impairment, change in body temperature regulation, suicidality, and dysphagia are possible adverse effects, with each agent having varying levels of risk (Young, Taylor, & Lawrie, 2015).

Methodological Limitations

Several methodological considerations warrant caution when interpreting results of the research discussed above. Among other concerns, there is no obvious definition of who "responds" to a trial and who does not; participants in randomized trials do not always represent the population of youth with psychosis, as many individuals are excluded based on strict entry criteria (see entry criteria for studies listed in Table 7.1; Guloksuz & van Os, 2017); follow-up is typically short; side effects are often not weighed in relation to benefits (Murray et al., 2016); how gains translate to school settings is unclear; and the role of industry sponsorship (see Siskind et al., 2016) is not usually discussed as a potential limitation in published research.

Combined Treatment for Youth with Psychosis

Very few studies have examined the efficacy of adjunctive psychosocial interventions for treatment of psychosis in youth, and the potential they may have in the school setting in particular. This is unfortunate given their demonstrated efficacy in adults with psychosis and in youth with serious, non-psychosis-spectrum mental health concerns (e.g., bipolar disorder; Vallariono et al., 2015). Psychosocial interventions in combination with pharmacotherapy may hold promise in engaging youth and their families, setting personalized goals, and developing a crisis-response plan. Such interventions could be administered at schools or at least involve important school personnel (e.g., teachers, counselors, mentors, and coaches), shortly following stabilization of acute psychotic symptoms with antipsychotics (Kline, Denenny, Reeves, & Schiffman, 2014). Psychosocial intervention can also help to address barriers to taking medications as prescribed, with medication and psychological interventions ultimately developing a synergistic relationship to improve functioning in the school. A recent review of studies of psychosocial intervention for youth with psychosis identified four trials of psychoeducational family-based intervention and one trial of cognitive behavioral therapy (Armando, Pontillo, & Vicari, 2015). The authors concluded that there is some evidence to support the use of psychosocial intervention for youth with psychosis (e.g., supported education), but significantly more research is needed.

Implications for School Personnel

Initial and Ongoing Assessment of Psychosis in Schools

Accurate identification of psychosis requires thorough assessment. Given the low prevalence of psychosis in school-age children, it is likely that emerging mental health concerns among youth are not related to psychosis. Therefore, it is important to rule out other mental health concerns and contributors to the behaviors before psychosis is deemed to be the diagnosis. The Kiddie Schedule for Affective Disorders and Schizophrenia is a semi-structured, clinician-administered interview designed to generate psychiatric diagnoses and is an excellent option for assessment of suspected psychosis (Kaufman et al., 1997). The interview is conducted with caregivers as respondents and then, separately, the child. Nonetheless, despite the value of gold-standard, semi-structured interviews, such a time- and training-intensive clinical assessment is often impractical in the school setting, and typically not part of routine practice.

As an alternative to semi-structured interviews, brief screening tools may be helpful. Student support staff, including school psychologists, social workers, and nurses, may administer screening for psychosis if other "red flag" signs are present that warrant further assessment. A number of self-report questionnaires are available to screen for the possibility of emerging psychosis. Cutoff scores can signal an appreciable likelihood of meeting criteria for a psychosis-spectrum disorder and thus can add to school-based clinicians' formulation as to whether the student may be appropriate for a referral to a psychiatrist or psychosis specialist.

No studies to our knowledge have examined the ability of school personnel reports to aid in identifying the prodromal phase of psychosis. Teacher reports, however, have been shown to identify social deficits among students (ages 10–13) without prodromal symptoms who would eventually develop psychosis as adults (Tsuji et al., 2013), suggesting that teachers could play a role in identifying students with emerging symptoms as well. Disclosure of psychosis-like symptoms can be challenging for young people who tend to feel scared, confused, and stigmatized by these experiences. Teachers and administrative staff with regular, close contact with students can foster a safe environment in which students can feel comfortable disclosing early symptoms, and can perhaps be trained to administer empirically supported screening questionnaires designed to identify emerging psychosis. Alerting school clinicians and/or family members of symptoms endorsed by students has the potential to mobilize youths' support network, initiating closer monitoring or intervention. At the same time, regardless of treatment initiation, school personnel should keep in mind that attenuated symptoms of psychosis do not necessarily mean that a more severe illness is inevitable. Adopting a positive, hopeful attitude with youth and their families can promote optimism and treatment engagement at a sensitive developmental phase.

Once students have made contact with a prescribing clinician for psychosis, baseline assessment and regular follow-up are important for several reasons, including monitoring of side effects, ongoing effectiveness, and changes in the environment or behavior (e.g., changes in schools, experimentation with substances), particularly as youth transition through adolescence. Consistent adherence to long-term antipsychotic medication is rare among youth with psychosis, and it should therefore be expected that there will be times when medication is not taken as prescribed. In these cases, clinicians are encouraged to engage nonjudgmentally, encourage honesty, and seek to understand the reasons for nonadherence. Again, schools offer an unparalleled setting for following up with students' mental health treatment progress, with a growing body of research demonstrating significantly higher rates of engagement and follow through in school-based mental health treatment than traditional outpatient care (see Kline, Denenny, Reeves, & Schiffman, 2014, for further discussion of school-based mental health for psychosis).

Symptom changes can be complex and difficult to assess, even for experienced clinicians. Standardized assessments of psychotic symptoms can therefore aid in accurate monitoring of treatment effectiveness. The Brief Psychiatric Rating Scale for Children assesses a range of symptoms commonly occurring in early psychosis within the past 2 weeks and is sensitive to treatment-related changes. As with the Kiddie Schedule for Affective Disorders and Schizophrenia, however, administration of semi-structured interviews such as these may not be routine practice in school settings. Self-report questionnaires completed by clients may be more compatible with the demands of school mental health and can be used as methods for systematic, ongoing symptom monitoring.

Psychoeducation

Psychoeducation is an important part of any intervention for a complex illness like psychosis. Educating students and their families involves providing information about the causes of psychosis in layperson and developmentally appropriate terms, why the medication chosen was chosen, and the potential side effects. Additionally, it is important to help individuals anticipate the short-term course of treatment, including the expected time to treatment response and the plan for symptom and side effect monitoring, so that students and their families can be more engaged in the intervention. Given the metabolic side effects, including weight gain, of many antipsychotics, education on a healthy diet may be an important part of psychoeducation, particularly for individuals with preexisting risk factors for metabolic problems (e.g., those who are currently overweight). Learning about the causes and treatment of psychosis, the high degree of variability in functional outcome, and ways that the client and family can be active participants in treatment can help to empower consumers, reduce feelings of stigma, and foster engagement in treatment.

In addition to direct psychoeducation of clients and their families, brief psychoeducational interventions administered by clinicians to teachers and administrative staff, or to classrooms directly, can be conducted at a low cost with potential to have a widespread and sustained impact on the school community. Studies have found that brief interventions (e.g., 2 hours) targeting attitudes and beliefs toward individuals with mental health concerns improved knowledge of the mental illnesses, reduced stigmatizing attitudes toward individuals with mental illness, and reduced a desire for social distancing. In a school setting, these interventions can be framed as "workshops" or "lesson plans," further emphasizing the educational aspect and normalizing discussion of mental illness. Psychoeducational interventions may also help teachers and administrative staff to be aware of medication side effects that might otherwise be interpreted as intentionally disruptive or withdrawn, such as akathisia and sedation or drowsiness. Watson and associates (2004) demonstrated improvement in knowledge and attitudes among middle school students through a five-session intervention titled "The Science of Mental Illness" that emphasized biopsychosocial causes of mental health concerns.

Collaboration Between School Practitioners

Collaboration among key school personnel is critical for optimizing treatment of students with psychosis. Given that sessions with teachers, counselors, psychologists, social workers, and psychiatry practitioners may all have different areas of focus, students may only disclose certain, important concerns (e.g., emerging psychosocial stressors) to select personnel. Scheduling periodic meetings or conference calls to discuss shared clients can help promote continuity of care between treatment providers. If possible, periodic joint sessions including clients and their families are optimal. Such sessions may help ensure that providers and consumers are aware of one another's expectations and can also promote a sense of cohesion among practitioners, clients, and their families.

Summary

Psychotic disorders can take a variety of forms among youth. These disorders are heterogeneous in their outcome and carry a unique personal meaning for every individual affected. Although they frequently disrupt individuals' ability to form stable friendships, to perform to their potential in school, and to achieve their life's goals, early intervention provides substantial hope of recovery and for living a life of the youth's choosing. Antipsychotic medications currently play an important role in this effort. As discussed in this chapter, randomized controlled trials of SGA treatment for youth with psychosis suggest that youth are likely to experience meaningful relief from psychiatric symptoms, at least in the short term. At the same time, medications do not solve the problem of psychosis in youth. Support from school personnel, friends, families, and psychosocial interventions are all important pieces of what is ideally a comprehensive treatment approach.

Academic institutions can formally support the health and education of youth with mental health concerns through brief psychoeducational interventions, assessment of psychotic disorders through use of screeners, and clinical interventions. Beyond these approaches, individual personnel can enhance the probability that early intervention is initiated rapidly and collaboratively when needed by fostering a supportive, non-stigmatizing environment in which students and their families feel comfortable disclosing emerging symptoms. The frequent contact with students, regular correspondence with families, and educational institutional orientation makes schools an ideal environment for educating communities on mental health and illness, reducing psychosocial stress, and identifying psychosis among school-age youth. In collaboration with families and outside providers, schools can have a significant impact on the long-term course of youth affected with these disorders.

Suggested Readings

- Kline, E., Denenny, D., Reeves, G., & Schiffman, J., 2014. Early identification of psychosis in schools. In *Handbook of School Mental Health* (pp. 323–338). Springer US.

  In-depth discussion of school-based assessment and psychosocial intervention strategies for youth with psychosis. The chapter is clinically focused and provides numerous recommendations for practice.

- Ballard, R. R. (Ed). 2015. *Helping parents, youth, and teachers understand medications for behavioral and emotional problems: A resource book of medication information handouts.* American Psychiatric Pub.

  Handouts for consumers and schoolteachers outlining important psychiatric medication information.

- Saks, E. R., 2007. *The center cannot hold: My journey through madness.* Hachette UK.

  A compelling memoir written by Elyn Saks, a law professor affected with schizophrenia from a young age. The book elegantly describes the intrapersonal, psychosocial, and academic challenges caused by her illness, as well as her heroic efforts to overcome these challenges and live a meaningful, productive life.

List of Websites

- http://www.marylandeip.com

  The Maryland Early Intervention Program is a multi-institutional collaborative designed to improve the lives of young people in the early phases of psychosis. Educational resources are available for professionals and consumers.

- http://www.nami.org

  The National Alliance on Mental Illness (NAMI) is a nationwide nonprofit organization designed to support individuals and families affected by mental illness. Community events, support groups, and more can be found at the website.

- http://www.schizophrenia.com

  Internet community designed to provide high quality information regarding psychotic disorders to individuals, caregivers, and families affected by psychosis.

References

American Psychiatric Association. (2013). *Diagnostic and statistical manual of mental disorders (DSM-5)*. Washington, DC: American Psychiatric Pub.

Addington, J., Addington, D., Abidi, S., Raedler, T., & Remington, G. (2017). CPA treatment guidelines for individuals at clinical high risk of psychosis. *The Canadian Journal of Psychiatry, 62*(9), 656–661. https://doi.org/10.1177/0706743717719895.

Armando, M., Pontillo, M., & Vicari, S. (2015). Psychosocial interventions for very early and early-onset schizophrenia: A review of treatment efficacy. *Current Opinion in Psychiatry, 28*(4), 312–323. https://doi.org/10.1097/YCO.0000000000000165.

Bo, S., & Haahr, U. H. (2016). Early-onset psychosis and child and adolescent schizophrenia. *Scandinavian Journal of Child and Adolescent Psychiatry and Psychology, 4*(1), 1–3.

Caccia, S. (2013). Safety and pharmacokinetics of atypical antipsychotics in children and adolescents. *Pediatric Drugs, 15*(3), 217–233. https://doi.org/10.1007/s40272-013-0024-6.

Correll, C. U. (2010). From receptor pharmacology to improved outcomes: individualising the selection, dosing, and switching of antipsychotics. *European Psychiatry, 25,* S12–S21. https://doi.org/10.1016/S00924-9338(10)71701-6.

Findling, R. L., Robb, A., Nyilas, M., Forbes, R. A., Jin, N., Ivanova, S., … & Carson, W. H. (2008). A multiple-center, randomized, double-blind, placebo-controlled study of oral aripiprazole for treatment of adolescents with schizophrenia. *American Journal of Psychiatry, 165*(11), 1432–1441. https://doi.org/10.1176/appi.ajp.2008.07061035.

Findling, R. L., McKenna, K., Earley, W. R., Stankowski, J., & Pathak, S. (2012). Efficacy and safety of quetiapine in adolescents with schizophrenia investigated in a 6-week, double-blind, placebo-controlled trial. *Journal of Child and Adolescent Psychopharmacology, 22*(5), 327–342. https://doi.org/10.1089/cap.2011.0092.

Findling, R. L., Çavuş, I., Pappadopulos, E., Vanderburg, D. G., Schwartz, J. H., Gundapaneni, B. K., et al. (2013). Ziprasidone in adolescents with schizophrenia: Results from a placebo-controlled efficacy and long-term open-extension study. *Journal of Child and Adolescent Psychopharmacology, 23*(8), 531–544. https://doi.org/10.1089/cap.2012.0068.

Findling, R. L., Landbloom, R. P., Mackle, M., Pallozzi, W., Braat, S., Hundt, C., … Mathews, M. (2015). Safety and efficacy from an 8 week double-blind trial and a 26 week open-label extension of asenapine in adolescents with schizophrenia. *Journal of Child and Adolescent Psychopharmacology, 25*(5), 384–396. https://doi.org/10.1089/cap.2015.0027.

Guloksuz, S., & van Os, J. (2017). The slow death of the concept of schizophrenia and the painful birth of the psychosis spectrum. *Psychological Medicine*, 1–16. https://doi.org/10.1017/s0033291717001775.

Haas, M., Eerdekens, M., Kushner, S., Singer, J., Augustyns, I., Quiroz, J., … Kusumakar, V. (2009a). Efficacy, safety and tolerability of two risperidone dosing regimens in adolescent schizophrenia: double-blind study. *The British Journal of Psychiatry, 194*(2), 158–164. https://doi.org/10.1089/cap.2008.0144.

Haas, M., Unis, A. S., Armenteros, J., Copenhaver, M. D., Quiroz, J. A., & Kushner, S. F. (2009b). A 6-week, randomized, double-blind, placebo-controlled study of the efficacy and safety of risperidone in adolescents with schizophrenia. *Journal of Child and Adolescent Psychopharmacology, 19*(6), 611–621. https://doi.org/10.1192/bjp.bp.107.046177.

Kaufman, J., Birmaher, B., Brent, D., Rao, U., Flynn, C., Moreci, P., … Ryan, N. (1997). Schedule for affective disorders and schizophrenia for school-age children-present and lifetime version (K-SADS-PL): Initial reliability and validity data. *Journal of the American Academy of Child and Adolescent Psychiatry, 36*(7), 980–988. https://doi.org/10.1097/00004583-199707000-00021.

Kline, E., Denenny, D., Reeves, G., & Schiffman, J. (2014). Early identification of psychosis in schools. In *Handbook of school mental health* (pp. 323–338). Springer US. https://doi.org/10.1007/978-1-4614-7624-5_24.

Kryzhanovskaya, L., Schulz, S.C., Mcdougle, C., Frazier, J., Dittmann, R., Robertson-Plouch, C., … Carlson, J. (2009). Olanzapine versus placebo in adolescents with schizophrenia: a 6-week, randomized, double-blind, placebo-controlled trial. *Journal of the American Academy of Child & Adolescent Psychiatry, 48*(1), 60–70. https://doi.org/10.1097/chi.0b013e3181900404.

Kumra, S., Kranzler, H., Gerbino-Rosen, G., Kester, H.M., DeThomas, C., Kafantaris, V., … Kane, J.M. (2008). Clozapine and "high-dose" olanzapine in refractory early-onset schizophrenia: a 12-week randomized and double-blind comparison. *Biological Psychiatry, 63*(5), 524–529. https://doi.org/10.1016/j.biopsych.2007.04.043.

Lehman, A. F., Lieberman, J. A., Dixon, L. B., McGlashan, T. H., Miller, A. L., Perkins, D. O., … Altshuler, K. (2004). Practice guideline for the treatment of partients with schizophrenia. *American Journal of Psychiatry, 161*(2 SUPPL).

Leucht, S., Tardy, M., Komossa, K., Heres, S., Kissling, W., Salanti, G., et al. (2012). Antipsychotic drugs versus placebo for relapse prevention in schizophrenia: A systematic review and meta-analysis. *The Lancet, 379*(9831), 2063–2071. https://doi.org/10.1016/S0140-6736(12)60239-6.

Murray, R. M., Quattrone, D., Natesan, S., van Os, J., Nordentoft, M., Howes, O., … Taylor, D. (2016). Should psychiatrists be more cautious about the long-term prophylactic use of antipsychotics? *The British Journal of Psychiatry, 209*(5), 361–365. https://doi.org/10.1192/bjp.bp.116.182683.

Nesvag, R., Hartz, I., Bramness, J. G., Hjellvik, V., Handal, M., & Skurtveit, S. (2016). Mental disorder diagnoses among children and adolescents who use antipsychotic drugs. *European Neuropsychopharmacology, 26*(9), 1412–1418. https://doi.org/10.1016/j.euroneuro.2016.07.001.

Olfson, M., King, M., & Schoenbaum, M. (2015). Treatment of young people with antipsychotic medications in the United States. *Journal of the American Medical Association, Psychiatry, 72*(9), 867–874. https://doi.org/10.1001/jamapsychiatry.2015.0500.

Pagsberg, A. K., Tarp, S., Glintborg, D., Stenstrom, A. D., Fink-Jensen, A., Correll, C. U., et al. (2017). Acute antipsychotic treatment of children and adolescents with schizophrenia—Sperctrum disorders: A systematic review and network meta-analysis. *Journal of the American Academy of Child and Adolescent Psychiatry, 56*(30), 191–202. https://doi.org/10.1016/j.jaac.2016.12.013.

Perälä, J., Suvisaari, J., Saarni, S. I., Kuoppasalmi, K., Isometsä, E., Pirkola, S., … Kieseppä, T. (2007). Lifetime prevalence of psychotic and bipolar I disorders in a general population. *Archives of General Psychiatry, 64*(1), 19–28. https://doi.org/10.1001/archpsyc.64.1.19.

Perkins, D. O., Gu, H., Boteva, K., & Lieberman, J. A. (2005). Relationship between duration of untreated psychosis and outcome in first-episode schizophrenia: A critical review and meta-analysis. *American Journal of Psychiatry, 162*(10), 1785–1804. https://doi.org/10.1176/appi.ajp.162.10.1785.

Savitz, A. J., Lane, R., Nuamah, I., Gopal, S., & Hough, D. (2015). Efficacy and safety of paliperidone extended release in adolescents with schizophrenia: a randomized, double-blind study. *Journal of the American Academy of Child and Adolescent Psychiatry, 54*(2), 126–137. e121. https://doi.org/10.1016/j.jaac.2014.11.009.

Schoeler, T., Monk, A., Sami, M. B., Klamerus, E., Foglia, E., Brown, R., … Bhattacharyya, S. (2016). Continued versus discontinued cannabis use in patients with psychosis: A systematic review and meta-analysis. *The Lancet Psychiatry, 3*(3), 215–225. https://doi.org/10.1016/S2215-0366(15)00363-6.

Shaw, P., Sporn, A., Gogtay, N., Overman, G. P., Greenstein, D., Gochman, P., … Rapoport, J. L. (2006). Childhood-onset schizophrenia: A double-blind, randomized clozapine-olanzapine comparison. *Archives of General Psychiatry, 63*(7), 721–730. https://doi.org/10.1001/archpsyc.63.7.721.

Sikich, L., Frazier, J. A., McClellan, J., Findling, R. L., Vitiello, B., Ritz, L. …Michael, E. (2008). Double-blind comparison of first-and second-generation antipsychotics in early-onset schizophrenia and schizo-affective disorder: Findings from the treatment of early-onset schizophrenia spectrum disorders (TEOSS) study. *American Journal of Psychiatry, 165*(11), 1420–1431. https://doi.org/10.1176/appi.ajp.2008.08050756.

Singh, J., Robb, A., Vijapurkar, U., Nuamah, I., & Hough, D. (2011). A randomized, double-blind study of paliperidone extended-release in treatment of acute schizophrenia in adolescents. *Biological Psychiatry, 70*(12), 1179–1187. https://doi.org/10.1016/j.biopsych.2011.06.021.

Siskind, D., McCartney, L., Goldschlager, R., & Kisely, S. (2016). Clozapine v. first-and second-generation antipsychotics in treatment-refractory schizophrenia: Systematic review and meta-analysis. *The British Journal of Psychiatry, 209*(5), 385–392. https://doi.org/10.1192/bjp.bp.115.17726.

Tempelaar, W. M., Termorshuizen, F., MacCabe, J. H., Boks, M. P., & Kahn, R. S. (2017). Educational achievement in psychiatric patients and their siblings: A register-based study in 30 000 individuals in The Netherlands. *Psychological Medicine, 47*(4), 776–784. https://doi.org/10.1017/S0033291716002877.

Thompson, E., Millman, Z. B., Okuzawa, N., Mittal, V., DeVylder, J., Skadberg, T., … Schiffman, J. (2015). Evidence-based early interventions for individuals at clinical high risk for psychosis: A review of treatment components. *The Journal of Nervous and Mental Disease, 203*(5), 342–351. https://doi.org/10.1097/nmd.0000000000000287.

Tsuji, T., Kline, E., Sorensen, H. J., Mortensen, E. L., Michelsen, N. M., Ekstrom, M., … Schiffman, J. (2013). Premorbid teacher-rated social functioning predicts adult schizophrenia-spectrum disorder: a high-risk prospective investigation. *Schizophrenia Research, 151*(1), 270–273. https://doi.org/10.1016/j.schres.2013.10.022.

Vallarino, M., Henry, C., Etain, B., Gehue, L. J., Macneil, C., Scott, E. M., … Scott, J. (2015). An evidence map of psychosocial interventions for the earliest stages of bipolar disorder. *The Lancet Psychiatry, 2*(6), 548–563. https://doi.org/10.1016/s2215-0366(15)00156-x.

Watson, A. C., Otey, E., Westbrook, A. L., Gardner, A. L., Lamb, T. A., Corrigan, P. W., et al. (2004). Changing middle schoolers' attitudes about mental illness through education. *Schizophrenia Bulletin, 30*(3), 563–572. https://doi.org/10.1093/oxfordjournals.schbul.a007100.

Young, S. L., Taylor, M., & Lawrie, S. M. (2015). First do no harm. A systematic review of the prevalence and management of antipsychotic adverse effects. *Journal of Psychopharmacology, 29*(4), 353–362.

Chapter 8
Effective Medications for Treating Mood Dysregulation Disorders in School-Aged Youth

Elizabeth C. Grier, Elizabeth H. Jeffords and Kristen E. Dewey

Bipolar disorder (BD) is a neurobiological disorder (APA, 2013; Strakowski, DelBello, & Adler, 2015) affecting mood. It is highly heritable, often considered progressive and characterized by distinct periods of manic (i.e., abnormally elevated or irritable mood with increased activity) and depressive (e.g., feelings of sadness or anhedonia) episodes leading to severe impairment in functioning (Goldstein et al., 2017). These impairments have an impact in the school setting. For example, adolescents diagnosed with BD are often hospitalized resulting in time away from academic instruction. They are at greater risk for substance abuse and suicidal behaviors. Finally, they often have poor peer relationships which may prevent them from successfully engaging with others in the school setting (Birmaher & Axelson, 2006). Early bipolar prevalence studies estimated that up to 3.3% of the general population of children experience this condition (Copeland, Angold, Costello, & Egger, 2013) while more recent ones suggest occurrences of 8.2% in the general population with rates up to 31% in the clinical population (Benarous et al., 2017).

There are two types of BD, with Bipolar 1 representing a more severe disturbance in mood than Bipolar 2. While the DSM-5 criteria identify children as potentially having depressive episodes, the benchmarks for manic and hypomanic episodes do not refer to children (APA, 2013). Children have been reported to manifest manic symptoms differently or to a lesser extent than adults (Rao, 2014) often showing severe irritability, lack of clear episodes, a mixed presentation, chronic course, and coexisting disorders (Margulies, Weintraub, Basile, Grover, & Carson, 2012). The current DSM-5 standards do not eliminate the possibility of a diagnosis of BD in children, but the guidelines are not clear in specifying the duration of the vacillating mood symptoms (APA, 2013). While more is being understood about BD in children,

E. C. Grier (✉) · E. H. Jeffords
Independent Private Practice, Columbia, SC, USA
e-mail: betsygrier@me.com

K. E. Dewey
The Ohio State University, Columbus, SC, USA

J. S. Carlson and J. A. Barterian (eds.), *School Psychopharmacology*,
Pediatric School Psychology, https://doi.org/10.1007/978-3-030-15541-4_8

uncertainties persist about the diagnostic criteria, clinical presentation, and treatment approaches for children (Goldstein et al., 2017; Parry & Levin, 2012).

The newer and equally controversial diagnostic category Disruptive Mood Dysregulation Disorder (DMDD; APA, 2013; Baweja et al., 2016b) evolved as a solution from the debate surrounding the BD diagnosis. Diagnostic criteria for DMDD include chronic irritability in combination with severe temper outbursts at least three times each week, which have been occurring for at least 12 months with no symptom-free period for 3 months, and interference with development in more than one setting. Symptoms typically begin before age 10; however, a child must be 6 years old before the diagnosis can be considered (APA, 2013). With the introduction of DMDD, researchers have been hopeful of the beneficial effects of offering a less severe diagnostic alternative to children whose symptoms of chronic irritability do not evolve into BD (Faheem, Petti, & Mellos 2017; Towbin & Leibenluft, 2015) as well as develop effective treatments for this population. The rate of BD diagnosis in children has declined since DMDD was introduced (Faheem, Petti, & Mellos, 2017; Goldstein et al., 2017). Current research suggests that DMDD does not seem to persist into adulthood, is different from episodic or cycling BD which presents in late adolescence and adulthood, is more associated with affect and likely to predict unipolar depression, and frequently coexists with emotional and behavioral disorders (APA, 2013; Dougherty et al., 2014; Goldstein et al., 2017; Lochman et al., 2015; Parry & Levin, 2012). The few studies available estimate that 3% of the population meet criteria for DMDD (Towbin & Leibenluft, 2015), while up to 8–9% of young children meet criteria for the disorder (Grau et al., 2017). Prevalence rates appear to decline as children get older. Functional impairments associated with the disorder can have a significant impact on academic progress and behavior at school. Children diagnosed with DMDD are more likely to be suspended and miss instruction time. Moreover, some research suggests that DMDD may negatively impact relationships between children and their teachers (Copeland et al., 2013).

Psychopharmacological Treatment of Mood Disorders in Children

Given the severity of symptoms exhibited by children with mood instability, the use of medication is a primary consideration and part of the broader treatment plan, which includes psychosocial treatments (Goldstein et al., 2017). The use of more than one medication is often required to stabilize symptoms when monotherapy is unsuccessful. A growing number of Randomized Controlled Studies (RCTs) support the use of psychopharmacological treatment in children with BD. However, there is a paucity of well-designed psychopharmacological treatment studies for DMDD (Tourian et al., 2014; Towbin & Leibenluft, 2015). In practice, the approach taken by prescribers has been similar between the two disorders (Faheem et al., 2017).

The most commonly prescribed classes of medication for BD are mood stabilizers and antipsychotics (Lytle, Moratschek, & Findling, 2015). Antipsychotics are typically used first due to more rapid symptom relief and a reduction in manic symptoms (Cullins, Call, & Joshi, 2016). For DMDD, which is classified as a depressive disorder, an antidepressant is typically the first choice (Chen, Wang, & Fang, 2016). Some other studies for DMDD have investigated stimulant monotherapy or an atypical antipsychotic in conjunction with a stimulant and antidepressant (Benarous et al., 2017; Lytle et al., 2015). Given the lack of available studies, medication treatment for DMDD is typically driven by the individual symptoms often associated with coexisting disorders affecting the child (Stringaris, Vidal-Ribas, Brotman, & Leinbenluft, 2017; Tourian et al., 2014).

Antipsychotics

Research has demonstrated that second-generation antipsychotics (SGAs; "atypical antipsychotics") control psychotic symptoms (e.g., delusions and hallucinations), stabilize mood, and decrease agitation (Goldstein et al., 2017) by blocking both dopamine and serotonin. The Food and Drug Administration (FDA) recently approved risperidone and aripiprazole to manage mania in youth. A randomized clinical trial examining aripiprazole in children and adolescents diagnosed with Bipolar 1 disorder across 30 weeks found the medication demonstrated long-term benefits for managing manic and mixed mood states; however, many families discontinued treatment prior to the completion of the study (Findling et al., 2013a). Moreover, a recent randomized control study conducted in multiple countries including 347 participants found that lurasidone significantly reduced symptoms of BD depression in children diagnosed with Bipolar 1 disorder (DelBello et al., 2017). Some research has demonstrated the utility of atypical antipsychotics for children who do not respond to mood stabilizers. For example, Walkup and colleagues (2015) found that children of ages 6–15 years old who did not respond well to initial treatment with lithium or divalproex showed benefits when switching to risperidone. They also may be used in combination with mood stabilizers to aid in controlling the aggression exhibited by some children with BD (Lytle, Moratschek, & Findling, 2015).

Preliminary findings also demonstrate that risperidone is particularly effective in minimizing the irritability often observed in DMDD (Benarous et al., 2017) and severe mood dysregulation (Krieger & Stringaris, 2013) as well as lessening aggression that persists after stimulant use for DMDD (Baweja et al., 2016b). Risperidone has also demonstrated utility in reducing aggression in children with ADHD and disruptive behavior disorders (Aman et al., 2014), which may be useful in mitigating these symptoms in DMDD (Chen, Wang, & Fan, 2016). Paliperidone is an SGA that is FDA approved for adolescents with schizoaffective disorder. As a monotherapy, it resulted in clinically significant reductions in manic symptoms as well as improvements in coexisting ADHD behaviors and psychosis; weight gain side effects were concerning but less so than with risperidone (Joshi et al., 2013). School mental health professionals should be aware of the possibility of weight gain and motor tremors when children are prescribed atypical antipsychotics, but the list of potential side effects for atypical antipsychotics is less daunting than those associated with lithium and anticonvulsants. See Table 8.1 for review.

Mood Stabilizers/Anticonvulsants

These medicines are used to alleviate alternating symptoms of mania or depression and to control mood cycling (Lytle et al., 2015). This class of medications may take a few weeks to demonstrate effectiveness and primarily includes lithium. The exact mechanism through which lithium works is unclear and is likely complex, involving numerous neurotransmitters (Rappaport, Kulick, & Phelps, 2013). The FDA has approved lithium for use only in children older than 12 years of age for symptoms of Bipolar I. Various studies have demonstrated the positive impact of lithium on mood for youth (Lytle et al., 2015); yet, complete remission of symptoms has not been found (Findling et al., 2013a) and considerable variability in symptom improvement is noted (Findling et al., 2013b). Lithium has been used in combination with other psychiatric medications. For example, one study found that quetiapine or risperidone in combination with lithium results in improvements in Bipolar 1 symptoms with quetiapine having fewer side effects (Habibi, Dodangi, & Nazeri, 2017). Despite the noted improvements in BD symptoms, a recent investigation indicated that lithium did not work better than placebo in a youth with severe mood dysregulation (Benarous et al., 2017) meaning this type of medicine would not be the first line of treatment for DMDD. Lithium has a range of side effects requiring close monitoring (Lytle et al., 2015) including increased thirst resulting in increased urination. Other side effects can be associated with lithium toxicity: blurred vision, excessive hand tremors that interfere with hand use and cause poor coordination, feeling ill, vomiting, diarrhea, and ataxia. See Table 8.2 for review.

Anticonvulsants also stabilize mood via enhanced GABA function. Divalproex (i.e., valproic acid, depakene, depakote, depakote XR) is an anticonvulsant medication used to treat seizures, prevent migraines, and manage mood cycling. In adults, divalproex has been effective in treating mixed episodes and rapid cycling (Lytle et al., 2015). Carbamazepine (i.e., Tegretol) is an anticonvulsant medication also used to treat BD, showing efficacy in adults with both euphoric and mixed manic episodes. Carbamazepine has shown some effectiveness in youth with bipolar mania, especially when combined with other medicines; as monotherapy, it did not show the benefits that divalproex and lithium showed (Nandagopal, DelBello, & Kowatch, 2009). Lamotrigine (Lamictal) may be beneficial for bipolar depression in children (Goldstein et al., 2017; Lytle et al., 2015), especially adolescents (Findling et al., 2015). However, carbamazepine and lamotrigine are not FDA-approved for BD treatment in children.

As with lithium, patients taking anticonvulsants may experience fatigue, dry mouth, tremor, and weight gain. There is also significant potential for negative

Table 8.1 Atypical antipsychotics

Generic	Brand	FDA approval	General benefits, mechanism of action, and side effects	Evidence and frequency of use in children and adolescents	
				BD	DMDD
Olanzapine	Zyprexa	BD 1: ages 13–17 BD 1 depression symptoms: ages 10 and up with combination of fluoxetine	• Atypical, second generation, antipsychotics can manage mood. • They block dopamine and serotonin • Side effects include weight gain and motor tremors	• High evidence • Often used	• Little/no evidence • Sometimes used for symptoms of aggression and irritability
Quetiapine	Seroquel	BD 1: ages 10–17			
Clozapine	Clozaril	Not approved for BD or DMDD in children/adolescents			
Aripiprazole	Abilify	BD 1: ages 10–17			
Ziprasidone	Geodon	Not approved for BD or DMDD in children/adolescents			
Paliperidone	Invega	Not approved for BDD or DMDD in children/adolescents			
Asenapine	Saphris	BD 1: ages 10–17			
Larasidone	Latuda	BD 1: ages 10–17			

BD Bipolar Disorder; *DMDD* Disruptive Mood Dysregulation Disorder; *FDA* Food and Drug Administration

Table 8.2 Mood stabilizer

Generic	Brand	FDA approval	General benefits, mechanism of action, and side effects	Evidence and frequency of use in children and adolescents	
				BD	DMDD
Lithium	Lithium salts	BD 1: ages 12–17	• It is a mineral and it is the most researched medication for BD in adults. • It evens temperament and calms mood. It reduces the risk of suicide • The mechanism of action is unclear, but it is believed to decrease norepinephrine and to increase the release of serotonin • Initial side effects include increased thirst and urination as well as hand shakiness, tiredness, and weight gain. Serious side effects include blurred vision, excessive hand trembling/poor coordination, feeling ill, vomiting, diarrhea, and ataxia. • Blood levels must be monitored closely to prevent lithium toxicity	• High evidence • Commonly used	• Little/no evidence • Infrequently used

BD Bipolar Disorder; *DMDD* Disruptive Mood Dysregulation Disorder; *FDA* Food and Drug Administration

drug interaction effects, and long-term use of these medications can impair liver and kidney function and interfere with blood platelet formation. Divalproex specifically may cause sedation as well as liver toxicity, thrombocytopenia, pancreatitis, and polycystic ovary disease. Patients are screened for these potential complications using periodic blood tests. Carbamazepine may cause sedation, dizziness as well as agranulocytosis (i.e., a deficiency in white blood cells). Lamotrigine may cause sedation and dizziness along with a severe reaction known as Stevens–Johnson syndrome (i.e., a serious skin disorder marked by a painful red rash), which requires immediate medical attention. See Table 8.3 for review.

Antidepressants

These medications primarily include Selective Serotonin Reuptake Inhibitors (SSRIs) and work by blocking the serotonin from leaving the synapse between the neurons. SSRIs have been effective in reducing depressive symptoms in BD after mood stabilization (Lytle et al., 2015). SSRIs have also been effective in treating anxiety disorders that may coexist with BD and DMDD. Healthcare providers must proceed with caution when using SSRIs as they can cause activation that may be misinterpreted as mania and/or ADHD. Two studies are in progress to determine the efficacy of treating irritability using SSRIs (Benarous et al., 2017), but little research is currently available about the effectiveness of these medications for DMDD. Even so, antidepressants are sometimes added to the medication regimen if the child is experiencing chronic symptoms of sadness, melancholy, or other symptoms of depressed mood. The two approved for children for treatment of depression, and/or OCD, fluoxetine, and sertraline can be very helpful but are not without significant side effects. There have been some reports of increased risk of suicidal ideation when children and adolescents first begin taking the medicine. Other side effects include stomachaches, headaches, agitation/activation, apathy, and issues with drug interactions. See Table 8.4 for a review.

Stimulants

Stimulants are the main class of medications used to treat ADHD in children and include medications such as methylphenidate (e.g., Ritalin) and amphetamine derivatives (e.g., Adderall). They work by increasing the levels of dopamine and norepinephrine in the prefrontal cortex. Extensive research has supported their safety and efficacy in treating ADHD, but some scholars believe that stimulants are ineffective in the treatment of BD and may actually induce mania in some children (Baweja et al., 2016; Barkley, 2015). However, if ADHD coexists with BD, the addition of a stimulant as adjunct therapy can be useful after mood stabilization has occurred (Lytle et al., 2015; Schneck, Chang, Singh, Delbello, & Miklowitz, 2017). Interest-

Table 8.3 Anticonvulsant/mood stabilizer

Generic	Brand	FDA approval	General benefits, mechanism of action, and side effects	Evidence and frequency of use in children and adolescents	
				BD	DMDD
Divalproex	Valproic acid Depakene Depakote	Not approved for BD or DMDD in children/adolescents	• Manage seizure activity by stopping the excessive firing of neurons, but they also stabilize mood by enhancing GABA function • Dizziness, drowsiness, fatigue, tremor, dry mouth, and weight gain can occur. These can have negative drug interaction effects. • Long-term this type of medication can affect kidney and liver function and development of blood platelets	• Moderate evidence • Commonly used	• Little/no evidence • Infrequently used
Carbamazepine	Tegretol	Not approved for BD or DMDD in children/adolescents			
Lamotrigine	Lamictal	Not approved for BD or DMDD in children/adolescents			

BD Bipolar Disorder; *DMDD* Disruptive Mood Dysregulation Disorder

Table 8.4 Antidepressant

Generic	Brand	FDA approval	General benefits, mechanism of action, and side effects	Evidence and frequency of use in children and adolescents	
				BD	DMDD
Fluoxetine	Prozac	BD 1 depression symptoms: ages 10 and up with combination of olanzapine	• In children and adolescents, Selective Serotonin Reuptake Inhibitors (SSRI) are commonly used. • These reduce depression, lessen irritability, and calm anxiety • Side effects include heightened risk for suicidal ideation initially, stomach distress, headaches, agitation/activation, apathy, and problems with drug interactions	• Some evidence for anxiety and depression management once mood is stable • Commonly used for secondary symptoms	• Medium evidence • Often used
Sertraline	Zoloft	Not approved for BD or DMDD in children/adolescents			
Escitalopram	Lexapro	Not approved for BD or DMDD in children/adolescents			

BD Bipolar Disorder; *DMDD* Disruptive Mood Dysregulation Disorder; *FDA* Food and Drug Administration

ingly, Benarous and colleagues (2017) describe stimulant medications as being partly efficacious for coexisting ADHD and Severe Mood Dysregulation (SMD) as well as beneficial in lessening irritability and aspects of aggression. Decreased externalizing symptoms and slightly improved mood were seen in children with DMDD with the use of stimulants only, but ongoing impairment suggested the need for additional medication treatments to support best functioning (Baweja et al., 2016). In regard to side effects, as mentioned, some children with BD may have manic symptoms triggered by these stimulant medicines; however, this is not the case for children diagnosed with DMDD (Baweja et al., 2016; Stringaris, DelBello, & Adler, 2017). Decreased appetite is a very common side effect. And, some children experience difficulty getting to sleep and increased anxiety. See Table 8.5 for review.

Contraindications

A combination of medications is often required to best manage mood disorder symptoms. Therefore, prescribers should be well versed in treating mood disorders when prescribing medications. Many potential adverse events can be avoided (e.g., manic activation) by ensuring mood symptoms are stabilized before another medication is added to improve depression or attention. Moreover, if BD is diagnosed, unipolar depressive versus manic/mixed mood guides the initial medication choice of mood stabilizer or antipsychotic used (AACAP, 2007) with careful attention to family history, coexisting symptoms, and activation of behaviors from other medications used previously. If DMDD is diagnosed, the most disruptive symptoms are typically treated first (e.g., chronic irritability, extreme emotional outbursts, or aggression).

Treatment Guidelines

Treatment guidelines for children with BD and depressive disorders are largely based on replicated research completed in adults, though researchers have been studying treatment algorithms to offer guidance for psychopharmacological treatment to better help youth with BD and DMDD (e.g., Kowatch et al., 2005; Stringaris et al., 2017) with clearly delineated practice parameters for BD provided by the American Academy of Child and Adolescent Psychiatry (AACAP) in 2007. Guidelines from AACAP for BD include: (1) psychological assessment to determine the presence of a mood disorder as well as comorbid issues (e.g., suicidality, medical problems); (2) treatment with an agent that is approved for bipolar disorder in adults given the limited evidence available for such treatments in children (e.g., lithium, aripiprazole, valproate, and lamotrigine); (3) psychopharmacological maintenance treatment if necessary to prevent relapse; (4) baseline and follow-up assessment, side effect monitoring, and lab monitoring ensure psychopharmacological treatment is effective and well tolerated; and (5) evidence-based psychosocial interventions. At the time

Table 8.5 Stimulant

Generic	Brand	FDA approval	General benefits, mechanism of action, and side effects	Evidence and frequency of use in children and adolescents	
				BD	DMDD
Methylphenidate	Ritalin, Ritalin, LA, Concerta, Focalin, Focalin XR, Daytrana Quillivant, Quillichew, Metadate, Aptensio, Contempla, and Methylin	Not approved for BD or DMDD in children/adolescents	• They increase neurotransmitter communication of dopamine and neuroepinephrine, especially in the frontal lobes. • Methylphenidates limit the reuptake of the neurotransmitters while amphetamines release them. • Stimulants enhance alertness, focus, and impulse control while calming hyperactivity • They can reduce appetite, interfere with sleep, and aggravate anxiety. In an individual with BD disorder, they may induce mania	• Commonly used for secondary symptoms • Some evidence for ADHD symptom improvement, after mood is stable	• High evidence for ADHD symptom improvement after irritability is addressed. • Often used
Amphetamine derivatives	Adderall, Procentra, Evekeo, Zenzedi, Vyvanse, Adzenys, Dexedrine, and Mydayis	Not approved for BD or DMDD in children/adolescents			

BD Bipolar Disorder; *DMDD* Disruptive Mood Dysregulation Disorder; *FDA* Food and Drug Administration

this chapter was written, the authors were not aware of any guidelines published by a professional organization for the treatment of DMDD.

Implications for School Personnel

Psychopharmacological treatment of mood disorders and behavioral symptoms in children with BD and DMDD is challenging given the complexities surrounding the initial diagnosis. A comprehensive assessment by a trained professional well versed in DMMD and BD is essential, as it reduces the possibility of negative side effects from medications that are not appropriate (Faheem et al., 2017). School mental health professionals and parents can play an important role by documenting behaviors, changes in mood, and sleep patterns, as medication and other interventions are initiated, to guide treatment. School mental health providers should be familiar with current diagnostic guidelines in the DSM-5, stay abreast of the research, and work collaboratively with all family members and professionals who are part of the treatment team. Diligent follow-up and progress monitoring are imperative due to potential side effects and individual variations in responses to medications. Medication contraindications should be routinely and systematically monitored. School mental health professionals are well positioned to collect this information and disseminate it to others on the treatment team (e.g., psychiatrists, parents, and teachers). See communication and tracking tool in Fig. 8.1 as an example of a communication tool for documenting and sharing this information with members of the treatment team.

School mental health professionals can provide support and resources to families and educators. Parents of children with mood disorders are an easy target of criticism from relatives, community members, and school personnel. Rather than assigning blame, the parents' efforts to seek help need to be supported and used as a foundation for building their resilience in caring for their child with special needs. Clinicians and educators must look for opportunities to support the family system so that parents can sustain the energy needed for the medication trials and new behavioral interventions that they will need to implement. Additionally, with consent, school mental health providers can provide psychoeducation to school staff (e.g., staff, teachers, and administrators) so these professionals have insight into behaviors a child may be exhibiting. Additionally, educating school professionals provides additional observers to watch for adverse events or signs that a medication is not improving functioning.

School mental health professionals can provide psychosocial treatments to children diagnosed with a mood disorder. At this time, the research base on specific therapeutic and psychosocial treatment protocols for children with DMDD and BD is still emerging. However, some guidelines do exist that outline treatment approaches and initial treatment effectiveness with individuals, groups, and families particularly for reducing symptoms of irritability (Waxmonsky et al., 2016) and improving emotional regulation while lessening aggression (Masi et al., 2016). Initial research has sug-

Pediatrician, Educator, & Parent Communication Tool

PEDIATRIC SCHOOL PSYCHOLOGY: EVALUATION AND CONSULTATION SERVICES, LLC

PEDIATRICIAN, EDUCATOR, & PARENT COMMUNICATION TOOL

Dear ______________________________: Your student, ____________________, is in my office today and his/her parents have expressed concern about his/her learning and/or behavior. I have asked for and received permission to communicate with you from the parents as indicated below:

PERMISSION TO DISCUSS CHILD'S PROGRESS

I, ______________________________, give permission for my child's teacher to talk back and forth with my child's
NAME OF PARENT OR LEGAL CAREGIVER

pediatrician, ______________________________, in order for us to work together to support my child's best learning
NAME OF PEDIATRICIAN

~~learning~~ and behavior in the classroom. Signed, ____,
SIGNATURE OF PARENT AND/OR LEGAL CAREGIVER

Parent or Legal Caregiver to ____. Date: ____________________.
CHILD'S FIRST & LAST NAME AND BIRTHDAY TODAY'S DATE

PEDIATRICIAN'S QUESTIONS & CONCERNS FOR CHILD

See circled information & notes below for a summary of my potential concerns and the parent (s) reports from today's appointment:

Potential Mood & Anxiety Issues	Potential Activity Level & Impulsivity Issues	At Home Parents ~~Report~~ Observe	
easily distracted	excessively talkative or fidgety	Attention in daily routine is:	poor fair good
difficulty staying focused	leaves chair when expected to sit	Attention for homework is:	poor fair good
does not listen well	interrupts or talks out in class	Activity level in play is:	too low average too high
Is irritable & whiny	climbs or always moving	Activity level during mealtime is:	too low average too high
easily frustrated when has to put more effort into things	difficulty interacting as positively as expected for age	Understanding of "rules" guiding social communication is:	poor fair good
Wants things his/her way	lack of self-control	Ability to follow through on directions is:	poor fair good
easily stressed	acts without thinking	Ability to deal with stress and disappointment is:	poor fair good
other	other	other	

EDUCATOR'S QUESTIONS & CONCERNS FOR CHILD

Please advise me of any issues you have concerns about by putting YOUR INITIALS beside the relevant behaviors listed in the table above. I would also appreciate feedback about what you, your school psychologist, etc. may have already done to support this child if you have had concerns (circle relevant items):

- parent-teacher meeting, *specify dates and results of meeting*______________________________
- general accommodations in the classroom, *such as preferential seating, frequent redirection, movement, other*____________
- student intervention team meeting
- RTI or response to intervention support for academics or behavior (*specific how much)*_______ ____________________
- 504 plan (*specify date started and details*______________________________
- IEP meeting (*specify date started and details*______________________________
- OTHER______________________________

Please fax this form directly back to my child's pediatrician to this number: ____________________________. Please keep this original
DIRECT FAX TO PEDIATRICIAN

form for your records, and please feel free to fax additional information or call my pediatrician's office at ______________. Ask for the pediatrician's nurse, ______________. **THANK YOU VERY MUCH FOR YOUR COMMUNICATION & COLLABORATION!**

September 2017 COMMUNICATION TOOL
Created By: Betsy C. Grier, Ph.D., NCSP
For More Information: betsygrier@me.com

Fig. 8.1 Pediatrician, educator, and parent communication tool

gested that cognitive-behavioral therapeutic strategies and family psychoeducational approaches may be effective in the treatment of BD and DMDD in school-aged youth (Benarous et al., 2017; Miklowitz, 2015; Waxmonsky et al., 2013). The involvement of the family in the child's treatment is critical (e.g., Goldstein et al., 2017).

Several avenues of school-based intervention are available for the child with mood dysregulation. These children are at risk to struggle to understand assignments because of issues such as their preoccupation with mood fluctuations, their fatigue, and their general distractibility. Others may actively avoid doing schoolwork and resist following directions when they are more irritable or sad. A number of education models can be considered. Children with mood disorders can be served in general education, special education, or a combination of these services. A formal plan can be developed under Section 504 of the Rehabilitation Act if the disorder substantially limits the child's potential to benefit from education. Generally, this type of plan is implemented through accommodations in the general education classroom and/or within the school environment, but it can also include behavior plans and school-based counseling. Under IDEA, an Individual Education Plan (IEP) can be created under the "Emotional Disability" or "Other Health Impaired" categories if the disorder adversely affects the child's learning.

A variety of professionals at school can support children with BD and DMDD including teachers, guidance counselors, social workers, school nurses, administrators, and school psychologists. All school personnel have the opportunity to provide beneficial support to the family members of the child with BD through efforts to provide a calm and caring environment. School psychologists should play a key role and are equipped with the basic skills necessary to be an advocate and direct service provider for students with challenging behaviors associated with BD or DMMD. The importance of a good teacher–student match cannot be overstated. Teachers must be aware of the child's issues (e.g., types of medications and nature of diagnostic pattern) so that they can help describe behaviors associated with school performance, energy level, mood, and social interactions to support treatment. Creating a safe "calm down" area in the room can provide a much-needed opportunity to support the student's self-regulation. School administrators' primary responsibility should involve establishing a collaborative intervention plan with the child's team (e.g., parents, teachers, mental health professionals, and medical providers) to encourage communication.

Summary

Disorders of mood dysregulation in children include BD and DMDD. Research continues to provide more data on the biology, onset, diagnostic profile, course, treatment efficacy, and outcome of these disorders with more information available for BD than DMDD at this time. Currently, best practice in intervention typically takes the form of a combination of psychotropic medication, family intervention, and school supports for the child. Medications include antipsychotics, mood stabilizers/anticonvulsants, antidepressants, and stimulants. Medication treatment for bipolar disorder has been modeled from efficacious treatments with adults; however, more research is necessary to establish the safety and efficacy of many of these medication treatments in the child and adolescent population. School mental health professionals are well positioned to play an integral role in the treatment of children with mood disorders, including conducting a comprehensive assessment, monitoring treatment outcomes including side effects, supporting families, educating teachers and other school staff, providing psychosocial interventions, and identifying appropriate educational settings/accommodations. While medication treatment especially has been highlighted in this chapter, it is vital to give equal attention to family education and active skill building via intervention, therapy, and counseling to best support the child's success in all areas.

List of Websites

https://www.nimh.nih.gov/health/publications/bipolar-disorder-in-children-and-teens/index.shtml

The National Institute for Mental Health is a federal agency focused on mental health research. The webpage on BD in children and teens provides an easy to read description of the symptoms and treatment options. Ideas for ways parents can support their children are included.

http://www.mentalhealthamerica.net/conditions/bipolar-disorder-children

Mental Health America is a community based non-profit association that focuses on early identification and well-coordinated treatment for individuals with mental health concerns. A brief description of BD in children with a focus on symptomology and links to other helpful websites is offered.

https://www.nimh.nih.gov/health/topics/disruptive-mood-dysregulation-disorder-dmdd/disruptive-mood-dysregulation-disorder.shtml

This is another information page from the National Institute for Mental Health, and it is one of the few research based sites that focuses on disruptive mood dysregulation disorder. Readers will find an excellent overview of DMDD symptoms and interventions including common classes of medications used to treat the symptoms.

Suggested Readings

Jamieson, P. E. 2006. *Mind race: A firsthand account of one teenager's experience with bipolar disorder.* Oxford US.

A fascinating window into the experience of having BD as a teenager and the journey towards finding effective treatment. The author also includes very informative descriptions of BD symptoms, treatment and ideas for navigating the daily routine more effectively.

Strakowski, S. M., DelBello, M. P., & Adler, C. M. (2015). *Bipolar Disorder in Youth: Presentation, Treatment, & Neurobiology.* Oxford US.

An excellent evidenced-based review of BD in children, including history of the disorder, differential diagnosis, treatment, and neurobiological understanding. A variety of researchers contribute to provide a comprehensive review.

References

Aman, M. G., Bukstein, O. G., Gadow, K. D., Arnold, L. E., Molina, B. S., McNamara, N. K., ... Butter, E. M. (2014). What does risperidone add to parent training and stimulant for severe aggression in child attention-deficit/hyperactivity disorder? *Journal of the American Academy of Child & Adolescent Psychiatry*, *53*(1), 47–60.

American Academy of Child and Adolescent Psychiatry. (2007). Practice parameter for the assessment and treatment of children and adolescents with bipolar disorder. *American Academy of Child and Adolescent Psychiatry, 46,* 107–125.

American Psychiatric Association. (2013). *Diagnostic and statistical manual of mental disorders* (5th ed.). Washington, DC: APA.

Barkley, R. A. (2015). *Attention-deficit hyperactivity disorder: A handbook for diagnosis and treatment* (4th ed.). New York: The Guilford Press.

Baweja, R., Belin, P. J., Humphrey, H. H., Babocsai, L., Pariseau, M. E., Waschbusch, D. A., ... Waxmonsky, J. G. (2016a). The effectiveness and tolerability of central nervous system stimulants in school-age children with attention-deficit/hyperactivity disorder and disruptive mood dysregulation disorder across home and school. *Journal of child and adolescent psychopharmacology*, *26*(2), 154–163.

Baweja, R., Mayes, S. D., Hameed, U., & Waxmonsky, J. G. (2016b). Disruptive mood dysregulation disorder: Current insights. *Neuropsychiatric Disease and Treatment, 12,* 2115.

Benarous, X., Consoli, A., Guile, J. M., Garny de La Riviere, S., Cohen, D., & Olliac, B. (2017). Evidence-based treatments for youths with severely dysregulated mood: a qualitative systematic review of trials for SMD and DMDD. *European Child and Adolescent Psychiatry*, *26,* 5–23.

Birmaher, B., & Axelson, D. (2006). Course and outcome of bipolar spectrum disorder in children and adolescents: A review of the existing literature. *Development and Psychopathology, 18*(4), 1023–1035.

Chen, J., Wang, Z., & Fang, Y. (2016). The history, diagnosis and treatment of disruptive mood dysregulation disorder. *Shanghai Archives of Psychiatry, 28*(5), 289–292.

Copeland, W. E., Angold, A., Costello, E. J., & Egger, H. (2013). Prevalence, comorbidity, and correlates of DSM-5 proposed disruptive mood dysregulation disorder. *The American Journal of Psychiatry, 170*(2), 173–179.

Cullins, L. M., Call, D. C., & Joshi, P. T. (2016). Pediatric bipolar disorders: Current understanding and management. In S. Malhotra & P. Santosh (Eds.), *Child and adolescent psychiatry* (pp. 3–17). New Delhi, India: Springer.

DelBello, M. P., Goldman, R., Phillips, D., Deng, L., Cucchiaro, J., & Loebel, A. (2017). Efficacy and safety of larasidone in children and adolescents with bipolar I depression: A double blind, placebo-controlled study. *Journal of the American Academy of Child and Adolescent Psychiatry, 56*(12), 1015–1025.

Dougherty, L. R., Smith, V. C., Bufferd, S. J., Carlson, G. A., Stringaris, A., Leibenluft, E., et al. (2014). DSM-5 disruptive mood dysregulation disorder: Correlates and predictors in young children. *Psychological Medicine, 44*(11), 2339–2350.
Goldstein, B. I., Birmaher, B., Carlson, G. A., Delbello, M. P., Findling, R. L., Fristad, M., et al. (2017). The international society for bipolar disorders task force report on pediatric bipolar disorder: Knowledge to date and directions for future research. *Bipolar Disorders, 19*(7), 524–543.
Grau, K., Plener, P. L., Hohmann, S., Fegert, J. M., Brähler, E., & Straub, J. (2017). Prevalence rate and course of symptoms of disruptive mood dysregulation disorder (DMDD). *Zeitschrift fur Kinder-und Jugendpsychiatriie und Psychotherapie,* 1–8.
Faheem, S., Petti, V., & Mellos, G. (2017). Disruptive mood dysregulation disorder and its effect on bipolar disorder. *Annals of Clinical Psychiatry, 29*(2), 84–91.
Findling, R. L., Chang, K., Robb, A., Foster, V. J., Horrigan, J., Krishen, A., et al. (2015). Adjunctive maintenance lamotrigine for pediatric bipolar I disorder: A placebo-controlled, randomized withdrawal study. *Journal of the American Academy of Child and Adolescent Psychiatry, 54*(12), 1020–1021.
Findling, R. L., Correll, C. U., Nyilas, M., Forbes, R. A., McQuade, R. D., Jin, N., … Carlson, G. A. (2013a). Aripiprazole for the treatment of pediatric bipolar I disorder: A 30-week, randomized placebo-controlled study. *Bipolar Disorders, 15*(2), 138–149.
Findling, R. L., Kafantaris, V., Pavuluri, M., McNamara, N. K., Frazier, J. A., Sikich, L., … & Taylor-Zapata, P. (2013b). Post-acute effectiveness of lithium in pediatric bipolar I disorder. *Journal of child and adolescent psychopharmacology, 23*(2), 80–90.
Habibi, N., Dodangi, N., & Nazeri, A. (2017). Comparison of the effect of lithium plus quetiapine with lithium plus risperidone in children and adolescents with bipolar I disorder: A randomized clinical trial. *Medical Journal of the Islamic Republic of Iran,* 1–7.
Joshi, G., Petty, C., Wozniak, J., Faraone, S., Spencer, A., Woodworth, K., et al. (2013). A prospective open-label trail of paliperidone monotherapy for the treatment of bipolar spectrum disorders in children and adolescents. *Psychopharmacology (Berl), 227*(3), 449–458.
Kowatch, R. A., Fristad, M., Birmaher, B., Wagner, K. D., Findling, R. L., & Hellander, M. (2005). Treatment guidelines for children and adolescents with bipolar disorder: Child psychiatric workgroup on bipolar disorder. *Journal of American Academy of Children and Adolescent Psychiatry, 4,* 213–235.
Krieger, F. V., & Stringaris, A. (2013). Bipolar disorder and disruptive mood dysregulation in children and adolescents: Assessment, diagnosis and treatment. *Evidenced Based Mental Health, 16,* 93–94.
Lochman, J. E., Evans, S. C., Burke, J. D., Roberts, M. C., Fite, P. J., Reed, G. M., et al. (2015). An empirically based alternative to DSM-5's disruptive mood dysregulation disorder for ICD-11. *World Psychiatry, 14*(1), 30–33.
Lytle, S. M., Moratschek, S. K., & Findling, R. L. (2015). Medical treatment strategies for young people with bipolar disorder. In S. M. Strakowski, M. P. DelBello, & C. M. Adler (Eds.), *Bipolar disorder in youth: Presentation, treatment, and neurobiology* (pp. 156–188). Oxford: Oxford University Press.
Margulies, D. M., Weintraub, S., Basile, J., Grover, P. J., & Carson, G. A. (2012). Will disruptive mood dysregulation disorder reduce false diagnosis of bipolar disorder in children? *Bipolar Disorders, 14,* 488–496.
Masi, G., Milone, A., Madfredi, A., Brovedi, P., Pisano, S., & Muratori, P. (2016). Combined pharmacotherapy-multimodal psychotherapy in children with disruptive behavior disorders. *Psychiatric Research, 238,* 8–13.
Miklowitz, D. J. (2015). Psychotherapeutic strategies for treating youth with or at risk for bipolar disorder. In S. M. Strakowski, M. P. DelBello, & C. M. Adler (Eds.), *Bipolar disorder in youth: Presentation, treatment, and neurobiology* (pp. 189–204). Oxford: Oxford University Press.
Nandagopal, J. J., Delbello, M. P., & Kowatch, R. (2009). Pharmacologic treatment of pediatric bipolar disorder. *Child and Adolescent Psychiatric Clinic, 18,* 455–469.

Parry, P. I., & Levin, E. C. (2012). Pediatric bipolar disorder in an era of "mindless psychiatry." *Journal of Trauma & Dissociation, 13*, 51–68.
Rao, U. (2014). DSM-5: Disruptive mood dysregulation disorder. *Asian Journal of Psychiatry, 11*, 119–123.
Rappaport, N., Kulick, D., & Phelps, L. (2013). Psychotropic medications: An update for school psychologists. *Psychology in the Schools, 50*(6), 589–600.
Schneck, C. D., Chang, K. D., Singh, M. K., Delbello, M. P., & Miklowitz, D. J. (2017). A pharmacologic algorithm for youth who are at high risk for bipolar disorder. *Journal of Child and Adolescent Psychopharmacology, 27*(9), 1–10.
Strakowski, S. M., DelBello, M. P., & Adler, C. M. (Eds.). (2015). *Bipolar disorder in youth: Presentation, treatment, and neurobiology*. Oxford: Oxford University Press.
Stringaris, A., Vidal-Ribas, P., Brotman, M. A., & Leibenluft, E. (2017). Practitioner review: Definition, recognition, and treatment challenges of irritability in young people. *Journal of Child Psychology & Psychiatry*, 1–19.
Tourian, L., LeBoeuf, A., Breton, J., Cohen, D., Gignac, M., Labelle, R., et al. (2014). Treatment options for the cardinal symptoms of disruptive mood dysregulation disorder. *Journal of the Canadian Academy of Child and Adolescent Psychiatry, 24*(1), 41–54.
Towbin, K. E., & Leibenluft, E. (2015). Differential diagnosis of bipolar disorder in children and youth. In S. M. Strakowski, M. P. DelBello, & C. M. Adler (Eds.), *Bipolar disorder in youth: Presentation, treatment, and neurobiology* (pp. 34–55). Oxford: Oxford University Press.
Walkup, J. T., Wagner, K. D., Miller, L., Yenokyan, G., Luby, J. L., Joshi, P. T., … Sanyal, A. (2015). Treatment of early-age mania: outcomes for partial and nonresponders to initial treatment. *Journal of the American Academy of Child & Adolescent Psychiatry, 54*(12), 1008–1019.
Waxmonsky, J. G., Waschbusch, D. A., Belin, P., Li, T., Babocsai, L., Humphery, H., … & Mazzant, J. R. (2016). A randomized clinical trial of an integrative group therapy for children with severe mood dysregulation. *Journal of the American Academy of Child & Adolescent Psychiatry, 55*(3), 196–207.
Waxmonsky, J. G., Wymbs, F. A., Pariseau, M. E., Belin, P. J., Waschbusch, D. A., Babocsai, L., … Pelham, W. E. (2013). A novel group therapy for children with ADHD and severe mood dysregulation. *Journal of attention disorders, 17*(6), 527–541.

Chapter 9
Psychotropic Medication Side Effects in School-Aged Populations

Thomas Kubiszyn, Sarah S. Mire and Allison Meinert

Introduction

The American Academy of Child and Adolescent Psychiatry (AACAP, 2015) recently identified safety concerns associated with pediatric psychotropic prescription practices (e.g., "off-label" prescribing, polypharmacy, underutilization of psychosocial treatments), and unintended and potentially dangerous medication side effects. In this chapter, we review the wide range of unwanted outcomes associated with drugs approved by the United States (US) Food and Drug Administration (FDA) and used to treat pediatric emotional and behavioral disorders (EBDs). The purpose of this chapter is to help inform risk-benefit analysis, treatment decision-making, and monitoring for unwanted outcomes. To help guide the thought processes that undergird risk-benefit analysis, we provide a framework for stakeholder's (e.g., prescribers, parents, school professionals) communications at the end of this chapter.

Risk-Benefit Analysis

Psychosocial treatments are often recommended as first-line treatments for pediatric EBDs, with psychotropic treatment recommended only after a failed psychosocial intervention trial that has been implemented with integrity (AACAP, 2015). Yet, for a variety of practical and financial reasons (e.g., urgency, ease of implementation, lack of access to appropriate psychosocial treatments, reimbursement issues) drug treatments often prevail as first-line treatments with pediatric patients (Rapoport, 2013).

T. Kubiszyn (✉) · S. S. Mire · A. Meinert
University of Houston, Houston, TX, USA
e-mail: TKubiszyn@Central.UH.EDU

J. S. Carlson and J. A. Barterian (eds.), *School Psychopharmacology*, Pediatric School Psychology, https://doi.org/10.1007/978-3-030-15541-4_9

Although solutions to practical and financial issues may not be readily available, stakeholders can help ensure that risk-benefit analysis occurs before treatment decisions are finalized, and that ongoing risk-benefit analysis is informed by evidence-based, systematic monitoring of both therapeutic and unwanted outcomes. The child's developing central nervous system (CNS) may be affected differently by drugs than the adult CNS, increasing or decreasing beneficial and/or harmful drug effects compared to adults and illustrating why the safety and efficacy of extrapolation from adult prescribing practices can be risky (Greenhill et al., 2006; Hazell & Mirzaie, 2013; Maayan & Correll, 2011). Children may also not understand or be able to accurately recognize or report side effects (i.e., they may deny, minimize or exaggerate symptoms), and may report side effects differently at home than in school or other settings. Those factors underscore the need to assess for unwanted outcomes beyond a pediatric patient's self-report, and across multiple settings.

Yet, the risk of harm from delaying drug treatment may pose safety concerns for the child or others, or effective psychosocial or other alternatives (e.g., hospitalization) may not exist or be unavailable. For example, should a drug treatment that may suppress self-destructive behavior (e.g., sexual promiscuity or aggressive behavior during a manic episode) be withheld because of the drug's possible side effects? The risk of withholding drug treatment could be judged to be unacceptably high, even if efficacy and safety data are lacking.

Scope and Nature of This Review

This chapter reviews drugs with pediatric indications (i.e., those approved by the FDA for specific conditions and age ranges) that are currently marketed in the US and prescribed for pediatric EBDs. They include four drug classes and are presented in order of frequency of use within pediatric populations (i.e., 18 years and younger) in the US (Olfson, Marcus, Weissman, & Jensen, 2002): ADHD drugs (stimulant and non-stimulant), antidepressants (ADs), second-generation antipsychotics (SGAs), and the antiepileptic drugs (AEDs) and lithium. Most of the drugs we review have indications for a variety of pediatric EBDs, but the AEDs are only FDA-approved for a medical condition (i.e., pediatric epilepsy).

This review focuses exclusively on FDA sources of information. Non-FDA sources (e.g., journal articles, web/media reports) are not used given the wide variation in inclusionary criteria, definitions, classifications, and assessment approaches across those sources. FDA data may be the most consistent, reliable, and evidence-based data we currently have about unwanted outcomes (Kubiszyn, Mire, Dutt, Papathopoulos, & Backsheider-Burridge, 2012).

The FDA safety data we summarize should not be considered to be exhaustive or predictive for any individual case. As with efficacy data, individual differences in genetic, environmental, developmental, and physiological factors may affect the safety of any drug. Notably, unwanted outcomes may not emerge during the Phase Three clinical trials that the FDA requires to evaluate safety and efficacy prior to drug approval, and the generalizability of findings from clinical trials to clinical practice may be limited by restrictive criteria applied to clinical trials (e.g., 3–13 weeks duration, single diagnoses without comorbidities, avoidance of multiple drugs or psychosocial treatments).

The FDA evaluates late-emerging outcomes (i.e., subsequent to a drug's approval after clinical trials) through its post-approval reporting systems. Sentinel, the FDA's electronic active surveillance system; https://www.sentinelinitiative.org/) became fully operational in 2016. Previously the FDA relied on a voluntary reporting system called Medwatch. Sentinel was developed because voluntary reporting resulted in underreporting of unwanted outcomes.

Our Data Source: The FDA Prescribing Information (PI)

The FDA requires that drug manufacturers publish and distribute Full Prescribing Information (PI) for each drug that is given an FDA indication or approval. Recently standardized, the PI begins with a summary called Highlights of Prescribing Information followed by more detailed information. This chapter reviews safety data from the Highlights section of the PI that are relevant to pediatric patients (e.g., Warnings about patients with dementia are not included).

Both the Highlights and Full PI sections are organized by corresponding numbers to facilitate access to desired information. The sections include Boxed Warnings (if any have been issued for a drug), (1) Indications and Usage, (2) Dosage and Administration, (3) Dosage Forms and Strengths, (4) Contraindications, (5) Warnings and Precautions, (6) Adverse Reactions, (7) Drug Interactions, and (8) Use in Specific Populations. Sections that may be most relevant to stakeholders concerned about safety risks include the Boxed Warnings, Contraindications, Warnings and Precautions, and Adverse Reactions sections.

An informed risk-benefit analysis considers data from the Highlights of the PI and proceeds to more detailed data included in the Full PI, and should always begin with a review of the Boxed Warnings section. A Warning is issued when a serious, post-approval public health risk has been identified (e.g., serious metabolic effects with SGAs, increased suicidality with ADs). The Contraindications section should be reviewed next because it may preclude further consideration of a drug (e.g., if preexisting conditions, concurrent drug usage, or prior allergic reactions pose significant risks). Further, the Warnings and Precautions section identifies serious post-approval adverse events that should be considered. The Adverse Reactions section lists unwanted outcomes from the clinical trials, as well as the inclusionary criteria for the unwanted outcomes (i.e., incidence threshold and whether the incidence must be greater than double the placebo [PBO] incidence). This section also indicates whether the clinical trials included purely pediatric or mixed age and diagnosis samples. Regularly updated FDA PIs are available from the FDA at (https://www.accessdata.fda.gov/scripts/cder/daf/).

Unwanted Outcomes: Adverse Events Versus Side Effects

Some unwanted outcomes are rare, but may be debilitating and significantly interfere with social and academic functioning. They may also be persistent, permanent, disfiguring, or even fatal. Such rare but serious outcomes emerge after clinical trials are completed and a drug has been approved. We refer to generally low frequency but serious, late-emerging, unwanted outcomes as adverse events (AEs). AEs appear in the PIs as Boxed Warnings and/or in the Warnings and Precautions section of the PI. Independent expert panels convened by the FDA have judged some of the AEs to be more serious risks than other AEs. The FDA informs the public about the most serious AEs through what is known as Drug Safety Communications (DSCs) that are issued separately from the PIs. In January 2010, the FDA introduced the term DSC to supersede a multitude of terms previously used to inform about public health threats (i.e., Warnings, advisories, "Dear Healthcare Professional" letters). To enhance consistency and readability, we refer to the Warnings, advisories, and letters issued prior to 2010 as DSCs, as well as the formal DSCs issued after January 2010. Kubiszyn and Mire (2014) provide additional detail about 22 DSCs issued between 1998 and 2011 for drugs used for pediatric EBDs. Additional details pertaining to those DSCs and more recent DSCs can be found on the FDA website (https://www.fda.gov/Drugs/DrugSafety/ucm199082.htm). This website is updated as new DSCs are issued. DSCs typically appear in the Boxed Warnings and/or Warnings and Precautions sections of the PIs.

Side effects (SEs) occur much more frequently (5–80% incidence) than AEs. Incidence of SEs can vary widely, even for drugs within the same drug class. SEs (e.g., headache, stomachache, fatigue) are typically less serious than the AEs and may be mild, manageable, or they may resolve on their own over time. SEs tend to emerge shortly after drug treatment is started or after a dosage adjustment. Because SEs manifest during clinical trials, specific inclusion, sample and incidence detail may be found in the Adverse Reactions section of the Full PI. Boxed Warnings, DSC AEs, other AEs, and SEs should all be considered integral to informed risk-benefit analysis.

How the Safety Data Are Organized

Our overall intent is to enhance risk-benefit analysis by presenting safety data for each class of drugs. We begin by discussing drugs with pediatric FDA indications within each of the four drug classes that we review. Next, we summarize data from the Contraindications sections of the PIs for the drugs we review because that data may preclude the need for further risk-benefit analysis.

We then present three consolidated tables. The tables list unwanted outcomes from the most serious and least common (AEs with DSCs in Table 9.1, and AEs without DSCs in Table 9.2) to the less serious and most common (SEs in Table 9.3). Table 9.1

includes incidence data when available from the DSCs (we use n.a. to indicate when data were not available). Accompanying Table 9.1 we include brief commentary to help contextualize some of the most salient DSC safety issues within each drug class.

Table 9.2 lists the AEs without DSCs from the Warnings and Precautions sections of the PIs. Brief commentary about those AEs accompanies Table 9.2. Table 9.3 lists the SEs from the Adverse Reactions sections of the PIs and also indicates the inclusionary criteria listed in the PIs for the SEs (e.g., incidence > 5% and >2 times placebo). Table 9.3 also indicates whether the samples were purely pediatric or mixed age, and the diagnoses included in the samples.

AEs and SEs by Drug Class

ADHD Drugs

Medications with FDA pediatric indications for ADHD also are prescribed off-label for externalizing disorders, autism, and other disorders, with or without ADHD symptoms. Our non-exhaustive review includes selected FDA-approved short- and long-acting methylphenidate-based (MPH) and amphetamine-based (AMP) stimulants. MPH-based drugs, include Ritalin, Focalin, Methylin, Quillivant, Daytrana, Concerta, and Metadate; and AMP-based drugs, include Adderall and Vyvanse. All are Schedule II/federally controlled substances because they can be abused or lead to dependence. Non-stimulant ADHD drugs include atomoxetine (Strattera), guanfacine (Intuniv), and clonidine (Kapvay). The non-stimulants are not controlled substances.

Contraindications. All ADHD drugs are contraindicated when drug hypersensitivity is known, and the stimulants and Strattera are contraindicated within two weeks of MAOI usage (a class of ADs seldom prescribed for pediatric use). MPH drugs are also contraindicated when marked anxiety, tension, or agitation; glaucoma; tics; or a family history or diagnosis of Tourette's syndrome is present. Metadate is contraindicated before surgery when halogenated anesthesia is to be used. AMP drugs are contraindicated when there is advanced arteriosclerosis, symptomatic cardiovascular disease, moderate to severe hypertension, hyperthyroidism, glaucoma, agitation, or a drug abuse history. Strattera is contraindicated with narrow-angle glaucoma, pheochromocytoma, and severe cardiovascular disorders.

Antidepressants (ADs)

Two SSRI (selective serotonin reuptake inhibitor) ADs, fluoxetine (Prozac) and escitalopram (Lexapro), have indications for pediatric depression, with escitalopram indicated only for ages 12 and up. Three SSRIs (fluvoxamine, or Luvox; sertraline, or Zoloft; and fluoxetine) and the tricyclic AD clomipramine (Anafranil) have indications for pediatric obsessive-compulsive disorder. Duloxetine (Cymbalta) is an SNRI (serotonin-norepinephrine reuptake inhibitor) with an indication for generalized anxiety disorder. The SSRIs are commonly prescribed off-label for other EBDs as well.

Contraindications. The PIs all caution against concurrent monoamine oxidase inhibitor (MAOI) usage and when hypersensitivity to the AD under consideration is known. Most also caution against concurrent use of pimozide, a first-generation antipsychotic.

Second-Generation Antipsychotics (SGAs)

SGAs with current pediatric FDA indications include risperidone (Risperdal), aripiprazole (Abilify), olanzapine (Zyprexa), quetiapine (Seroquel), asenapine (Saphris), paliperidone (Invega), and lurasidone (Latuda). With the exception of asenapine, all have FDA indications for pediatric schizophrenia. Except for lurasidone and paliperidone, they all have indications for pediatric mania or bipolar disorder. Risperidone and aripiprazole are also indicated for irritability associated with autism, and olanzapine has an indication for pediatric depression associated with bipolar disorder.

Contraindications. SGAs are contraindicated when a patient has a known sensitivity (e.g., allergy) to the drug under consideration. Asenapine is contraindicated if liver function is impaired, and lurasidone is contraindicated with concurrent use of a strong inhibitor or inducer of CYP3A4 (an enzyme that may increase/decrease the drug's serum levels). If quetiapine is administered with lithium, valproate acid (Depakote), or fluoxetine (Prozac), the Contraindications sections for those drugs should be reviewed.

Antiepileptic Drugs (AEDs) and Lithium

AEDs and lithium are commonly prescribed for bipolar disorder, aggression, and other EBDs as part of a polypharmacy regimen. We include lithium with the AED class of drugs because lithium is often considered as an alternative to the AEDs for EBDs.

None of the 24 AEDs with pediatric epilepsy indications reviewed by Sirven, Noe, Hoerth, and Drazkowski (2012) had an FDA indication for pediatric EBDs. Nevertheless, off-label use of many AEDs for pediatric bipolar, psychotic disorders, and other EBDs doubled between 1996 and 2009 (Tran, Zito, Safer, & Hundley, 2012), with increased pediatric usage of lamotrigine (Lamictal) significantly higher than other AEDs studied. We review five AEDs included in Tran et al. that are commonly prescribed for pediatric EBDs (lamotrigine, or Lamictal; divalproex sodium, or Depakote; carbamazepine, or Tegretol; oxcarbazepine, or Tripleptal; and topiramate, or Topamax).

Lithium received an FDA indication for pediatric mania and bipolar disorder (ages 12 and up) in 1970. It has been prescribed off-label for depression, aggression, comorbid substance use disorder, OCD, and autism symptoms. Its popularity has been limited because of its troubling side-effect profile and the need for careful invasive monitoring to avoid toxic levels, which are close to therapeutic levels. Both factors have led to high nonadherence rates (Advokat, Comaty, & Julien, 2014).

Contraindications. Except for topiramate, the AEDs and lithium are contraindicated when a patient has a known sensitivity to the drug under consideration. Divalproex sodium Contraindications include hepatic disease, mitochondrial disorders, urea cycle disorders, and pregnancy. Carbamazepine Contraindications include bone marrow suppression, sensitivity to tricyclic antidepressants, and concurrent use of MAOIs, nefazodone, delavirdine or other non-nucleoside reverse transcriptase inhibitors that are CYP3A6 substrates (an enzyme that affects drug serum levels). Lithium is contraindicated for patients with renal and cardiovascular disease, and patients with dehydration or taking diuretics.

Unwanted Outcomes Tables

Tables 9.1, 9.2, and 9.3 list the unwanted outcomes that the FDA has identified for four classes of drugs: the ADHD drugs, ADs, SGAs, and the AEDs and lithium. Table 9.1 includes the AEs for which DSCs have been issued by the FDA. Table 9.2 includes the AEs for which DSCs have not been issued, and Table 9.3 lists the SEs.

Each of the tables follows the same order. We list outcomes associated with the entire drug class first, followed by outcomes associated with multiple drugs within a drug class. Finally, we alphabetically list specific drugs and their unwanted outcomes.

Drug Safety Communications by Drug Class (Table 9.1)

Table 9.1 lists the AEs for which DSCs have been issued. The dates the DSCs were issued are included, along with incidence estimates, when available from the FDA. Commentary about the DSCs, by drug class, accompanies Table 9.1.

ADHD Drugs. Unwanted outcomes are more similar for the stimulants (i.e., DSCs, other AEs, and SEs) than within other drug classes, although there are differences between amphetamine (AMP) and methylphenidate (MPH) based stimulants. More differences are evident between stimulant and non-stimulant ADHD drugs. Abuse and diversion are concerns with the stimulants, especially with adolescents. DSCs about Sudden Unexplained Death (SUD) with ADHD drugs have been controversial. The subsequent SUD Safety Review by the FDA in 2011 was a cohort study of 1,200,438 children and young adults (ages 2–24 years). It revealed seven serious

Table 9.1 AEs with DSCs (for drugs with FDA pediatric indications used to treat pediatric EBDs)

Drug class/name	DSC date	Adverse events	Incidence
ADHD drugs			
All ADHD drugs	2007	Expanded 2005 Adderall DSC for Sudden Unexplained Death (SUD) and significant cardiovascular events; psychiatric symptoms (i.e., psychotic symptoms, mania)	No incidence data
All ADHD drugs	2011	FDA Safety Review—failed to find an association between ADHD drugs and SUD; blood pressure (BP) and heart rate (HR) monitoring is recommended, avoid prescribing if HR and BP increases may be harmful	n.a.
All stimulants	n.a.	Drug dependence/diversion	n.a.
All MPH	2013	Priapism (long-lasting erections)	12 reports
Adderall products	2005	Sudden Unexplained Death (SUD)	0.0003%
Atomoxetine	2004	Liver damage and liver failure	8 reports
Atomoxetine	2005	Suicidality (extension of 2004 boxed warning of pediatric suicidality for all antidepressants)	0.4%
MPH transdermal patch	2015	Chemical leukoderma (permanent loss of skin color)	51 reports
ADs			
All antidepressants	2004	Black box warning about increased pediatric suicidality	4%/2% PBO
All antidepressants	2007	Expanded 2004 warning for patients up to age 24	4%/2% PBO
7 SSRIs and 3 other ADs	2003	Increased risk of suicidality with pediatric use	n.a.
Triptans (migraine drugs) used with SSRI or SNRI ADs	2006	Serotonin syndrome	27 reports
SGAs			
All SGAs	2004	Metabolic issues (i.e., weight gain, glucose intolerance, hyperglycemia, diabetes mellitus, hyperlipidemia [high cholesterol], hypertension, stroke, premature mortality)	Very common
Aripiprazole, lurasidone, quetiapine,	2007	Increased risk of suicidality (extension of 2004 AD suicidality DSC)	n.a. for SGAs
Aripiprazole	2016	New compulsive behaviors (i.e., gambling, shopping, eating, sexual behavior)	169 reports

(continued)

Table 9.1 (continued)

Drug class/name	DSC date	Adverse events	Incidence
Asenapine	2011	Serious allergic reactions (i.e., anaphylaxis, angioedema, difficulty breathing, hypertension, rash, swollen tongue, tachycardia, wheezing)	52 reports
Olanzapine	2010	Weight gain, hyperlipidemia greater for adolescents than adults	Very common
Olanzapine	2016	Drug reaction with Eosinophilia and Systemic Symptoms (DRESS; fever plus rash or face swelling and swollen lymph glands)	23 reports
Olanzapine injectable	2015	FDA Safety Review—no change in prescription or use but reinforced need to follow the FDA Risk Evaluation and Mitigation Strategy (REMS)	n.a.
Risperidone	2011	Confusion with ropinirole (drug for Parkinson's and restless leg syndrome in adults; no pediatric indication)	223 reports
AEDs and lithium			
All AEDs	2008	Suicidality	0.43%/0.24% PBO
Carbamazepine	2007	Higher risk of life-threatening rash (SJS[a] and TEN[a]) for Asian compared to non-Asian patients	10x higher if Asian
Divalproex sodium	2006	Liver damage when used with multiple antiepileptics and in children under 2 with congenital metabolic and mitochondrial disorders, intellectual disability with seizures, or an organic brain syndrome; possibility of life-threatening pancreatitis	Liver: n.a. Pancreatitis: 2/2416
Lamotrigine	1998	Life-threatening rash (e.g., SJS and TEN)	0.8%
Lamotrigine	2010	Aseptic meningitis (nonbacterial inflammation of the protective membranes that cover the brain and spinal cord)	0.0001%

(continued)

Table 9.1 (continued)

Drug class/name	DSC date	Adverse events	Incidence
Lithium	1970	Toxic at close to therapeutic levels, close accurate serum level needed	n.a.
Oxcarbazepine	2005	Life-threatening rash (e.g., SJS and TEN), multi-organ sensitivity (e.g., multi-systemic complaints, such as profound fatigue, mental confusion, myalgia, depression, anxiety, dizziness, headache, insomnia, loss of appetite, numbness of the extremities)	n.a.

[a]SJS: Stevens–Johnson Syndrome; TEN: Toxic epidermal necrolysis

cardiovascular events (four strokes and three sudden cardiac deaths) in current users. In comparison to nonuse, no association was observed between serious cardiovascular events with ADHD drug use. However, the low cardiac event incidence limited the power of statistical comparisons, indicating that caution should continue to be exercised, especially in patients with known cardiac issues.

ADs. The 2004 suicidality DSC may be the best known of the pediatric Boxed Warning DSCs issued for this drug class. The FDA aggregated data from 24 AD clinical trials (4,400 subjects, 24 clinical trials, multiple diagnoses), which revealed an incidence roughly twice as high as the placebo group (no completed suicides were reported) and reported an incidence of about 4% for the ADs, compared to 2% for placebo. No completed suicides were found. The AD suicidality DSC also has the highest incidence after the metabolic effects associated with the SGAs.

Like the SUD warning for the ADHD drugs, the AD suicidality warning has been controversial. Although the 4% risk of suicidality (i.e., ideation and actions) was twice that of placebo in the FDA study, there also were no completed suicides, in spite of the fact that, paradoxically, ADs are often prescribed when suicidality is suspected or an attempt has been made. Studies published after the DSC was issued have not resolved the controversy (Noel, 2015), suggesting again the importance of informed risk-benefit analysis when pediatric ADs are under consideration or use. Because triptans and SSRI and SNRI ADs both enhance availability of serotonin, concurrent use risks serious high serotonin levels of serotonin and the potential emergence of dangerous serotonin syndrome.

SGAs. Most SGAs are prescribed off-label for pediatric aggressive and disruptive behavior or for depression (Olfson et al., 2015) and AEs associated with SGAs result in thousands of pediatric emergency room visits every year (Hampton, Duabresse, Chang, Alexander, & Budnitz, 2015). The many AEs and SEs associated with SGAs all suggest that informed risk-benefit analysis may be most important when considering pediatric SGA usage.

Table 9.1 indicates metabolic issues (e.g., endocrine changes, weight gain) that are common and expected with the SGAs, unlike almost all other DSCs. Pediatric metabolic issues are serious and have been associated with later cardiovascular complications, stroke, and premature mortality (Maayan & Correll, 2011). Pisano et al. (2016) concluded that the frequency of pediatric SGA metabolic and endocrine effects (e.g., weight gain, hyperlipidemia, diabetes, prolactin elevation) made them the AEs of greatest concern. Weight gain and other metabolic effects were greatest with olanzapine, followed by quetiapine, risperidone, and aripiprazole; but risperidone was most often associated with prolactin elevation, menstrual irregularities and amenorrhea, gynecomastia (development of abnormally large breasts in males), and sexual dysfunction. The Boxed Warning DSCs about increased suicidality for aripiprazole, quetiapine and lurasidone are extensions of the 2004 AD suicidality Boxed Warning. They were issued because those SGAs are increasingly used off-label as adjunctive treatment for pediatric depression.

AEDs and lithium. Off-label usage of AEDs for pediatric EBDs has substantially increased in recent years, often in combination with other drugs (i.e., polypharmacy) (Tran et al., 2012). Three DSCs were issued for the AEDs for life-threatening rash (SJS or TEN). Although SJS or TEN can occur with any drug, no DSCs have been issued for the other drug classes we reviewed. The 2008 suicidality warning applied to all ages and indicated nearly double the risk for AED users over nonusers. The relevance of the FDA AE and SE data may be more limited for AED risk-benefit analysis than for the other drug classes for several reasons. Specifically, the samples varied widely, consisting almost entirely of patients with epilepsy; pediatric subjects were often mixed with adults; inclusion criteria for SEs varied; and the trials were commonly part of a polypharmacy/augmentation/transition regimen (Tran et al., 2012).

Adverse Events (Non-DSC) by Drug Class (Table 9.2)

Table 9.2 lists the serious AEs in the Warnings and Precautions sections of the PIs that have not been identified through DSCs. The dates of the relevant PIs are included, but incidence data are not available in the PIs. Commentary about the AEs, by drug class, accompanies Table 9.2.

ADHD Drugs. Growth suppression of about 2–3 cm over time and HR and BP increases are expected with the stimulants. An increased risk of a dangerous serotonin syndrome exists with the AMP drugs because they can enhance serotonin availability. Somnolence/sedation are common AEs with the non-stimulants, with hypotension and other cardiac issues evident for guanfacine and clonidine.

ADs. Caution is urged when initiating AD treatment when bipolar disorder is suspected because of increased potential for mania, behavioral activation, and disinhibition. In addition to the AEs common to most of the ADs, the PIs for duloxetine (an SNRI) and clomipramine (a tricyclic AD) listed several more AEs than did the PIs for the SSRI ADs.

SGAs. The metabolic issues highlighted in the 2004 SGA DSC were also the most common AEs across the SGAs, with variable incidence across the SGAs. Although

Table 9.2 AEs without DSCs (for drugs with FDA pediatric indications used to treat pediatric EBDs)

Drug class/name	Non-DSC AEs	PI date
ADHD drugs		
All stimulants	Growth suppression, BP and HR increases, seizures, peripheral vasculopathy (including Raynaud's Phenomenon), visual disturbances, aggression	Various
All non-stimulants	Sedation/somnolence/fatigue	Various
All AMP	Serotonin syndrome	Various
Guanfacine, clonidine	Hypotension, slowed heart rate, cardiac conduction abnormalities, and allergic reactions	2/2013, 3/2016
Atomoxetine	Growth suppression, aggression, allergic reactions, urine retention, and priapism	4/2015
OROS MPH	Gastrointestinal obstruction (with preexistent narrowing)	1/2017
ADs		
All ADs	Activation of mania, serotonin syndrome, appetite and weight changes, angle-closure glaucoma, sexual dysfunction, nausea (except sertraline), abnormal bleeding and hyponatremia (except clomipramine), discontinuation/withdrawal syndrome (except fluoxetine), seizures (except sertraline and duloxetine)	Various
Clomipramine	Cardiovascular events, psychosis/confusion, hepatotoxicity, hyperthermia, hematologic changes, discontinue before surgery, caution with concurrent illness and electroconvulsive therapy	6/2014
Duloxetine	Hepatotoxicity, orthostatic hypotension, and syncope, severe skin reaction, blood pressure changes, glucose control in diabetes, slowed gastric emptying, urinary hesitation/retention, do not administer with CYP1A2 inhibitors or thioridazine	1/2017
Escitalopram	Interference with cognitive/motor performance, caution in patients with altered metabolism or hemodynamic responses	1/2017
Fluoxetine	Qt prolongation, long half-life	1/2017
Fluvoxamine	Caution with drugs that affect metabolism and liver function	1/2017
SGAs		
All SGAs	Metabolic changes (hyperglycemia, diabetes, dyslipidemia, and weight gain); neuroleptic malignant syndrome (NMS); extrapyramidal symptoms (EPS); orthostatic hypotension; leukopenia, neutropenia, agranulocytosis; cognitive and motor impairment (except for quetiapine and lurasidone)	Various
Aripiprazole	Pathological gambling, seizures/convulsions, suicide	8/2016
Asenapine	Qt prolongation, seizures, suicide	3/2015

(continued)

Table 9.2 (continued)

Drug class/name	Non-DSC AEs	PI date
Lurasidone	Hyperprolactinemia	1/2017
Olanzapine	Suicide, DRESS (Drug Reaction with Eosinophilia and Systemic Symptoms: fever plus rash or face swelling and swollen lymph glands), seizures, hyperprolactinemia	1/2017
Paliperidone	Qt prolongation, hyperprolatinemia, gastrointestinal narrowing, seizures, suicide	2/2017
Quetiapine	Increased BP, cataracts	2/2017
Risperidone	Hyperprolactinemia, seizures	2/2017
AEDs and lithium		
Carbamazepine	DRESS, embryofetal toxicity, seizure risk with abrupt discontinuation, hyponatremia, cognitive and motor impairment, liver damage, hepatic porphyria	9/2016
Divalproex sodium	Hepatotoxicity, birth defects/decreased IQ after in utero exposure, excessive bleeding, hyperammonemia, hypothermia, DRESS	3/2017
Lamotrigine	DRESS, blood dyscrasias, suicidal behavior and ideation, clinical worsening when treating bipolar disorder, medication errors due to name confusion	3/2015
Lithium	Lithium-Induced polyuria, hyponatremia, lithium-induced chronic kidney disease, encephalopathic syndrome, hypothyroidism and hyperthyroidism, hypercalcemia and hyperparathyroidism	10/2016
Oxcarbazepine	Hyponatremia, anaphylactic reactions, and angioedema, increased seizure risk on discontinuation, cognitive/neuropsychiatric adverse events, multi-organ hypersensitivity, agranulocytosis, pancytopenia and leukopenia, altered seizure control during pregnancy, low sodium levels on lab tests	6/2014
Topiramate	Acute myopia and secondary angle closure glaucoma, visual field defects, decreased sweating and hyperthermia, metabolic acidosis, cognitive dysfunction, fetal toxicity, withdrawal must be gradual, hyperammonemia and encephalopathy, kidney stones, hypothermia	12/2014

less frequent overall than the metabolic issues, Pisano et al. (2016) found that the incidence of cardiovascular (e.g., Qt prolongation, an abnormal heart rhythm associated with serious cardiac complications) and neurological complications (e.g., extrapyramidal symptoms, or EPS) also varied across the SGAs. Yet, Qt prolongation only appears in the asenapine and lurasidone Warnings and Precautions sections of the respective PIs.

AEDs and lithium. There were no non-DSC AEs in common for these drugs; they have largely idiosyncratic AE profiles. None have FDA indications for pediatric

EBDs (except lithium). The lack of indications for pediatric EBDs and the diverse AE profiles may indicate the need for more careful risk-benefit analysis and treatment outcome monitoring for this class than with the other classes.

Side Effects (SEs) by Drug Class (Table 9.3)

Table 9.3 lists SEs for each drug class. The SEs are drawn from the Adverse Reactions sections of the relevant PIs (PI dates included). Because these data emerged from pre-approval clinical trials, we include brief descriptions of the inclusion thresholds (incidence and/or drug–placebo ratios that must be exceeded), and indicate how the samples were characterized in the Highlights for each drug class. Full PIs provide more specific incidence data, which can be as high as 50–80% for some SEs.

Implications of SEs for School Functioning

It is obvious that the severity of the DSCs and some of the other non-DSC AEs can negatively impact many aspects of school functioning (e.g., attendance, achievement, social development) albeit for a small number of students. However, the more common but less serious SEs (e.g., somnolence/sedation, insomnia, blurred vision, and dizziness) also can negatively affect school functioning, and for a much larger number of students. In this section, we consider the implications for school and social functioning of those common SEs.

The SGAs, ADs, and non-stimulant ADHD drugs are most frequently associated with somnolence/sedation, with stimulant ADHD drugs most frequently associated with insomnia. These SEs influence arousal, attention, and concentration. Thus, the behavioral manifestations of somnolence/sedation and insomnia are comparable (sleeping in class, drowsiness, inattention, and disorientation in extreme cases). Comprehension problems, decreased time-on-task, failure to complete seat work, and lack of engagement may be expected. Performance on tests and assessments may be significantly impaired as well. Somnolent or sedated students also may experience rejection, bullying, or other social, emotional, or behavioral consequences and may fall behind alert, engaged peers in multiple domains.

Blurred vision and visual disturbances were most often associated with the SGAs, lithium, and the AEDs. Vision can be key to school success. Blurred vision can both distract from and directly impair visual perception, attention and concentration, and participation in class. Together these limitations may negatively affect multiple core academic areas (e.g., reading, math) and elective subjects (e.g., keyboarding, art, physical education), as well as social interaction and development. Like somnolence, blurred vision may lead to deficits in multiple aspects of school functioning, including test/assessment performance.

Table 9.3 SEs (for drugs with FDA pediatric indications used to treat pediatric EBDs)

Drug class/name	Inclusion criteria, sample constellation and SEs	PI date
ADHD drugs	*(>5% and >2X PBO, all pediatric samples)*	
All stimulants	Appetite decrease/weight loss, insomnia, dizziness, irritability, emotional lability, nausea, anxiety, abdominal pain, vomiting	Various
All AMP	Dry mouth, diarrhea	Various
All MPH	Headache, dyspepsia, tachycardia, and blood pressure increase	Various
All non-stim.	Dizziness, dry mouth, irritability	Various
Atomoxetine	Nausea, appetite decrease, vomiting, constipation	5/2017
Clonidine	Insomnia, nightmares, constipation, dry mouth	8/2016
Guanfacine	Hypotension, fatigue, nausea, and lethargy, abdominal pain, insomnia, irritability, vomiting, and bradycardia	3/2016
ADs	*(>5% and >2X PBO, except >PBO for clomipramine; samples were mixed ages and diagnoses, except pediatric-only for clomipramine)*	
All ADs	Nausea, sexual dysfunction, somnolence, and fatigue (except sertraline), hyperhidrosis (except clomipramine)	Various
Clomipramine	Dry mouth, constipation, dyspepsia, tremor, dizziness, nervousness, weight gain, visual changes	6/2014
Duloxetine	Dry mouth, constipation, decreased appetite	1/2017
Escitalopram	Insomnia	1/2017
Fluoxetine	Abnormal dreams, anorexia, anxiety, asthenia, diarrhea, dry mouth, dyspepsia, flu syndrome, insomnia, nervousness, pharyngitis, rash, sinusitis, tremor, vasodilatation, and yawn	1/2017
Fluvoxamine	Insomnia, asthenia, nervousness, dyspepsia, anorexia, tremor, vomiting, agitation, depression, dysmenorrhea, flatulence, hyperkinesia, and rash	1/2017
Sertraline	Diarrhea/loose stool, tremor, dyspepsia, decreased appetite	12/2016
SGAs	*(>5% and >2X PBO, samples not described in highlights)*	
All SGAs	Somnolence/sedation, appetite and weight increase, fatigue, nausea (except olanzapine and paliperidone), dizziness (except lurasidone and paliperidone), nausea and vomiting (except aripiprazole, olanzapine, and paliperidone)	Various
Aripiprazole	EPS, tremor, blurred vision, akathisia, excess saliva, drooling, pyrexia headache, decreased (i.e., for patients with ASD) appetite, nasopharyngitis	8/2016
Asenapine	Dysgeusia, oral paresthesia	3/2015
Lurasidone	Akathisia, extrapyramidal symptoms, rhinitis/rhinorrhea (80 mg dosage only)	1/2017
Olanzapine	Headache, abdominal pain, pain in extremity, dry mouth	1/2017

(continued)

Table 9.3 (continued)

Drug class/name	Inclusion criteria, sample constellation and SEs	PI date
Paliperidone	Akathisia, tremor, dystonia, cogwheel rigidity, anxiety, tachycardia	2/2017
Quetiapine	Dry mouth, tachycardia	2/2017
Risperidone	Parkinsonism, akathisia, dystonia, tremor, blurred vision, anxiety, upper abdominal pain, stomach discomfort, dyspepsia, diarrhea, salivary hypersecretion, constipation, dry mouth, rash, nasal congestion, URI tract infection, nasopharyngitis, pharyngolaryngeal pain	2/2017
AEDs and lithium	*(lithium n.a., lamotrigine, topiramate > 10%, oxcarbazepine, divalproex > 5%, carbamazepine > 5%, >2X PBO, mixed samples, epilepsy only except topiramate included migraine)*	
All AEDs and lithium	Nausea, vomiting, somnolence, visual disturbance and dizziness (except lithium and lamotrigine)	Various
Carbamazepine	Ataxia, constipation, pruritus, dry mouth, asthenia, and speech disorder	9/2016
Divalproex sodium	Abdominal pain, alopecia, amnesia, anorexia, asthenia, ataxia, bronchitis, constipation, depression, diarrhea, dyspepsia, dyspnea, subcutaneous bleeding, decreased blood platelets, emotional lability, fever, flu syndrome, headache, infection, insomnia, nervousness, nystagmus, peripheral edema, pharyngitis, rhinitis, abnormal thinking, tinnitus, tremor, weight gain or loss	3/2017
Lamotrigine	*Epilepsy*: fever, infection, accidental injury, diarrhea, abdominal pain. *Bipolar*: insomnia, back pain, fatigue, rash, rhinitis, abdominal pain, and xerostomia	3/2015
Lithium	Fine hand tremor, polyuria, thirst, general discomfort during initial treatment	10/2016
Oxcarbazepine	Fatigue, ataxia, abdominal pain, tremor, dyspepsia, abnormal gait, <4 years old: infections and infestations	6/2014
Topiramate	*Epilepsy*: paresthesias, anorexia/weight decrease, speech disorders and related speech problems, fatigue, nervousness, psychomotor slowing, fever. *Migraine*: paresthesias, anorexia/weight decrease, difficulty with memory, taste perversion, upper respiratory tract infection, abdominal pain, diarrhea, hypoesthesia	12/2014

Dizziness was common to the SGAs, ADHD drugs, lithium, and the AEDs. Dizziness can limit students' capacity to attend to academic tasks because of the distracting and potentially anxiety-inducing impact of visual and proprioceptive sensations that accompany dizziness. Depending on severity, attendance may suffer, and performance on tests and assessments may also be affected. Dizziness may affect many nonacademic domains (e.g., physical education, social activities, meal time, transitioning from class to class), potentially interfering with social and personal development.

Given that SEs are common, stakeholders (e.g., prescribers, school professionals) can help monitor and manage them by consulting with parents, teachers, coaches, and others to develop monitoring strategies and accommodations that may mitigate the impact of the SEs on school functioning. Because SEs often vary in their frequency and severity over time, continual assessment (i.e., progress monitoring) can provide prescribers and other stakeholders with data they need to inform ongoing risk-benefit analysis and subsequent psychotropic dosage adjustments, medication changes, or adjunctive or alternative treatments.

Practice Implications

In this section, we offer suggestions to consider when assisting stakeholders (e.g., prescribers, parents) with initial risk-benefit analysis and ongoing data-based risk-benefit decision-making about pediatric psychotropic usage.

Informing risk-benefit analysis. Figure 9.1 identifies several fundamental questions that can systematically guide stakeholders through risk-benefit analysis, as well as potentially stimulate additional questions and discussion. The questions prompt consideration of (a) the problem or the specific symptoms to be addressed by the medication; (b) both the *risks* (e.g., Contraindications, DSCs, other serious AEs, and SEs identified in this chapter, in the relevant PIs, and in other scientific sources) and the *benefits* of potential drug treatment (e.g., improved attendance, attention, or school and social functioning); (c) psychosocial treatment alternatives (e.g., evidence-based interventions); and (d) reasons for choosing a medication. Another useful risk-benefit resource is a free brochure developed by the FDA. The webpage for that brochure can be found in the Web Resources sections of this chapter.

Monitoring safety and efficacy. Pediatric psychotropic efficacy studies have become increasingly sophisticated and rigorous over the last two decades, stimulating the development of a variety of useful rating scales and observation approaches for data-based efficacy monitoring (see Carlson & Shahidullah, 2014 for example). Although not as advanced as efficacy monitoring, assessment and monitoring of safety issues in research (e.g., clinical trials) has become more rigorous over time as well, providing us with evidence-based SE and AE data from FDA clinical trials and post-approval systems like those that we have summarized in this chapter. In clinical practice, though, safety monitoring tends to be less systematic.

Monitoring for AEs and SEs may be limited to broad, informal, retrospective questions to caregivers ("How has her dizziness been?") or to the child, or to the inspection of simple AE/SE frequency counts or percentages. However, AE/SE assessment can be enhanced by encouraging parents, educators, and others to systematically monitor AEs/SEs in school, home, and other settings using formal measures that are specific to the psychotropic being monitored, when available.

For example, measures like the Stimulant Drug Side Effect Rating Scale (Barkley, 1998) can focus observers in multiple settings on a common set of AEs/SEs associated with stimulants. Other examples of measures that can help systematize AE/SE

RISK-BENEFIT ANALYSIS: A WORKSHEET GUIDE TO WEIGHING PEDIATRIC PSYCHOTROPIC USE	
Note for user: This risk-benefit worksheet is intended to guide thinking processes for decision-making when medication use is being considered. It is intended to help ensure that various risks, benefits and medication alternatives are systematically considered before decisions are finalized.	
Medication name:	
What is the **problem** this medication is intended to address?	
What are the **specific symptoms** targeted by this medication?	

RISKS		BENEFITS	
What are the **contraindications listed in the PI** for this medication?	☐ None ☐ not sure ☐ yes, including:	What are the **positive aspects** of using this medication for school and social functioning? Family and other functioning?	
What **DSCs, Boxed Warnings, other AEs, and SEs** are listed in the PI with this medication and how will these be monitored?			

ALTERNATIVES			
Are there **other treatment options** available to address this problem and these symptoms?	☐ No ☐ not sure ☐ yes, including:	*Pros*	*Cons*

Based on my risk-benefit analysis, at this time, I believe it is in the best interest of my child to :	
	☐ try this medication ☐ decline this medication ☐ unsure, I will seek additional information

Fig. 9.1 A worksheet to guide psychotropic risk-benefit analysis

collection across settings include the Psychotropic Medication Monitoring Checklists (PMMC) (Ninan et al., 2014). There are 10 PMMC measures specific to various psychotropics. Although promising, the aforementioned measures are not exhaustive of all medications, or measures, and their evidentiary support is emerging. Further psychometric study of AE and SE monitoring approaches is called for.

In summary, it is clear that the prescription of psychotropic drugs for pediatric EBDs is widespread and increasing, and the FDA data indicate clearly that those drugs are not without risk. The FDA data we have provided, coupled with the vast additional information available from the FDA itself and from other scientific sources such as those we list at the end of this chapter, can be used by stakeholders to support enhanced safety and child outcomes. Careful initial and ongoing systematic consideration of the risks and benefits of both psychotropic and psychosocial treatments for pediatric EBDs should be considered a best practice when informed by systematic ongoing monitoring for unwanted outcomes and efficacy.

Web Resources

https://www.fda.gov/Drugs/DrugSafety/PostmarketDrugSafetyInformationforPatientsandProviders/ucm111085.htm

Up-to-date drug safety information for patients and providers may be accessed at the website of the FDA. Because post-approval data are continually emerging the website changes often and readers should be aware that at times dead links and other issues may complicate searches.

https://www.fda.gov/Drugs/DrugSafety/ucm085729.htm

Medication Guides issued by the FDA for consumers are updated regularly.

https://www.fda.gov/Drugs/ResourcesForYou/ucm079492.htm

The FDA recently made available a free brochure on its website entitled “Think it Through: A Guide to Managing the Risks and Benefits of Medicines” (United States Food and Drug Administration, 2016).

Additional Readings

Advokat, C., Comaty, J. & Julien, R. (2014). *Julien’s Primer of Drug Action: A Comprehensive Guide to the Actions, Uses and Side Effects of Psychoactive Drugs* (13th ed.)

A widely adopted textbook, encyclopedic coverage of drug efficacy and safety and basic pharmacokinetics, pharmacodynamics, and mechanisms of action.

Preston, J., O'Neal, J. & Talaga, M. (2015). *Child and Adolescent Clinical Psychopharmacology Made Simple* (3rd ed.)

Much less detailed and considerably more reader friendly than *Julien's Primer of Drug Action*. Organized by disorder and designed for clinicians.

Wilens, T. & Hammerness, P. (2016). *Straight Talk about Psychiatric Medications for Kids.* (3rd ed.)

This parent-friendly book is intended to familiarize nonprofessionals about pediatric psychotropic efficacy, safety, and controversies.

References

Advokat, C. D., Comaty, J. E., & Julien, R. M. (2014). *A primer of drug action* (13th ed.). New York, NY: Worth.

American Academy of Child and Adolescent Psychiatry. (2015). *Recommendations about the use of psychotropic medications for children and adolescents involved in child-serving systems.* Retrieved from https://www.aacap.org/App_Themes/AACAP/docs/clinical_practice_center/systems_of_care/AACAP_Psychotropic_Medication_Recommendations_2015_FINAL.pdf.

Barkley, R. A. (Ed.). (1998). Attention-deficit hyperactivity disorder. In *A handbook for diagnosis and treatment* (2nd ed.). New York: Guilford.

Carlson, J. S., & Shahidullah, J. D. (2014). Best practices in assessing the effects of psychotropic medications on student performance. In P. L. Harrison & A. Thomas (Eds.), *Best practices in school psychology: Systems-level services* (pp. 361–374). Bethesda, MD: National Association of School Psychologists.

Greenhill, L., Kollins, S., Abikoff, H., McCracken, J., Riddle, M., Swanson, J., … Skrobala, A. (2006). Efficacy and safety of immediate-release methylphenidate treatment for preschoolers with ADHD. *Journal of the American Academy of Child & Adolescent Psychiatry, 45,* 1284–1293.

Hampton, L., Duabresse, M., Chang, H., Alexander, G., & Budnitz, D. (2015). Emergency department visits by children and adolescent for antipsychotic drug adverse events. *JAMA Psychiatry, 72,* 292–294.

Hazell, P., & Mirzaie, M. (2013). Tricyclic drugs for depression in children and adolescents. *Cochrane Database Systematic Reviews, 18,* CD002317. https://doi.org/10.1002/14651858.cd002317.pub2.

Kubiszyn, T., & Mire, S. S. (2014). Recent FDA drug safety communications for pediatric psychotropics. *Journal of Child and Family Studies, 23,* 716–727.

Kubiszyn, T., Mire, S., Dutt, S., Papathopoulos, K., & Backsheider-Burridge, A. (2012). Significant differences in pediatric psychotropic sides effects: Implications for school behavior and performance. *School Psychology Quarterly, 27,* 4–28.

Maayan, L., & Correll, C. (2011). Weight gain and metabolic risks associated with antipsychotic medications in children and adolescents. *Journal of Child and Adolescent Psychopharmacology, 21,* 517–535.

Ninan, A., Stewart, S. L., Theall, L., King, G., Evans, R., Baiden, P., & Brown, A. (2014). Psychotropic medication monitoring checklists: Use and utility for children in residential care. *Journal of the Canadian Academy of Child and Adolescent Psychiatry, 23,* 38–47.

Noel, C. (2015). Antidepressants and suicidality: History, the black-box warning, consequences, and current evidence. *Mental Health Clinician, 5,* 202–211.

Olfson, M., King, M., & Schoenbaum, M. (2015). Treatment of young people with antipsychotic medications in the United States. *JAMA Psychiatry, 72,* 867–874.

Olfson, M., Marcus, S. C., Weissman, M. M., & Jensen, P. S. (2002). National trends in the use of psychotropic medications in children. *Journal of the American Academy of Child and Adolescent Psychiatry, 41,* 514–521.

Pisano, S., Catone, G., Lanzaro, V., Pozzi, M., Clementi, E., Iuliano, R., … Masi, G. (2016). Update on the safety of second generation antipsychotics in youths: A call for collaboration among paediatricians and child psychiatrists. *Italian Journal of Pediatrics, 42*. https://doi.org/10.1186/s13052-016-0259-2.

Rapoport, J. (2013). Pediatric psychopharmacology: Too much or too little? *World Psychiatry, 12,* 118–123.

Sirven, J. I., Noe, K., Hoerth, M., & Drazkowski, J. (2012). Antiepileptic drugs 2012: Recent advances and trends. *Mayo Clinic Proceedings, 87,* 879–889.

Tran, A. R., Zito, J. M., Safer, D. J., & Hundley, S. D. (2012). National trends in pediatric use of anticonvulsants. *Psychiatric Services, 63,* 1095–1101.

United States Food and Drug Administration. (2016). *Think it through: A guide to managing the risks and benefits of medicines.* Retrieved from https://www.fda.gov/Drugs/ResourcesForYou/ucm079492.htm.

Chapter 10
Psychopharmacology: Special Considerations When Working with Young Children

Justin A. Barterian

When young children, ages 2–5, experience mental health problems, special care is needed to identify an appropriate treatment plan that maximizes benefits and minimizes risks (Gleason et al., 2007). In a review of the available literature, Egger and Angold (2006) found the prevalence rates for any mental health disorder in young children ranged from 14 to 26%. Depression is observed at a notably lower rate (prevalence: 0–2%) than other mental health disorders such as anxiety (prevalence: 10–20%), oppositional defiant disorder: (ODD; prevalence: 4–16.7%) and attention deficit hyperactivity disorder (ADHD; prevalence: 2–5.7%; Egger & Angold, 2006; Whalen, Sylveter, & Luby, 2017). In the United States, the diagnosis of mental health problems in young children appears to be on the rise. For example, Chirdkiatgumchai and colleagues (2013) reviewed the data from greater than 40,000 children from the National Ambulatory and National Hospital Ambulatory Medical Care Surveys. Of the office-based visits surveyed, 1.56% included the diagnosis of behavioral disorder in a child between the ages of 2 and 5, with a 56% increase between 1994 and 2009. Demographic factors appeared to be related to the rate of diagnosis, with boys and children who did not have private insurance receiving diagnoses more frequently. While diagnostic trends need to be further explored in order to identify occurrences of overdiagnosis or underdiagnosis (Whalen et al., 2017), the evidence clearly indicated that young children do experience mental health problems, necessitating the development of efficacious and safe treatment approaches.

Mental health problems experienced in preschool have detrimental effects on children as they progress into school. For example, preschool children diagnosed with mental health disorders were more likely to experience that same disorder when reaching school age, including conduct disorder (odds ratio: 4.56:1), oppositional defiant disorder (odds ratio: 4.62:1), attention deficit hyperactivity disorder (ADHD; odds ratio: 3:1), and depression (odds ratio: 2.7:1). Preschool depression

J. A. Barterian (✉)
Department of Psychiatry and Behavioral Health, Ohio State University Wexner Medical Center, Columbus, OH, USA
e-mail: Justin.Barterian@osumc.edu

J. S. Carlson and J. A. Barterian (eds.), *School Psychopharmacology*,
Pediatric School Psychology, https://doi.org/10.1007/978-3-030-15541-4_10

and preschool anxiety both predict school-age anxiety disorders (depression odds ratio 3.48:1; anxiety odds ratio: 1.91:1; Luby, Gaffrey, Tillman, April, & Belden, 2014). Mental health problems in preschool can have an impact on academic performance. For example, preschool children diagnosed with ADHD have demonstrated more challenges on tests of school-readiness than their peers (DuPaul, McGoey, Eckert, & Van Brakle, 2001). Additionally, given the negative academic effects of mental health problems in school-age children (discussed more thoroughly in Chaps. 4–8) and the increased likelihood that preschool children with mental health problems will experience the same difficulties as school-age children, addressing these mental health concerns is essential in order to improve socioemotional and academic outcomes for students.

Fontanella, Hiance, Phillips, Bridge, and Campo (2014), examined the trends of psychotropic medication prescriptions in 559,275 preschool children continuously enrolled in Ohio's Medicaid program from 2002 to 2008. Results indicated that the rate of prescription medication only increased slightly (1.7–1.9%) during this time; however, the prevalence of prescriptions for stimulants, alpha-agonist medications, and antipsychotics significantly increased. Antipsychotic prescriptions in preschool children rose from 2000 to 2007, with the annualized rate of antipsychotic use per 1,000 children between the ages of two and five, increasing from 0.78 to 1.59. Primary diagnoses being treated in this sample included pervasive developmental disorder or intellectual disability, ADHD, and disruptive behavior disorders (e.g., ODD, CD; Olfson, Crystal, Huang, & Gerhard, 2010). Despite this, overall trends of psychotropic medications in preschool children have stabilized, with the highest rate of prescriptions occurring from 2002 to 2005, and then reducing to levels seen in the 1990s from 2006 to 2009 (Chirdkiatgumchai et al., 2013).

Psychopharmacological Treatment of Young Children

To date, there have been no psychopharmacological medications marketed and labeled for preschoolers (i.e., ages 2–5); however, this is likely to change in the near future. Currently, many of the medications that are approved for children and adults are provided to preschoolers "off-label" (i.e., unapproved by the FDA). One particular problem in receiving FDA approval status for medications in preschool children is the ethical considerations associated with developing a study in this population given the unknown and potential risks associated with introducing a new medication to a developing brain and nervous system (Gleason et al., 2007).

Externalizing Disorders

Stimulants. A majority of the medications prescribed to young children are for the treatment of externalizing disorders, such as ADHD. Stimulant medications, such as methylphenidate (e.g., Concerta, Daytrana, Ritalin), are the most studied medications for this population. In a review completed by Ghuman, Arnold, and Anthony (2008), the authors found 20 published studies examining the use of stimulants for the treatment of ADHD including preschool children, with 12 of these studies including a double-blind treatment design. However, many of these studies incorporated the outcomes of preschool children with those of school-age children. Overall, at the time of the review, 417 preschool children have been included in studies examining the efficacy of stimulants for ADHD. Seven blinded studies of stimulant medications for the treatment of ADHD *specifically for preschool children* have been completed, with the first two occurring in the 1970s (Conners, 1975; Schleifer et al., 1975), and the most recent and comprehensive, completed by Greenhill and colleagues (2006; i.e., Preschool ADHD Treatment Study (PATS)). The PATS study was necessary due to the flaws in the methodological designs of prior studies examining the use of stimulants solely for preschool children. These flaws included: (1) only using one research site (i.e., not a multisite trial); (2) brief treatment duration; (3) inconsistent diagnostic methods; (4) small sample sizes; (5) lack of teacher data; and (6) lack of follow-up.

During the PATS study (Greenhill et al., 2006), a randomized control trial, multisite, design was used in order to examine the efficacy of immediate-release methylphenidate for the treatment of ADHD in children between the ages of 2 and 5 (see Table 10.1 for details on this study and other relevant studies of psychotropic medications in young children). Participants were 165 preschool children, who were treated across five sites throughout the United States. Outcome data demonstrated that immediate release methylphenidate was efficacious, with an optimal total daily dose ranging from 7.5 to 30 mg/day. The investigators started children on low doses, and then slowly increased until an optimal dose was achieved based on clinical response and side effects. The overall effect sizes were lower for preschool children in this study (ES = 0.35 (parent); ES = 0.43 (teacher)) when compared to the effect sizes in school-age children in the Multimodal Treatment for ADHD (MTA) study. Interestingly, moderator analysis demonstrated that preschool children with comorbid mental health diagnoses, such as oppositional defiant disorder, had diminished responses to methylphenidate when compared to children with ADHD alone (Ghuman et al., 2007). In addition to examining outcomes associated with symptomology, the investigators also examined the role of methylphenidate in the improvement of functioning in other domains of preschool children with ADHD. Of note, improvements in functioning associated with methylphenidate treatment in preschool children were not similar to the improvements found in school-age children. Specifically, children who received the active methylphenidate treatment had similar parent ratings of social competence and social skills compared to those children who received placebo. However, examination of teacher ratings revealed that children who received methylphenidate were significantly more improved compared to those who received placebo in the domains of social competence and social skills, despite no difference in parent ratings of social competence. Parents of children who received methylphenidate did report a significant improvement in mood associated with methylphenidate treatment compared to those children who received placebo. Overall, during the PATS study, approximately 30% of children experienced a moderate to severe adverse event, including emotional outburst, difficulty falling asleep, repetitive behaviors/thoughts, reduction of appetite, and irritability, and 11% of children discontinued treatment because of these side effects. Taking these findings in conjunction with treatment outcomes, methylphenidate appears to be a safe and efficacious treatment for ADHD in preschool children (Wigal et al., 2006).

Extension and follow-up studies have been completed with the children who participated in PATS. Vitiello and colleagues (2007) examined the utility of methylphenidate in a 10-month open-label extension, including 95 participants. After 10 months of treatment, children continued to improve on clinical global impression ratings completed by the prescribing provider. Additionally, improved ratings of ADHD symptomology were maintained across the 10 months. Overall, the authors note that the maximum effect of methylphenidate treatment occurs quickly after the onset of treatment; however, improvements in functioning, such as social skills, gradually improve over time. Mild symptoms still persisted across the 10-months based on parent and teacher ratings. During the 10-month extension, only 5% of children discontinued treatment due to adverse events. Recently, Vitiello and colleagues (2015) conducted a systematic, prospective, naturalistic follow-up study of 68% (N = 206) of the children who participated in the PATS study to examine continued medication use. At 3 and 6 years post-treatment, approximately 40% of children remained on stimulant medication. A notable percentage of children were receiving stimulant treatment plus an atypical antipsychotic (i.e., year three: 8.3%; year six: 13.4%). After 6 years, approximately a quarter of the participants were receiving no psychopharmacological treatment.

Norepinephrine Reuptake Inhibitors. Atomoxetine (*Brand Name: Strattera*) is approved by the FDA for school-age children as a non-stimulant psychotropic intervention for the treatment of ADHD. Given some children are not able to tolerate stimulants, non-stimulant options, such as atomoxetine, become attractive. Despite this, only a few studies have examined the use of this medication in young children; however, the results are positive. Ghuman et al. (2009) completed a naturalistic open-label study of atomoxetine in 3 to 5-year-old children (N = 12) in order to examine effectiveness and tolerability. Children showed significant improvements in the domains of parent-rated hyperactivity/impulsivity. However, teachers did not report improvements in any domain of ADHD symptomology. A majority of participants (n = 8) displayed side effects such as defiance, tantrums, aggression, irritability, and a "chest ache;" however, most of these side effects were only mild to moderate and not concerning to parents.

Kratochvil and colleagues (2011) completed a randomized control trial examining the efficacy of atomoxetine to treat ADHD symptoms from 5- to 6-year-old children (N = 101). Atomoxetine treatment significantly reduced parent ratings of overall inattention, hyperactivity/impulsivity, and overall ADHD symptoms (ES = 0.70) after 8 weeks of treatment. Teachers also reported significant improvements in the domains of inattention and overall ADHD symptoms (ES = 0.60). Significant adverse events included reduced appetite, gastrointestinal upset, and sedation. The effect sizes seen in this study are comparable with the effect sizes observed in older children treated with atomoxetine. Despite the significant effect of atomoxetine on ratings of behavior, only 40% of the children were rated as "much" or "very much" approved

Table 10.1 Select studies examining the use of psychotropic medications in preschool children (N ≥ 10; published 2000 or later)

First author (Year)	Trial type	Sample size (Age range: years)	Diagnoses	Medication(s)	Outcomes	Adverse events
Greenhill et al. (2006)	RCT	N = 165 (3–5)	ADHD	Methylphenidate	• Significant improvement of parent (ES = 0.35) and teacher (ES = 0.43) ratings of ADHD symptoms	• 92% of participants tolerated methylphenidate treatment. • Common side effects included: appetite loss, insomnia, gastrointestinal upset, social withdrawal, and lethargy
Ghuman et al. (2009)	Open-label	N = 12 (3–5)	ADHD	Atomoxetine	• 75% of participants were identified as responders. Significant improvements of parent-rated hyperactivity/impulsivity (ES = 1.54), inattention (ES = 1.34), overall ADHD (ES = 1.70), oppositional behaviors (ES = 0.83), peer conflict (ES = 0.99), sleep problems (ES = 0.44) and anxiety (ES = 0.75), and clinician rated symptom severity (ES = 1.64)	• 66.7% of participants experienced side effects, including defiance, tantrums, aggression, irritability, and gastrointestinal complaints
Kratochvil et al. (2011)	RCT	N = 101 (5–6)	ADHD	Atomoxetine	• 40% of participants were identified as responders. Significant improvement of parent (ES = 0.70) and teacher ratings (ES = 0.60) of ADHD symptoms	• Common side effects included: decreased appetite, gastrointestinal upset, and sedation

(continued)

Table 10.1 (continued)

First author (Year)	Trial type	Sample size (Age range: years)	Diagnoses	Medication(s)	Outcomes	Adverse events
Arabgol et al. (2015)	RCT	N = 33 (3–6)	ADHD	Methylphenidate (N = 15); Risperidone (N = 18)	• Improvements in ADHD symptoms were found for both groups • No significant differences between groups regarding reduction in ADHD symptoms	• 20% of children in the risperidone group experienced daytime drowsiness and reduced appetite • Children in the methylphenidate group experienced reduced appetite (55.55%), nervousness (33.33%) and trouble sleeping (27.77%)
Masi et al. (2001a)	Open-label	N = 24 (3–6)	Autism/PDD	Risperidone	• Improvements in ratings of hyperactivity, fidgetiness, angry affect, lability of affect, withdrawal, negative and uncooperative behaviors, non-spontaneous relation to examiner, rhythmic motions, and autism symptoms	• 45% of children reported side effects with the most common including appetite disturbance, weight gain, modest agitation, and enuresis. • One child experienced dystonia
Masi et al. (2003)	Open-label	N = 53 (3–6)	Autism/PDD	Risperidone	• Significant improvement in multiple domains on the children's psychiatric rating scale and the children's global assessment scale	• Common side effects included: increased prolactin levels, increased appetite, agitation, enuresis, decreased appetite, sedation, hypoactivity, tremors, and increased levels of liver enzymes
Luby et al. (2006)	RCT	N = 24 (2–6)	Autism/PDD	Risperidone	• Improvements in autism symptoms ratings (ES = 0.95), and emotional response	• Common side effects included: sedation, increased appetite, hypersalivation, increased prolactin, and weight gain

(continued)

Table 10.1 (continued)

First author (Year)	Trial type	Sample size (Age range: years)	Diagnoses	Medication(s)	Outcomes	Adverse events
Biederman et al. (2005)	Open-label	N = 31(4-6)	Bipolar disorder	Olanzapine (n = 15); Risperidone (n = 16)	• Significant reduction in mania and psychotic symptoms for both medications. Risperidone resulted in greater improvements in motor activity, pressured speech, and depression	• There were not statistical differences for most side effects between the two medications. • Common adverse events, included: increased appetite, headache, weight gain and sedation. • Risperidone resulted in increase in prolactin levels
Ercan et al. (2011)	Open-label	N = 12 (2–6)	Conduct disorder	Risperidone	• 78% reduction in CGI—Severity ratings; improvement in parent and teacher ratings of behavior disorder symptoms	• Sedation (n = 2); significant increase in prolactin levels across all participants

by clinicians, and clinically significant symptoms were still present for a majority of the participants at the end of treatment.

Atypical antipsychotics. According to medication prevalence studies, atypical antipsychotics, such as risperidone (*Brand Name: Risperdal*), are being prescribed to preschool children in clinical practice at increasing numbers (Fontanella et al., 2014). There are significant gaps in the literature in regards to the use of atypical antipsychotic medications in preschool children. A recent review completed by Memarzia, Tracy, and Giaroli (2014) found that eight studies have included preschool children and examined the use of atypical antipsychotics for ADHD or disruptive behavior disorders. However, in a majority of these studies, outcomes for preschool children were included with outcomes for school-age children.

Only a few studies have examined the outcomes of atypical antipsychotics for the treatment of disruptive behavior disorders exclusively in preschool children. Ercan, Basay, Basay, Durak, and Ozbaran (Ercan et al. 2011) conducted an 8-week, open-label, trial to examine the tolerability and efficacy of risperidone monotherapy in preschool children (n = 12), ages two to six, with conduct disorder and severe behavioral problems in Turkey. Participants showed clinically significant improvement as rated by the study physicians. Additionally, participants demonstrated improvements on the parent and clinician completed ratings of inattention, hyperactivity–impulsivity, opposition-defiance, and conduct disorder. All participants were considered responders and parents reported minimal adverse events. These adverse events included mild to moderate sedation (n = 2) and increased prolactin levels (n = 6). Arabgol, Panaghi, and Nikzad (2015) examined the comparative efficacy of methylphenidate and risperidone in 33 preschool children, age 3 to 6 years old. Results indicated that both medications were equally effective in treating ADHD symptoms after a 6-week trial, based on parent report of symptoms on standardized rating scales. In this study, risperidone was generally well-tolerated with approximately 20% of children reporting minor side effects such as drowsiness and loss of appetite. Taking all of the available research into consideration, there is clearly a need for more high-quality research, such as randomized control trials, examining the safety, and efficacy of using atypical antipsychotics for the treatment of preschool children with externalizing disorders.

Internalizing disorders. There are very few studies examining the efficacy and safety of psychotropic medications for the treatment of internalizing disorders (i.e., anxiety and depressive disorders) in young children. Unfortunately, to date, there have been no randomized control trials, such as the PATS study, that examined the utility of any medication for the treatment of internalizing disorders in preschool children. Instead, only a handful of small studies and case studies are available. Barterian and colleagues (2014) completed a systematic review of the literature in order to identify studies that examined the use of psychotropic medications for the treatment of mental health disorders in preschool children. Selective serotonin reuptake inhibitors (SSRIs) were identified as the most common medications prescribed for internalizing disorders in young children with fluoxetine (*Brand Name: Prozac*) having the most published studies (n = 8) followed by sertraline (n = 2; *Brand Name: Zoloft*).

All of the publications were derived from case studies or individual participant data from small quasi-experimental studies examining both preschool and school-age children. Disorders addressed included selective mutism, obsessive-compulsive disorder (OCD), and specific phobia/feeding anxiety. Overall, regardless of disorder, all participants demonstrated improvements in symptomology. Side effects were mild across studies and included: increased oppositionality, self-harming behaviors, weight loss, sleep difficulty, headache, gastrointestinal upset, drowsiness, and tooth grinding. Behavioral disinhibition was observed across multiple studies and required some participants discontinue treatment due to the severity of this adverse event (Barterian et al., 2014). Since the Barterian and colleagues review article, only one more study has been completed examining the use of an SSRI for the treatment of selective mutism in a preschool child, who experienced improvements in symptomology with minimal adverse events (Barterian et al., 2018). Interestingly, to date, there have been no studies examining the utility of SSRIs for the treatment of depression in preschool children and this remains an area where much research continues to be needed. Clearly, there is a need for randomized clinical trials to examine the utility of SSRI medications for this population.

Mood disorders. The diagnosis of mood disorders (e.g., Bipolar Disorder) in children, especially preschool children, is outside of the scope of this chapter (for more information regarding pediatric bipolar disorder see Birmaher, 2013). Aside from small case studies, only atypical antipsychotics have been examined in a systematic nature for the treatment of preschool children with bipolar disorder. A review completed by Memarzia, Tracy, and Giaroli (2014) identified four studies examining the use of atypical antipsychotics for the treatment of bipolar disorder. Only two of these studies reported results specifically for preschool children. Biederman and colleagues (2005) completed an open-label study investigating the use of risperidone (n = 16) or olanzapine (n = 15) in preschool children diagnosed with bipolar 1 or bipolar disorder NOS. Results indicated that risperidone and olanzapine were effective in reducing symptoms of mania, while only risperidone was effective for improving symptoms of depression. Side effects were minimal with only one child dropping out of the study due to adverse events. Joshi and colleagues (2012) examined the utility of quetiapine (*Brand Name: Seroquel*) in an open-label study, which reported the results for 30 preschool children. Preschool children demonstrated a significant improvement in mania and depression symptoms. Additionally, preschool children demonstrated improvements in symptoms of psychosis, anxiety, and ADHD. Side effects included increased pulse, increased blood pressure, abnormal heart rhythm, decreases in some blood values (i.e., creatine, HCT, HGB, RBC), sedation, gastrointestinal upset, headache, and decreased energy.

Autism Spectrum Disorder

First generation antipsychotics. First generation antipsychotics have been used in the past to treat young children with autism. However, the last of the studies examining this class of medication for the treatment of autism in preschool children occurred in the 1980s. Given the reduced risk for extrapyramidal side effects of second-generation antipsychotics (i.e., atypical antipsychotics) compared to first-generation antipsychotics (Leucht et al., 2009), it is not surprising that the most recent studies have focused on these newer agents. Briefly, three studies examined the use of haloperidol for the treatment of autism in young children (ages 2–7; n = 118 total; Anderson et al., 1984, 1989; Campbell, Anderson, Small, Green, & Caplan, 1982). Participants demonstrated significant improvements in withdrawal, stereoptypic behaviors, abnormal object relationships, fidgetiness, and hyperactivity. Significant improvements were also noted on clinician ratings of improvement and severity. Adverse events included acute dystonia, sedation, and increased irritability.

Atypical antipsychotics. Similar to other disorders, there are several studies investigating atypical antipsychotics for the treatment of autism spectrum disorder; however, only a handful of studies (n = 4) report specifically on the outcomes for preschool children (Memarzia et al., 2014). Luby and colleagues (2006) completed a double-blind, randomized trial of risperidone for the treatment of autism spectrum disorders in preschool children (N = 24). Results indicated that children who received risperidone showed significant improvements over the placebo group after six months of treatment on the *Childhood Autism Rating Scale* total score (*CARS*; ES = 0.95; Schopler, Reichler, & Rochen, 1988) and the emotional response subscale. Despite these improvements, there were no significant improvements in autism core symptoms including communicative language, restricted interests, stereotypic behavior, and social competence/reciprocity. Children tolerated risperidone treatment well, and there were no problematic changes in EKG or dystonic or dyskinetic movements. Side effects experienced included sedation, increased appetite, hypersalivation, constipation, increased prolactin blood serum levels, increased leptin blood serum levels, and weight gain. Despite the positive findings, this study was small; therefore, replication with larger sample sizes is needed.

The remaining reports that examine the use of atypical antipsychotics for preschool children with ASD, include two open-label studies and one naturalistic study. Together, the two open-label studies (Masi, Cosenza, Mucci, & Brovedani, 2001a, Masi, Cosenza, Mucci, Brovedani, & De Vito, 2001b) examined the use of risperidone in 24 preschool children over the course of 16-weeks. At the end of treatment, children demonstrated significant improvements on the *CARS* (Schopler, Reichler, & Rochen, 1988) total score (14%) and the Children's Psychiatric Rating Scale (CPRS; 21%; Fish, 1985) total score, and demonstrated improvements in the following domains: negative and uncooperative behaviors, relationship to others, interaction with objects, emotional lability, withdrawal, fidgetiness, rhythmic motions, angry affect, and verbal and nonverbal communication. Clinical global impression ratings for all participants ranged from very much improved to minimally improved. Two participants discontinued due to adverse events, including frequent crying, fever, and tachycardia. The same research group conducted a 3-year naturalistic study of risperidone for the treatment of preschoolers (N = 53) with ASD (Masi, Cosenza, Mucci, & Brovedani, 2003). Fifty-three percent of participants took risperidone for the entire three years. Significant improvements were noted on ratings of overall psychiatric symptoms and global functioning and 46.8% of children were deemed responders based on an a priori definition. Of note, 22.6% of children discontinued treatment due to side effects. Common side effects included increased prolactin levels and weight gain. Adverse events included sedation, increased irritability, and acute dystonic reaction (n = 9).

Stimulants. Stimulants have been examined in several studies to treat autism spectrum disorders in school-age children; however, there is very little evidence examining the use of stimulants in preschool children with autism. One study that reports on outcomes specifically for preschoolers were completed by Handen, Feldman, Lurier, and Murray (1999). They conducted a very small, randomized, double-blind, placebo-controlled, study of methylphenidate in 11 preschool children who met criteria for a developmental disability as well as ADHD. Children demonstrated improvements on teacher-rated symptoms of hyperactivity and inattention-passivity. However, no changes in conduct problems or anxiety were noted. During laboratory tasks, children demonstrated a reduction in getting out of their seat and disruptive behavior. Of note, approximately 45% of the participants experienced an adverse event, which is higher than what was found in studies examining the use of methylphenidate in school-age children and typically developing preschool children with ADHD. The authors reported that five children experienced significant side effects and one child withdrew from the study due to the severity. Adverse events included social withdrawal, increased crying, irritability, and increased anxiety.

Opiate agonists. Naltrexone, an opiate agonist, has been examined in preschool children and older children for the treatment of symptoms related to autism. Willemson-Swinkels, Buitelaar, Weijnen, and van Engeland (1995) conducted a double-blind placebo-controlled study of naltrexone in young children (ages 3–7) diagnosed with autism (n = 20). In contrast to the authors' hypothesis, naltrexone did not lead to an improvement in social behaviors. However, participants did demonstrate improvements in behavior, including a reduction in irritability and improvements in attention. Side effects included sedation and increased stereotypic behaviors. However, the small sample size associated with this study is a significant limitation.

Selective serotonin reuptake inhibitors. Limited data exists regarding the use of SSRIs for the treatment of symptoms associated with autism. DeLong, Teague, and Kamron (1998) examined the use of fluoxetine for the treatment of autism in children ages two to seven years old using an open-label design (N = 37). Approximately 60% of the children had some positive response to fluoxetine treatment. More specifically, children demonstrated improvements in language learning, mood, and temperament, increased ability to relate to others, increased desire to talk, cognition, and reduced anxiety surrounding transitions. However, given the open-label nature of this study, replication of these findings is imperative.

Long-Term Adverse Events

One of the most prominent concerns regarding the use of psychotropic medications in preschool children is the impact that these medications have on the developing brain, given several neurodevelopmental processes occur during this time (Gleason et al., 2007). These processes include an increase in synaptic density, the refinement of monoaminergic pathways, vital changes in the number of dopamine and norepinephrine receptors, synaptic pruning, and myelination (Memarzia et al., 2014). The impact of psychotropic medications on these processes in preschool children is unknown and likely to remain so for some time given the ethical concerns and design requirements a study investigating this issue would require. Evidence from animal models suggests psychotropic medication exposure in utero can alter neural pathways throughout life (Maciag et al., 2006). Therefore, caution is needed whenever a treatment team considers the addition of psychotropic medication for a preschool child with a severe mental health issue, as the severity of the functional impairment and suffering must be weighed against potential unknown future harm/changes. In addition to potential interference with the developing brain, research has demonstrated the impact of these medications on other developmental processes (See Chap. 9). For example, long-term research on stimulant medications in school-age children has demonstrated that adults who were treated with stimulants on a regular basis as a child tend to be approximately one to two centimeters shorter than their peers (Swanson et al., 2017), and it is likely that children who start the medication in preschool will experience similar outcomes, Despite these concerns, untreated mental health issues in preschool often go on to cause problems during school and beyond causing deleterious effects; therefore, medication may be a suitable treatment option in some cases.

Ethics and Treatment Guidelines

Ethical questions abound when considering the use of a psychopharmacological medication for the treatment of a young child with a mental health problem. Many practitioners, such as school professionals, become rightly concerned when a psychotropic medication is considered for a young child with mental health issues. The knee-jerk reaction of many professionals is to avoid or discourage medications for this age group. However, this reaction may be depriving a child from much-needed relief from a serious mental health condition, such as severe anxiety or it may be putting a child at risk who displays dangerous impulsive behaviors (Jensen, 1998). Additionally, medication may better allow children who display serious symptoms to better access and participate in psychosocial treatments. For example, Avci, Diler, and Tamam (1998) report a case of a 2.5-year-old girl who could not ride in cars due to debilitating panic attacks. However, after brief treatment with fluoxetine, the child was able to ride in cars and the panic attacks stopped even when the medication was discontinued. A thorough risk-to-benefit calculation needs to be made with the unique characteristics of the preschool child in mind (Gleason et al., 2007).

The decision to treat a preschool child with a psychotropic medication must be carefully deliberated by a prescribing provider and/or a mental health treatment team in close collaboration with the child's parent(s). School psychologists and other mental health practitioners who work with young children at early childhood centers, such as Head Start, can play a critical role in data gathering and assessment regarding the child's functioning in preschool and/or at daycare. In 2007, the Preschool Psychopharmacology Working Group (PPWG; Gleason et al., 2007) commissioned by the American Academy of Child and Adolescent Psychopharmacology drafted treatment algorithms based on the little available evidence on the efficacy and safety of psychotropic medications for various disorders experienced by preschool children. While specific to each disorder, each treatment algorithm had consistent elements across diagnoses, which included: (1) a thorough diagnostic assessment, (2) implementation of evidence-based psychosocial treatment, (3) treatment of parental psychopathology if it is impacting childhood symptoms (e.g., parent training for disruptive behavior disorders), and (4) initiate medication treatment for a 6-month trial with consistent monitoring if prior interventions did not alleviate symptoms. School professionals are optimally positioned to play a role in each of these domains (see Fig. 10.1). Concerningly, at this time, it appears that very few children receive adequate mental health care prior to receiving medication, with only 28.4% receiving a mental health assessment, 23.7% meeting with a psychiatrist, and 29.7% receiving a psychosocial treatment (Fontanella et al., 2014).

As noted, the PPWG (Gleason et al., 2007) calls for the implementation of psychosocial treatments prior to the use of psychotropic medications with preschool children in order to maximize benefit and minimize risk. However, child and adolescent psychiatrists providing treatment to preschool children with ADHD reported that barriers to implementing this provision include concerns that the behavior of the child causes immediate danger (e.g., severe impulsivity) and lack of access to professionals who provide psychosocial treatment (Olfson, King, & Schoenbaum, 2016). Despite these barriers, there are evidence-based psychosocial treatments for preschool children who exhibit mental health difficulties in preschool, and school mental health practitioners can play a role in the facilitation of these programs for parents and children, especially when these types of services are not available in the surrounding community. Additionally, psychosocial interventions can be provided concurrently to augment medication treatment. For example, parent behavior training, such as the Positive Parenting Program (Triple P; Sanders, Bor, & Morawska, 2007) and the Incredible Years Parenting Program (Webster-Stratton, Reid, & Stoolmiller, 2008) have a wealth of evidence supporting their efficacy for children with externalizing behaviors. Moreover, Parent–Child Interaction Therapy-Emotion Development (PCIT-ED) treatment for childhood mood disorders (Lenze, Pautsch, & Luby, 2011) and the Fun FRIENDS (FF) program for childhood anxiety disorders (Barrett, Fisak, & Cooper, 2015) are promising treatments for internalizing disorders in this population.

Another challenge in ensuring appropriate, efficacious, and safe care for preschool children diagnosed with mental health disorders is the shortage of child psychiatrists. While primary care providers (PCPs) will often treat mental health issues, they are often reluctant to treat these issues in preschool children due to lack of expertise. A model to address these systemic challenges was developed in Michigan. The Michigan Child Collaborative Care Program (MC3; Marcus et al., 2017) provides consultation to PCPs across the state of Michigan. PCPs report high levels of satisfaction

Assist Psychiatrist and/or Treatment Team in Establishing Diagnosis
1. Conduct preschool/early childhood center/day care observations
2. Gather information from important stakeholders via interviews (e.g., teachers, day care providers, parents).
3. Distribute, score, and interpret psychometrically validated school/daycare based rating scales (e.g., Child Behavior Checklist 1.5-5; Caregiver-Teacher Report Form; Devereux Early Childhood Assessment)
4. Conduct any necessary psychological testing to establish cognitive ability and school readiness (e.g., Wechsler Preschool and Primary Scale of Intelligence – Fourth Edition; Mullen Scales of Early Learning)

Provide Evidence Based Psychosocial Treatment to the Child Prior to Medication Treatment
1. Treatments for preschool children with behavior disorders include programs/strategies such as: Positive Behavior Supports, Incredible Years, positive reinforcement (e.g., sticker charts), Daily Behavior Report Cards, parent behavior training, social skills training
2. Treatments for preschool children with internalizing disorders, include: systematic desensitization, positive reinforcement, contingency management, age-adapted cognitive behavioral therapy, and Parent-Child Interaction Therapy – Emotional Development (PCIT-ED)

Identifying and/or Providing Appropriate Treatment for Relevant Parent Psychopathology and Providing Parents with Support
1. Refer parents to clinicians who provide evidence-based treatments for parent mental health problems such as ADHD, anxiety, depression, and anger
2. Link families to appropriate agencies who may be able to help with systemic stressors (e.g., food banks, social work services)
3. Provide parent training (e.g., Incredible Years) and psychoeducation to address harmful or unhelpful parenting practices

Progress Monitoring of Symptoms During Medication Treatment
1. Routinely assess child's progress and side effects in the school/daycare setting through observation, formal rating scales, and teacher/caregiver interviews
2. Regularly connect with treatment team, including prescribing provider, regarding child's progress or possible side effects

Fig. 10.1 School professionals participation in the psychiatric treatment of young children. Adapted from Gleason and colleagues (2007)

with the MC3 program and used the services for diagnostic clarification, referral information, and pharmacological consultation. Utilization of collaborative models to ensure preschool children receive adequate mental health care is imperative given the ramifications that untreated mental health issues and psychopharmacological medications have on the developing brain.

Conclusions

Young children (ages 2–5) experience mental health problems, indicating a need for evidence-based treatments (Egger & Angold, 2006). Mental health problems in preschool are likely to continue when the child moves on to elementary school (Luby et al., 2014), compromising academic performance (DuPaul et al., 2001). Parents and teachers are essential members of the treatment team, given the young age of these children and the role that they play in children's lives. The prevalence of the use of psychotropic medications for the treatment of mental health disorders in preschool children increased substantially, beginning in the early 1990s, but stabilized between 2006 and 2009 (Chirdkiatgumchai et al., 2013). Despite this, there are very few randomized control trials examining the use of psychotropic medications in this population. The largest randomized treatment study for preschool children was the PATS study that examined the use of methylphenidate for the treatment of ADHD in young children (Greenhill et al., 2006). Most of the research regarding psychotropic medications for the treatment of preschool children has been conducted for externalizing disorders, resulting in a scarcity of research regarding the use of psychotropic medications for preschool children diagnosed with internalizing disorders (e.g., anxiety, depression). A thorough risk-to-benefit analysis should be conducted before preschool children are treated with a psychotropic medication given the unknown impact these medications may have on the developing brain (Gleason et al., 2007). School professionals can play an essential role in the treatment of preschool children who are being prescribed psychotropic medications by assisting the psychiatrist and treatment team in establishing diagnosis, implementing evidence-based psychosocial interventions prior to and during psychopharmacological treatment, connecting parents to psychosocial resources for their mental health problems, and monitoring treatment outcomes in the school setting.

Suggested Readings

Gleason et al., (2007). Psychopharmacological treatment for very young children: contexts and guidelines. *Journal of the American Academy of Child and Adolescent Psychiatry, 46,* 1532–1572. https://doi.org/10.1097/chi.0b013e3181570d9e

This articles provides an in depth discussion of the risks and benefits of treating preschool children with psychotropic medications and discusses recommended treatment algorithms.

Luby, J. (Ed). (2016). *Handbook of preschool mental health: Development, disorders, and treatment* (2nd ed.). New York: Guilford Press

This book reviews risk factors associated with preschool mental health issues as well as information specific to the presentation of mental health disorders in this population and evidence-based treatments.

Zero to Three (2016). *Diagnostic and classification of mental health and developmental disorders of infancy and early childhood: DC:0–5.* Washington D.C.: Author

This book provides a review of mental health problems in children ages 0–5 and discusses risk factors, case formulation, and intervention.

Websites

www.zerotothree.org

This organization provides resources for parents, professionals, and policymakers to promote the healthy development of young children.

www.developingchild.harvard.edu

This site provides information on current research, innovation, and policy regarding early childhood. Additionally, the site provides resources for professionals.

www.ecmhc.org

Head Start funds the Center for Early Childhood Mental Health Consultation. The center develops and disseminates resources for Head Start professionals in order to promote mental health.

References

Anderson, L., Campbell, M., Adams, P., Small, A., Perry, R., & Shell, J. (1989). The effects of haloperidol on discrimination learning and behavioral symptoms in autistic children. *Journal of Autism and Developmental Disorders, 19,* 227–239. https://doi.org/10.1007/BF02211843.

Anderson, L., Campbell, M., Grega, D., Perry, R., Small, A., & Green, W. (1984). Haloperidol in the treatment of infantile autism: Effects on learning and behavior symptoms. *The American Journal of Psychiatry, 141,* 1195–1202. https://doi.org/10.1176/ajp.141.10.1195.

Arabgol, F., Panaghi, L., & Nikzad, V. (2015). Risperidone versus methylphenidate in treatment of preschool children with attention-deficit hyperactivity disorder. *Iranian Journal of Pediatrics, 25,* e265. https://doi.org/10.5812/ijp.265.

Avci, A., Diler, R., & Tamam, L. (1998). Fluoxetine treatment in a 2.5 year-old-girl. *Journal of the American Academy of Child and Adolescent Psychiatry, 37,* 901–902. https://doi.org/10.1097/00004583-199809000-00005.

Barrett, P., Fisak, B., & Cooper, M. (2015). The treatment of anxiety in young children: Results of an open trial of the fun FRIENDS program. *Behaviour Change, 32*(4), 231–242.

Barterian, J., Rappuhn, E., Seif, E., Watson, G., Ham, H., & Carlson, J. (2014). Current state of evidence for medication treatment of preschool internalizing disorders. *Scientific World Journal, 2014,* 286085. https://doi.org/10.1155/2014/286085.

Barterian, J. A., Sanchez, J. M., Magen, J., Siroky, A. K., Mash, B. L., & Carlson, J. S. (2018). An examination of fluoxetine for the treatment of selective mutism using a nonconcurrent multiple-baseline single-case design across 5 cases. *Journal of Psychiatric Practice, 24,* 2–14.

Biederman, J., Mick, E., Hammerness, P., Harpold, T., Aleardi, M., Dougherty, M., et al. (2005). Open-label, 8-week trial of olanzapine and risperidone for the treatment of bipolar disorder in preschool-age children. *Biological Psychiatry, 58,* 589–594. https://doi.org/10.1016/j.biopsych.2005.03.019.

Birmaher, B. (2013). Bipolar disorder in children and adolescents. *Child and Adolescent Mental Health, 18,* 140–148. https://doi.org/10.1111/camh.12021.

Campbell, M., Anderson, L., Small, P., Green, W., & Caplan, R. (1982). The effects of haloperidol on learning and behavior in autistic children. *Journal of Autism and Developmental Disorders, 12,* 167–175. https://doi.org/10.1007/BF01531306.

Chirdkiatgumchai, V., Xiao, H., Fredstrom, B. K., Adams, R. E., Epstein, J. N., Shah, S. S., … & Froehlich, T. E. (2013). National trends in psychotropic medication use in young children: 1994–2009. *Pediatrics, 132*(4), 615–623.

Conners, K. (1975). Controlled trial of methylphenidate in preschool children with minimal brain dysfunction. *International Journal of Mental Health, 4,* 61–74. https://doi.org/10.1080/00207411.1975.11448675.

DeLong, G. R., Teague, L. A., & Kamran, M. M. (1998). Effects of fluoxetine treatment in young children with idiopathic autism. *Developmental Medicine and Child Neurology, 40*(8), 551–562.

DuPaul, G., McGoey, K., Eckert, T., & VanBrakle, J. (2001). Preschool children with attention-deficit/hyperactivity disorder: Impairments in behavioral, social, and school functioning. *Journal of the American Academy of Child and Adolescent Psychiatry, 40,* 508–515.

Egger, H., & Angold, A. (2006). Common emotional and behavioral disorders in preschool children: Presentation, nosology, and epidemiology. *Journal of Child Psychology and Psychiatry, 47,* 313–337. https://doi.org/10.1111/j.1469-7610.2006.01618.x.

Ercan, E., Basay, B., Basay, O., Durak, S., & Ozbaran, B. (2011). Risperidone in the treatment of conduct disorder in preschool children without intellectual disability. *Child and Adolescent Psychiatry and Mental Health, 5,* 10–22. https://doi.org/10.1186/1753-2000-5-10.

Fish, B. (1985). Children's psychiatric rating scale. *Psychopharmacology Bulletin, 21,* 753–764.

Fontanella, C., Hiance, D., Phillips, G., Bridge, J., & Campo, J. (2014). Trends in psychotropic medication use for medicaid enrolled preschool children. *Journal of Child and Family Studies, 23,* 617–631. https://doi.org/10.1007/s10826-013-9761-y.

Ghuman, J., Aman, M., Ghuman, H., Reichenbacher, T., Gelenberg, A., … Fort, C. (2009). Prospective, naturalistic, pilot study of open-label atomoxetine treatment in preschool children with attention-deficit/hyperactivity disorder. *Journal of Child and Adolescent Psychopharmacology, 19,* 155–166. https://doi.org/10.1089/cap.2008.054.

Ghuman, J., Arnold, L., & Anthony, B. (2008). Psychopharmacological and other treatments in preschool children with attention-deficit/hyperactivity disorder: Current evidence and practice. *Journal of Child and Adolescent Psychopharmacology, 18,* 413–447. https://doi.org/10.1089/cap.2008.022.

Ghuman, J., Riddle, M., Vitiello, B., Greenhill, L., Chuang, S., … Skrobala, A. (2007). Comorbidity moderates response to methylphenidate in the preschoolers with attention-deficit/hyperactivity disorder treatment study (PATS). *Journal of Child and Adolescent Psychopharmacology, 17,* 563–579. https://doi.org/10.1089/cap.2007.0071.

Gleason, M., Egger, H., Emslie, G., Greenhill, L., Kowatch, R. Lieberman, A., … Zeanah, C. (2007). Psychopharmacological treatment for very young children: Contexts and guidelines. *Journal of the American Academy of Child and Adolescent Psychiatry, 46,* 1532–1572. https://doi.org/10.1097/chi.0b013e3181570d9e.

Greenhill, L., Kollins, S., Abikoff, H., McCracken, J., Riddle, M., … Cooper, T. (2006). Efficacy and safety of immediate-release methylphenidate treatment for preschoolers with ADHD. *Journal of the American Academy of Child and Adolescent Psychiatry, 45,* 1284–1293. https://doi.org/10.1097/01.chi.0000235077.32661.61.

Handen, B., Feldman, H., Lurier, A., & Murray, P. (1999). Efficacy of methylphenidate among preschool children with developmental disabilities and ADHD. *Journal of the American Academy of Child and Adolescent Psychiatry, 38,* 805–812. https://doi.org/10.1097/00004583-199907000-00009.

Jensen, P. S. (1998). Ethical and pragmatic issues in the use of psychotropic agents in young children. *The Canadian Journal of Psychiatry, 43*(6), 585–588.

Joshi, G., Petty, C., Wozniak, J., Faraone, S. V., Doyle, R., Georgiopoulos, A., … & Yorks, D. (2012). A prospective open-label trial of quetiapine monotherapy in preschool and school age children with bipolar spectrum disorder. *Journal of affective disorders, 136*(3), 1143–1153.

Kratochvil, C., Vaughan, B., Stoner, J., Daughton, J., Lubberstedt, B., … March, J. (2011). A double-blind, placebo-controlled study of atomoxetine in young children with ADHD. *Pediatrics, 127,* e862–e868. https://doi.org/10.1542/peds.2010-0825.

Lenze, S. N., Pautsch, J., & Luby, J. (2011). Parent–child interaction therapy emotion development: A novel treatment for depression in preschool children. *Depression and Anxiety, 28*(2), 153–159.

Leucht, S., Corves, C., Arbter, D., Engel, R., Li, C., & Davis, J. (2009). Second-generation versus first-generation antipsychotic drugs for schizophrenia: A meta-analysis. *The Lancet, 373*(9657), 31–41. https://doi.org/10.1016/S0140-6736(08)61764-X.

Luby, J., Gaffrey, M., Tillman, R., April, L., & Belden, A. (2014). Trajectories of preschool disorders to full DSM depression at school age and early adolescent: Continuity of preschool depression. *American Journal of Psychiatry, 171,* 776–778. https://doi.org/10.1176/appi.ajp.2014.13091198.

Luby, J., Mrakotsky, C., Stalets, M., Belden, A., Heffelfinger, A., Williams, M., et al. (2006). Risperidone in preschool children with autistic spectrum disorders: An investigation of safety and efficacy. *Journal of Child and Adolescent Psychopharmacology, 16,* 575–587. https://doi.org/10.1089/cap.2006.16.575.

Maciag, D., Simpson, K. L., Coppinger, D., Lu, Y., Wang, Y., Lin, R. C., et al. (2006). Neonatal antidepressant exposure has lasting effects on behavior and serotonin circuitry. *Neuropsychopharmacology, 31*(1), 47.

Marcus, S. M., Malas, N. M., Quigley, J. M., Rosenblum, K. L., Muzik, M., LePlatte-Ogini, D. J., et al. (2017). Partnerships with primary care for the treatment of preschoolers. *Child and Adolescent Psychiatric Clinics, 26*(3), 597–609.

Masi, G., Cosenza, A., Mucci, M., & Brovedani, P. (2001a). Open trial of risperidone in 24 young children with pervasive developmental disorders. *Journal of the American Academy of Child and Adolescent Psychiatry, 40,* 1206–1214. https://doi.org/10.1097/00004583-200110000-00015.

Masi, G., Cosenza, A., Mucci, M., & Brovedani, P. (2003). A 3-year naturalistic study of 53 preschool children with pervasive developmental disorders treated with risperidone. *The Journal of Clinical Psychiatry, 64,* 1039–1047. Retrieved from http://europepmc.org/abstract/med/14628979.

Masi, G., Cosenz, A., Mucci, M., & De Vito, G. (2001b). Risperidone monotherapy in preschool children with pervasive developmental disorders. *Journal of Child Neurology, 16,* 395–400. https://doi.org/10.1177/088307380101600602.

Memarzia, J., Tracy, D., & Giaroli, G. (2014). The use of antipsychotics in preschoolers: A veto or a sensible last option. *Journal of Psychopharmacology, 28,* 303–319. https://doi.org/10.1177/0269881113519506.

Olfson, M., Crystal, S., Huang, C., & Gerhard, T. (2010). Trends in antipsychotic drug use by very young, privately insured children. *Journal of the American Academy of Child and Adolescent Psychiatry, 49,* 13–23. https://doi.org/10.1097/00004583-201001000-00005.

Olfson, M., King, M., & Schoenbaum, M. (2016). Stimulant treatment of young people in the United States. *Journal of Child and Adolescent Psychopharmacology, 26*(6), 520–526.

Sanders, M. R., Bor, W., & Morawska, A. (2007). Maintenance of treatment gains: A comparison of enhanced, standard, and self-directed Triple P-Positive Parenting Program. *Journal of Abnormal Child Psychology, 35*(6), 983.

Schleifer, M., Wiss, G., Cohen, N., Elman, M., Cvejic, H., & Kruger, E. (1975). Hyperactivity in preschoolers and the effect of methylphenidate. *American Journal of Orthopsychiatry, 45.* https://doi.org/10.111/j.1939-0025.1975.tb01164.x.

Schopler, E., Reichler, R., & Rochen, R. (1988). *The childhood autism rating scale*. Los Angeles, CA: Western Psychological Services.

Swanson, J., Arnold, L., Molina, B., Sibley, M., Hechtman, L., Hinshaw, S., … & Nichols, Q. (2017). Young adult outcomes in the follow-up of the multimodal treatment study of attention-deficit/hyperactivity disorder: symptom persistence, source discrepancy, and height suppression. *Journal of Child Psychology and Psychiatry, 58,* 663–678. https://doi.org/10.1111/jcpp.12684.

Vitiello, B., Abikoff, H., Chuange, S., Kollins, S., McCracken, J., Riddle, M., … Greenhill, L. (2007). Effectiveness of methylphenidate in the 10-month continuation phase of the preschoolers with ADHD treatment study (PATS). *Journal of Child and Adolescent Psychopharmacology, 17,* 593–603. https://doi.org/10.1089/cap.2007.0058.

Vitiello, B., Lazzaretto, D., Yershova, K., Abikoff, H., Paykina, N., McCracken, J, … Riddle, M. (2015). Pharmacotherapy of the preschool ADHD treatment study (PATS) children growing up. *Journal of the American Academy of Child and Adolescent Psychiatry, 54,* 550–556. https://doi.org/10.1016/j.jaac.2015.04.004.

Webster-Stratton, C., Jamila Reid, M., & Stoolmiller, M. (2008). Preventing conduct problems and improving school readiness: Evaluation of the incredible years teacher and child training programs in high-risk schools. *Journal of Child Psychology and Psychiatry, 49*(5), 471–488.

Whalen, D. J., Sylvester, C. M., & Luby, J. L. (2017). Depression and anxiety in preschoolers: A review of the past 7 years. *Child and Adolescent Psychiatric Clinics, 26*(3), 503–522.

Wigal, T., Greenhill., L., Chuange, S., McGough, J., Vitiello, B., … Stehli, A. (2006). Safety and tolerability of methylphenidate in preschool children with ADHD. *Journal of the American Academy of Child and Adolescent Psychiatry, 45,* 1294–1303. https://doi.org/10.1097/01.chi.0000235082.63156.27.

Willemsen-Swinkels, S., Buitelaar, J., Weijnen, F., & van Engeland, H. (1995). Placebo-controlled acute dosage naltrexone study in young autistic children. *Psychiatry Research, 58*(3), 203–215. https://doi.org/10.1016/0165-1781(95)02749-M.

Chapter 11
Cultural Considerations in School Psychopharmacology

Anisa N. Goforth, Andy V. Pham and Olivia G. Holter

Cultural Considerations in School Psychopharmacology

As schools become more culturally and linguistically diverse, school- and community-based mental health professionals are expected to provide culturally responsive services to address children's emotional, behavioral, and social needs. Recent estimates suggest that nearly 18 million children in the United States live with at least one immigrant parent (Zong & Batalova, 2015). Furthermore, the racial composition and language diversity of individuals in the United States are expected to increase within the next decade (Colby & Ortman, 2015). These demographic changes suggest that children in schools require culturally responsive mental health services that may include psychosocial and/or psychopharmacological interventions (e.g., medication).

There also has been increasing attention on addressing barriers to mental health treatments and reducing ethnic and racial disparities nationwide (United States Department of Health and Human Services, 2001). African American and Latina/o children living in urban cities utilized mental health services at approximately half the rate of White children, despite having similar socioeconomic conditions (Coker et al., 2009). Many minority and immigrant families experience challenges to mental health care, including poorer quality of care than White families, leading to disparities in mental health, and medication treatments (United States Department of Health and Human Services, 2001). Minorities and immigrants also experience more help-seeking barriers than White individuals, which include financial difficulties, stigma, and conflicting views of the causes of, and ways of coping with, mental health problems (Pham, Goforth, Chun, Castro-Olivo, & Costa, 2017).

A. N. Goforth (✉) · O. G. Holter
University of Montana, Missoula, MT, USA
e-mail: Anisa.Goforth@umontana.edu

A. V. Pham
Florida International University, Miami, FL, USA

J. S. Carlson and J. A. Barterian (eds.), *School Psychopharmacology*,
Pediatric School Psychology, https://doi.org/10.1007/978-3-030-15541-4_11

Mental health providers who use multimodal treatment approaches that combine both psychosocial and psychopharmacological treatments should take into consideration sociocultural factors when addressing mental health disparities. Using an integrative ecological model of development (Garcia Coll et al., 1996), this chapter highlights the sociocultural context of the child and family when developing treatment plans that involve psychopharmacological intervention. First, we provide an overview of notable sociocultural factors that should be considered when working with ethnic minority and/or immigrant children and families. Second, we include a brief primer on cultural psychiatry and the integration of clinical services with school support. Lastly, we discuss recommendations for school personnel when providing mental health services to diverse children and families, with a focus on psychopharmacological treatment for children.

Sociocultural Factors in Multimodal Treatment

There are a number of sociocultural factors to consider when using psychosocial and psychopharmacological treatments for diverse youth, particularly given the significant barriers to treatment for this group. The sources of these barriers and the subsequent health disparities can be described from three levels: the patient (e.g., child/parent), the provider, and the healthcare system (Smedley, Stith, & Nelson, 2012). Examples of relevant challenges from these levels include (a) conflicting parent perceptions of mental health and perceived need, (b) distrust of authority and/or systems, (c) stigma of mental health services, and (d) acculturative stress and language barriers (Pham, 2015). By understanding these barriers, as well as the multiple systems influencing a child's development (Garcia Coll et al., 1996) that influence parent treatment decision-making, providers can implement culturally responsive treatments that meet the child's individual needs.

Perceptions of Mental Health and Perceived Need

Several primary sociocultural factors to consider are the perceived need for treatment, the decision-making processes for treatment, and cultural/environmental concerns. There are often different perceptions among parents of disease etiology and healing processes based on the parent's cultures, as people from different societies vary in their perceptions of the origin and outcomes of mental health (Schlosser & Ninnemann, 2012). For instance, while mainstream United States (US) culture generally considers primarily biological causes of mental health disorders, Bangladeshi and Ethiopian cultures consider primarily fate or cosmic forces as the cause of mental health problems (Berry, Poortinga, Segall, & Dasen, 2002). In fact, in some cultures, such as the Lakota of the Northern Plains, there is no language for mental illness and "wellness" is defined more broadly to incorporate a number of "life forces" (Todd-Bazemore, 1999, p. 141). These cultural variations in definitions or conceptualizations of mental health are particularly important when considering psychopharmacological treatments.

Parental perceptions of psychopharmacological treatments. Parents' judgments of treatment, or treatment acceptability, is another factor that can influence treatment adherence (Kazdin, 1981). It is also defined as the degree to which stakeholders perceive the intervention to be fair, reasonable, appropriate, and consistent with expectations of treatment. Several studies have examined parents' perceptions and acceptability of Attention -Deficit/Hyperactivity Disorder (ADHD) interventions (Eiraldi & Diaz, 2010). ADHD is one of the most common childhood neurobehavioral disorders where treatment typically involves behavioral intervention, parent training, and/or psychotropic medication (e.g., psychostimulants; Visser et al., 2014). Although earlier research indicated that minority parents were less knowledgeable about ADHD etiology and treatments than nonminority parents (Bussing, Gary, Mills, & Garvan, 2003), more recent research indicated that this knowledge gap across ethnicities has narrowed over the past decade (Pham, Carlson, & Kosciulek, 2010).

Parental views of medication treatment have been investigated via several attributes including (1) duration and degree of symptom control (i.e., efficacy), (2) frequency of dosage, (3) potential for treatment abuse or dependence, (4) modes of administration, (5) side effects, and (6) treatment acceptability (Nafees et al., 2014). In one study, parents of adolescents from six different European countries rated "degree of symptom control" as the most important attribute when determining treatment choice, and there were also cultural variations among parents about medication side effects (Nafees et al., 2014). Pham and colleagues (2010) also found that minority parents (e.g., Latina/o and African American parents) in the US were most concerned about medication side effects, and rated this treatment option (e.g., psychostimulant treatment) less favorably than non-pharmacological treatment (e.g., counseling) for children with ADHD. However, the same parents also believed that medication was more efficacious in controlling symptoms quickly than counseling alone (Pham et al., 2010). Similarly, Latina mothers with children referred for behavior problems reported that medication was not even considered an option for treating their child because of concerns about long-term effects of medication on their child's physical and mental functioning (Arcia, Fernandez, & Jaquez, 2004). Thus, treatment acceptability and treatment adherence of medication may be low when the family's cultural beliefs do not align with Western medicine.

Distrust of Authority and Western Culture

For minority, refugee, or indigenous families, practitioners must be mindful of the history and experience of these populations to develop trusting relationships with parents and their communities (Ellis, Miller, Baldwin, & Abdi, 2011). Due to factors such as the political climate, families may have developed a distrust of authority and government, particularly among communities who have experienced historical trauma, racism, discrimination, and potential deportation (Ellis et al., 2011; Pham et al., 2017). Moreover, inequities stemming from social, economic, and environmental disadvantage also make it difficult for immigrant and indigenous families to trust service providers from Western cultures that represent a more socially empowered group. Effective services include authentic efforts to understand the family's personal, acculturation, or immigration experiences, cultural perceptions of mental health, and histories in order to build and establish relationships with underserved communities.

Mental Health Stigma

Mental health stigma may also impede families from seeking help for their child. For example, among some primarily White families in rural communities, one of the most cited barriers to receiving mental health care is stigma associated with accessing a mental health professional because of concerns of other community members' views (Hastings & Cohn, 2013). In rural communities where cultural values of autonomy and self-reliance may influence their willingness to seek mental health care, there is often a "stigma by association" in which parents with children with behavioral problems were concerned about the public stigma toward them by neighbors as well as by teachers in the schools (Heflinger, Wallston, Mukolo, & Brannan, 2014).

Similarly, some ethnically diverse parents who perceived their child's problems as being due to physical causes or trauma, rather than spirituality or disharmony, were more likely to seek mental health services for their children (Yeh et al., 2005). These families that attribute mental health issues to physical causes may be more likely to seek help because it may be less stigmatizing. Help-seeking behavior may, therefore, be affected by family's perceptions and beliefs of mental health.

Acculturation and Language Barriers

Acculturation, defined as the psychological, social, and behavioral change that results from participating in a variety of cultural environments (Berry et al., 2002), is another sociocultural factor to consider when developing treatment plans that involve medications. Acculturation is a multidimensional construct, in which an individual is adapting and negotiating with multiple cultural contexts, including the mainstream culture (e.g., American culture) as well as the heritage culture (e.g., ethnic or national origin). Further, acculturative stress may occur during the process of acculturation and can result in a number of negative outcomes for children and adolescents, such as higher internalizing symptoms (Sirin, Ryce, Gupta, & Rogers-Sirin, 2013) or conduct problems (Hurwich-Reiss & Gudiño, 2016).

Some families may experience acculturative stress when seeking healthcare services, particularly when the providers do not understand their cultural beliefs (Jin &

Acharya, 2016). Some families, such as those of Chinese descent who have maintained their heritage culture, may be less willing to incorporate Western medicine practices for their children because they do not trust the American medical system due to their lack of knowledge of Western medicine (Jin & Acharya, 2016). These participants also noted that they did not feel comfortable communicating with physicians, which affected their understanding of the purpose of medication. Overall, acculturation and acculturative stress may need to be considered when developing treatment plans involving medications, particularly for immigrant children.

The lack of linguistic services presents a further challenge for parents, as they may find it difficult to communicate with practitioners about concerns, personal experiences, or their worldview. Parents who are non-English speaking experience greater barriers to healthcare services, even when taking into account socioeconomic background, US nativity, and length of time in the US, or insurance status (Sentell, Shumway, & Snowden, 2007). Thus, for services to be accessible, practitioners, or at least translators, must demonstrate language fluency for both the child and parents. Given the potential differences in acculturation levels and language proficiency between immigrant youth and their parents, practitioners need to incorporate this understanding when developing treatment plans and monitoring medication outcomes.

Cultural Psychiatry: A Primer for School-Based Professionals

Mental health promotion among culturally diverse youth requires an understanding of the various sociocultural factors outlined above, as well as an integrated response to treatment barriers. Cultural (or transcultural) psychiatry seeks to determine how sociocultural factors create, determine, or influence mental illness in individuals, families, and communities (Measham, Heidenreich-Dutray, Rousseau, & Nadeau, 2014). With influences in psychological and social sciences, transcultural psychiatry is rooted in a biopsychosocial model. Transcultural psychiatry, therefore, fosters an integrated and interdisciplinary approach to mental health care with the focus on delivering culturally responsive assessment, consultation, and treatment services that are accessible to families. The Cultural Formulation Interview (CFI), which was included in the *Diagnostic and Statistical Manual, Fifth Edition* (DSM-5; American Psychiatric Association, 2013) is one method of collecting culturally relevant information from individuals and family members in order for clinicians to assess their worldview of the concern and aid in treatment planning (see Table 11.1). Ultimately, strategies employed from these programs using a multitiered system of support include engaging family and the community, developing partnerships with school-based professionals and staff, and integrating behavioral and mental health services with schools.

Table 11.1 Cultural Formulation Interview from the Diagnostic and Statistical Manual of Mental Disorders, Fifth Edition (American Psychiatric Association, 2013)

1. *Cultural definition of the problem*
Problem definition Questions to consider: How did the family describe the overall problem during the interview? Are there discrepancies between family members regarding the definition of the problem?
2. *Cultural perceptions of cause, context, and support*
Causes of the problem Questions to consider: What are the perceived causes of the problem according to family members (in terms of physical, spiritual, biological, or environmental causes)? Are these perceptions based on heritage or mainstream culture? Are there discrepancies between family members regarding the causes of the problem? *Stressors and supports* Questions to consider: Considering sociocultural norms and family structure, what unique stressors are the child and family experiencing? What are the child's and family's past and current sources of support? *Role of cultural identity* Questions to consider: What are the language, cultural, and religious backgrounds of which the child and family self-identify? What backgrounds do they not explicitly self-identify? Do the child and family have friends and/or reside in communities of their heritage or mainstream culture? Does the child interact with extended family members?
3. *Cultural factors affecting self-coping and past help seeking*
Self-coping Questions to consider: How and when does the child cope with challenges or difficulties? How often does this occur? *Past help seeking* Questions to consider: What kinds of help, services, or support have been sought in the past to address the problem? Did this occur in church, school, community, or with physician? What is the family's perception of the services sought? What were their expectations of the child's outcome after seeking help? *Barriers* Questions to consider: What has prevented the child or family from getting the help, services, and/or support that they need? Do language barriers, stigma, work and family commitments, racial/systemic discrimination, and lack of financial resources play a role?
4. *Cultural factors affecting current help seeking*
Preferences Questions to consider: What are the child's and family's perceived needs? What types of help would be most useful for the child and family currently and in the future? What is the timeframe that the family members hope to resolve the child's problem? *Clinician–patient relationship* Questions to consider: What are the child's and family's goals and expected results when meeting with the clinician? Are there discrepancies between clinician, child, and family members regarding goals and expectations?

Engaging Family and Community (Tier 1)

Engagement with family and community can help to establish trust between practitioners and families, and thus enhancing the cultural appropriateness of mental health services. Given that children often do not seek out mental health services themselves, "gateway providers" (e.g., parents, teachers, and school-based professionals) are important in initiating mental health services (Berger-Jenkins, McKay, Newcorn, Bannon, & Laraque, 2011). Services for children with significant mental health needs, therefore, must be built on a broader platform of community, schools, and youth and community engagement that seek to educate and support families (Ellis et al., 2011).

One approach is to develop parent outreach programs and community advisory boards that provide means of networking and disseminating resources with meaningful involvement of parents (Ellis et al., 2011). Partnerships with community-based organizations that serve immigrant or minority populations, along with the development of an interdisciplinary team, can help ensure that a diversity of perspectives and expertise is represented when addressing barriers or implementing services. For example, the Division of Social and Transcultural Psychiatry at McGill University, Jewish General Hospital, and Montreal Children's Hospital consist of a transcultural team of psychiatrists, anthropologists, psychologists, and clinicians who specialize in providing culturally responsive assessment, consultation, and treatment services to refugee and immigrant families in inner-city neighborhoods. With strong ties to community organizations and schools, the community-based team addresses issues related to risk and protective factors of refugee children and families, cultural adaptation and identity, war or migration trauma, and evaluation of school-based programs for refugee children (Measham et al., 2014).

Partnerships with School-Based Providers and Staff (Tier 2)

Partnerships with schools should be a core component of mental health services. School-related difficulties are typically more acceptable targets for services than problems related to mental illness (Ellis et al., 2011); however, parents, may have little or no involvement with their children's school. In some cultures, school-related issues are in the purview of teachers, rather than the parents (Birman & Espino, 2007). Thus, parent involvement with the school regarding child behavior can be a cultural shift for many families. Providing open houses, community-based workshops, English-learning classes, or computer literacy courses for parents can help reframe parents' perception of the school as a less stigmatizing environment.

To address children's mental health in schools, one school- and community-based program, Supporting the Health of Immigrant Families and Adolescents (SHIFA), provided weekly support groups for Somali refugee children in Boston Public School classrooms (Ellis et al., 2011). Because many Somali refugees have experienced significant exposure to trauma and acculturative stress, providing supports in the school system can help students recognize stressors and learn to use emotional regulation skills in applied settings (Ellis et al., 2011). In an attempt to streamline psychosocial services and behavioral supports into the school culture, school-based professionals can monitor academic and behavioral outcomes over the course of treatment. Teachers can also monitor these outcomes, and provide reinforcement or incentives, such as organizing class- or school-wide events (e.g., pizza parties) to promote children's positive behavior and successes.

Integrating Behavioral and Mental Health Services with Schools (Tier 3)

For children with significant mental health needs, intensive services may be warranted that often include pharmacological treatment. School-based medical evaluations and integrated healthcare centers are uniquely positioned to provide these services alongside preventive and psychosocial treatments. Psychosocial treatments may include school-based individual and group psychotherapy or home-based care in addition to educational supports, social services, and family therapies. If parents perceive these services as stigmatizing or unwanted, the interdisciplinary team should provide a space for dialogue to address parental and professional concerns and identify areas of common ground centered on the best interests of children (Measham et al., 2014).

Pharmacological treatment may also be needed for treating symptoms; however, for many families, medication may be the least preferred choice of treatment. Depending on the severity of the concern, psychosocial treatments that target stressors or changes in the social environment, along with teaching coping skills and techniques, can be effective alternatives to medication. However, school psychologists and other trained healthcare professionals can closely monitor and evaluate medication outcomes for severe externalizing or internalizing disorders. Nevertheless, providers should first provide an open dialogue with parents exploring potential benefits and drawbacks of medication intervention (e.g., child's age, cultural perceptions of treatment, medication titration, side effects), if behavioral or emotional concerns are not remediated by psychosocial intervention alone.

Implications and Recommendations for School Personnel

There are a number of implications for school personnel given the various sociocultural factors in treatment and barriers to mental health for immigrant and/or ethnic minority families, including providing culturally responsive assessment and treatment (see Fig. 11.1).

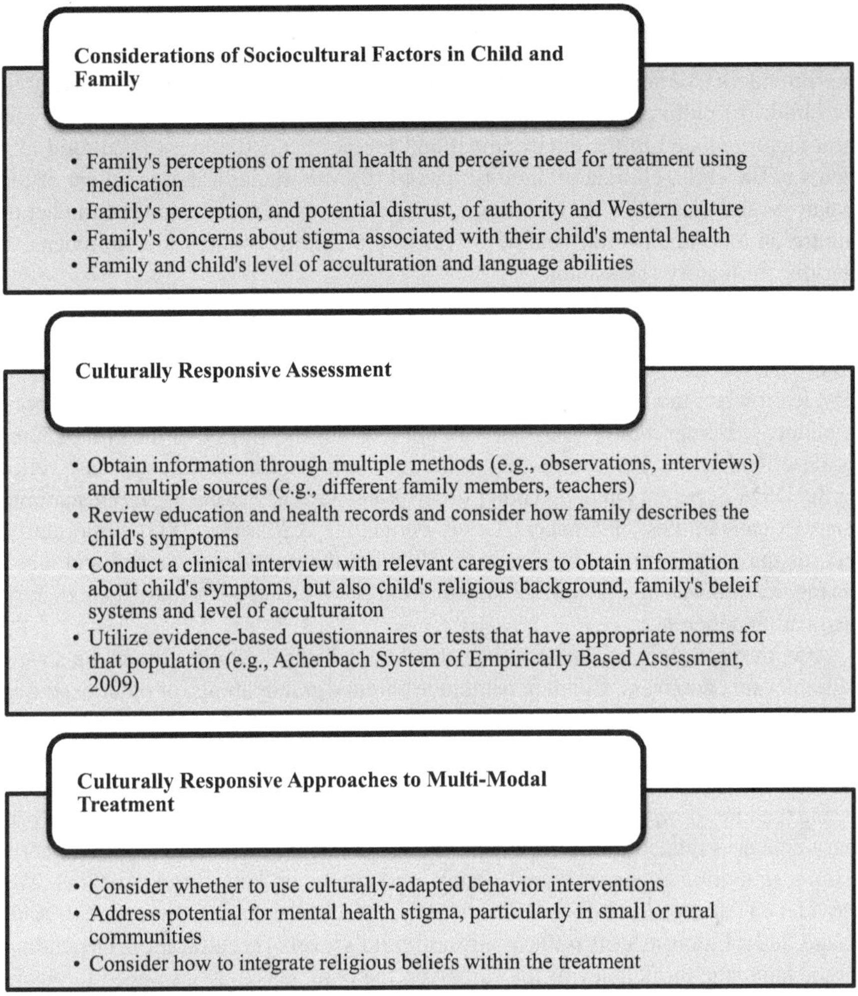

Fig. 11.1 Considerations for providing culturally responsive evidence-based assessment and multimodal treatment to diverse children

Culturally Responsive Evidence-Based Practices in Assessment

When working with ethnic minority and/or immigrant families, mental health providers should consider how to provide a non-discriminatory assessment to inform treatment, particularly when the treatment plan involves psychopharmacological treatment. It is important that a multi-method, multisource non-discriminatory assessment is conducted that examines a child within various ecological systems (e.g., home, school; Rhodes, Ochoa, & Ortiz, 2005). Providers should develop a cultural formulation of the child's pattern of symptoms beyond the diagnoses from the DSM-5. Specifically, Mezzich, Caracci, Fabrega, and Kirmayer (2009) suggest that providers examine the individual across five domains: (a) cultural identity of the child, (b) cultural explanation of the child's mental health problems, (c) cultural factors related to the environment and levels of functioning, (d) cultural elements of the child–clinician relationship, and (e) overall cultural assessment of the diagnosis and treatment. By examining these elements of culture and the impact of culture on a child's mental health, providers are able to conduct a comprehensive non-discriminatory assessment.

First, providers should conduct a review of the child's educational and health records to gather preliminary data on the child's history of mental health problems. Through a record review, the provider can understand the child's mental health history, learn when those problems first occurred, and the interventions that have been implemented. Importantly, providers should look for the ways that the child's family described his or her symptoms. Although American mental health care relies on the DSM-5, parents may use other descriptors, such as *ataque de nervios* among Puerto Rican families (Guarnaccia, Lewis-Fernández, & Marano, 2003). Importantly, records may also note any medications, allowing the provider to understand when the medication was first prescribed, medication dosage, and potentially the extent of medication adherence.

After the record review, the provider should conduct a thorough clinical interview with relevant caregivers, which may include parents, grandparents, or other extended family members. In many cultural groups, there may be multiple generations of family members within a household and each caregiver may share different perspectives on the child's behavioral problems and preferred treatment modalities. Furthermore, during the interview, the mental health provider can gather information about the primary concerns related to the child's problems, including the child's developmental history, schooling experience, and social, emotional, and behavioral concerns. The provider can also gather information about the family's heritage culture, beliefs, language, and religion, as well as the family and child's level of acculturation. Depending on the language proficiency of the caregiver, the clinicians may also need to obtain an interpreter that is equally fluent in English and the family's native language, and ideally, has no prior relationship with the family (Rhodes et al., 2005).

The clinical interview should be conducted with an understanding that language, culture, and social context can play a role in symptom expression (Alcántara & Gone, 2014). Among some ethnic minority groups, such as Arab Americans, caregivers may express concerns about the psychological symptoms using physical or somatic terms (Melhem & Chemali, 2014). The interview may also facilitate a better understanding of the family's explanatory model of mental health. The provider can ask questions such as, "Tell me some reasons why [child] is having these concerns" or "What do you believe are the causes of these problems?" to get a sense of the family's perspectives on etiological factors. The provider can explicitly ask, "Some families choose to provide medication to their child. What are your thoughts on medication?" Overall, the provider can ask relevant questions about their cultural beliefs related to the cause, nature, and effect of the child's mental health problems.

In addition, questionnaires, tests and behavior observations may be helpful in developing treatment plans as well as for progress monitoring. There are a number of measures, such as the Achenbach System of Empirically Based Assessment (2009) that have been normed with culturally and linguistically diverse children. Obtaining these scores from these measures can provide baseline data prior for physicians related to the administration of medication to the child. That is, pre- and post-treatment data can be gathered to understand the effectiveness of the medication. Similarly, observations of social, emotional, and behavioral functioning can be helpful in examining the effectiveness of the medication, as well as examining any potential side effects from the medication.

Culturally Responsive Approaches to Multimodal Treatment

Multimodal treatments that include psychosocial and psychopharmacological approaches have extensive research support for a variety of child disorders. Combined treatment approaches have been shown to be effective for children with ADHD (Hinshaw, Arnold, & M. T. A. Cooperative Group, 2015), anxiety (Piacentini et al., 2014), as well as preliminary research for reducing aggression in children with Autism Spectrum Disorder (Frazier et al., 2010). Thus, using multiple approaches may address issues for a variety of referral problems.

Providers who implement culturally responsive treatments should consider whether to implement evidence-based interventions with fidelity or to implement culturally-adapted interventions that may more appropriately meet the individual needs of culturally diverse youth. For example, cognitive-behavioral therapy is a highly effective treatment for a number of internalizing symptoms (Adler Nevo et al., 2014); however, culturally-adapted therapies, such as *cuento therapy* that uses storytelling techniques, has also been shown to be effective with specific populations (e.g., Puerto Rican children; Costantino, Malgady, & Rogler, 1986). Further, providers may also need to consider culturally-specific treatments, such as those among many indigenous American cultures such as the Lakota, in which treatment for a variety of ailments may be conducted through Sweatlodge ceremonies (Todd-Bazemore, 1999). During these ceremonies, temperatures are very high, leading to an increase in an individual's core body temperature; physicians and other providers may need to be aware of how psychopharmacological medications may interact with those participating in these traditional ceremonies.

Multimodal treatment approaches that include medication should also be considered within rural populations. Historically, delivering behavioral health services, including psychopharmacological interventions, in rural communities has been difficult. There are many barriers that have been identified, including fewer available medical centers (i.e., a significant shortage of child psychiatrists, primary care physicians with knowledge of mental health treatments) and psychologists (Amundson, 2001). Further, mental health providers may want to consider how to address psychosocial interventions overall given high stigma associated with mental health.

Providers may want to emphasize his or her responsibility to confidentiality and privacy, and provide many opportunities for the family to ask questions.

Mental health providers should also take into consideration religion and religious practices when considering psychotropic and psychosocial treatments with children and their families. For instance, among some Evangelical Christians, research suggests that evangelicals are less likely to perceive ADHD as a real disease and that children should not be treated with medication (Li, 2013). Furthermore, there may be perceptions that children's behavior problems are associated with them being "bad" rather than "sick," and thus children should be held accountable for their actions or behaviors. Other religious minorities, such as Muslims, integrate spiritual, physical, and mental aspects of help, and believe that God can provide an important role in the healing process (Padela, Killawi, Forman, DeMonner, & Heisler, 2012). Thus, mental health providers may want to ask the families whether or how religion or spirituality is important in their children's treatment.

Summary

School-based professionals can promote the academic and social success of culturally and linguistically-diverse children by understanding culturally-responsive approaches to providing psychosocial and psychopharmacological treatment. Overall, mental health providers should consider sociocultural factors beyond race when providing culturally-responsive treatment. By recognizing the interplay of such factors as perceptions of disease etiology, acculturation, cultural background, or religion, mental health providers can collaborate with families to improve the child's psychological well-being. Further, mental health providers should take into consideration the various sociocultural factors that may affect treatment acceptability and adherence, including perceptions of mental health and psychopharmacological treatment, distrust of authority and Western culture, and acculturation and language barriers. Using an interdisciplinary, tiered approach, providers can implement an integrated response to treatment barriers. By working within these systems, and collaborating with professionals within each system, mental health providers can better able to serve culturally diverse children to help them succeed in school.

List of Readings

Jones, J. (2014). Best practices in providing culturally responsive interventions. In P. L. Harrison & A. Thomas (Eds.), *Best practices in school psychology* (pp. 49–60). Bethesda, MD: National Association of School Psychologists.

This chapter provides a brief overview of best practice in school-based culturally-responsive interventions for children from different cultural and linguistic backgrounds. Additionally, this author asks the reader to question how to adapt practices to be culturally-responsive.

Lewis-Fernández, R., Aggarwal, N. K., Hinton, L., Hinton, D. E., In Kirmayer, L. J., & American Psychiatric Association (Eds.). (2015). *DSM-5 handbook on the cultural formulation interview.*

The Cultural Formation Interview (CFI) is an interview aimed to give clinicians an introduction to the cultural background of their clients. This tool can help clinicians pinpoint important cultural factors in order to best help their clients.

Lin, K. (2010). Cultural and ethnic issues in psychopharmacology. Psychiatric Times. Retrieved from http://www.psychiatrictimes.com/articles/cultural-and-ethnic-issues-psychopharmacology

This article considers the differences in effects of psychotropic medications across cultures. Additionally, this article describes how medical providers should take in considering a person's ethnic background in treating behavioral health conditions with medications.

List of Websites

Centers for Disease Control and Prevention. CDC Health Disparities & Inequalities Report (CHDIR). https://www.cdc.gov/minorityhealth/chdireport.html

This report provides information that clinicians may find useful for practice related to health disparities among individuals from ethnic minority and/or immigrant backgrounds. The CDC website also provides links to resources that summarize strategies for reducing health disparities.

Dimensions of Culture: Cross-Cultural Communications for Healthcare Professionals. http://www.dimensionsofculture.com/2014/03/cross-cultural-considerations-in-prescribing-medication/ http://www.dimensionsofculture.com/2014/03/cross-cultural-considerations-in-prescribing-medication/

This resource provides an overview of questions clinicians may want to consider when speaking with diverse clients about using medications in treating behavioral health conditions. Additionally, this website has additional resources specific to minority cultures within the United States.

Mental Health America. Minority Mental Health. http://www.mentalhealthamerica.net/conditions/minority-mental-health

This resource helps individuals understand behavioral health issues among a number of minority groups within the US. This web page also links to current policy issues and provides mental health resources in Spanish.

References

Achenbach System of Empircally Based Assessment (ASEBA). (2009). Group 1, 2, and 3 societies for CBCL, TRF, and YSR problem scales. Retrieved May 12, 2009, from http://www.aseba.org/products/Groups.html.

Adler Nevo, G. W., Avery, D., Fiksenbaum, L., Kiss, A., Mendlowitz, S., Monga, S., et al. (2014). Eight years later: Outcomes of CBT-treated versus untreated anxious children. *Brain and Behavior, 4,* 765–774. https://doi.org/10.1002/brb3.274.

Alcántara, C., & Gone, J. P. (2014). Multicultural issues in the clinical interview and diagnostic process. In F. T. Leong, L. Comas-Díaz, G. C. Nagayama Hall, V. C. McLoyd & J. E. Trimble (Eds.), *APA handbook of multicultural psychology* (Vol. 2: Applications and Training). Washington, D.C.: American Psychological Association.

American Psychiatric Association. (2013). *Diagnostic and statistical manual of mental disorders* (5th ed.). Washington, D.C.: American Psychiatric Association.

Amundson, B. (2001). America's rural communities as crucibles for clinical reform: Establishing collaborative care teams in rural communities. *Families, Systems, and Health, 19,* 3–33.

Arcia, E., Fernandez, M. C., & Jaquez, M. (2004). Latina mothers' stances on stimulant medication: Complexity, conflict, and compromise. *Developmental and Behavioral Pediatrics, 25,* 311–317.

Berger-Jenkins, E., McKay, M., Newcorn, J., Bannon, W., & Laraque, D. (2011). Parent medication concerns predict underutilization of mental health services for minority children with ADHD. *Clinical Pediatrics, 51,* 65–76. https://doi.org/10.1177/0009922811417286.

Berry, J. W., Poortinga, Y. H., Segall, M. H., & Dasen, P. R. (2002). *Cross-cultural psychology: Research and applications* (2nd ed.). Cambridge: Cambridge University Press.

Birman, D., & Espino, S. R. (2007). The relationship of parental practices and knowledge to school adaptation for immigrant and nonimmigrant high school students. *Canadian Journal of School Psychology, 22,* 152–166. https://doi.org/10.1177/0829573507307803.

Bussing, R., Gary, F. A., Mills, T. L., & Garvan, C. W. (2003). Parental explanatory models of ADHD. *Social Psychiatry and Psychiatric Epidemiology, 38,* 563-575. https://doi.org/10.1007/s00127-003-0674-8.

Coker, T. R., Elliott, M. N., Kanouse, D. E., Grunbaum, J. A., Schwebel, D. C., Gilliland, M. J., et al. (2009). Perceived racial/ethnic discrimination among fifth-grade students and its association with mental health. *American Journal of Public Health, 99,* 878–884. https://doi.org/10.2105/AJPH.2008.144329.

Colby, S. L., & Ortman, J. M. (2015). Projections of the size and composition of the U.S. population: 2014 and 2060. Retrieved from https://www.census.gov/content/dam/Census/library/publications/2015/demo/p25-1143.pdf.

Costantino, G., Malgady, R. G., & Rogler, L. H. (1986). Cuento therapy: A culturally sensitive modality for Puerto Rican children. *Journal of Consulting and Clinical Psychology, 54,* 639–645.

Eiraldi, R., & Diaz, Y. (2010). Use of treatment services for Attention-Deficit/hyperactivity Disorder in Latino children. *Current Psychiatry Reports, 12,* 403–408. https://doi.org/10.1007/s11920-010-0139-1.

Ellis, B. H., Miller, A. B., Baldwin, H., & Abdi, S. (2011). New directions in refugee youth mental health services: Overcoming barriers to engagement. *Journal of Child & Adolescent Trauma, 4,* 69–85. https://doi.org/10.1080/19361521.2011.545047.

Frazier, T. W., Youngstrom, E. A., Haycook, T., Sinoff, A., Dimitriou, F., Knapp, J., et al. (2010). Effectiveness of medication combined with intensive behavioral intervention for reducing aggression in youth with autism spectrum disorder. *Journal of Child and Adolescent Psychopharmacology, 20,* 167–177.

Garcia Coll, C., Lamberty, G., Jenkins, R., McAdoo, H. P., Crnic, K., Wasik, B. H., et al. (1996). An Integrative model for the study of developmental competencies in minority children. *Child Development, 67,* 1891–1914.

Guarnaccia, P. J., Lewis-Fernández, R., & Marano, M. R. (2003). Toward a Puerto Rican popular nosology: Nervios and Ataque de Nervios. *Culture, Medicine and Psychiatry, 27*, 339–366. https://doi.org/10.1023/a:1025303315932.

Hastings, S. L., & Cohn, T. J. (2013). Challenges and opportunities associated with rural mental health practice. *Journal of Rural Mental Health, 37*, 37–49. https://doi.org/10.1037/rmh0000002.

Heflinger, C. A., Wallston, K. A., Mukolo, A., & Brannan, A. M. (2014). Perceived stigma toward children with emotional and behavioral problems and their families: The Attitudes about Child Mental Health Questionnaire (ACMHQ). *Journal of Rural Mental Health, 38*, 9–19. https://doi.org/10.1037/rmh0000010.

Hinshaw, S. P., Arnold, L. E., & M. T. A. Cooperative Group. (2015). Attention-Deficit Hyperactivity Disorder, multimodal treatment, and longitudinal outcome: Evidence, paradox, and challenge. *Wiley Interdisciplinary Reviews: Cognitive Science, 6*, 39–52. https://doi.org/10.1002/wcs.1324.

Hurwich-Reiss, E., & Gudiño, O. G. (2016). Acculturation stress and conduct problems among Latino adolescents: The impact of family factors. *Journal of Latina/o Psychology, 4*, 218–231. https://doi.org/10.1037/lat0000052.

Jin, L., & Acharya, L. (2016). Cultural beliefs underlying medication adherence in people of Chinese descent in the United States. *Health Communication, 31*, 513–521. https://doi.org/10.1080/10410236.2014.974121.

Kazdin, A. E. (1981). Acceptability of child treatment techniques: The influence of treatment efficacy and adverse side effects. *Behavior Therapy, 12*, 493–506.

Li, K. (2013). Religion and medicalization: The case of ADHD. *Journal for the Scientific Study of Religion, 52*, 309–327. https://doi.org/10.1111/jssr.12023.

Measham, T., Heidenreich-Dutray, F., Rousseau, C., & Nadeau, L. (2014). Cultural consultation in child psychiatry. In J. G. L. J. Kirmayer & C. Rousseau (Eds.), *Cultural consultation* (pp. 71–87). New York: Springer.

Melhem, I., & Chemali, Z. (2014). Mental health of Arab Americans: Cultural considerations for excellence of care. In P. Ranna (Ed.), *The Massachusetts General Hospital textbook on diversity and cultural sensitivity in mental health* (pp. 3–30). Totowa, NJ: Humana Press.

Mezzich, J. E., Caracci, G., Fabrega, H., & Kirmayer, L. J. (2009). Cultural formulation guidelines. *Transcultural Psychiatry, 46*, 383–405. https://doi.org/10.1177/1363461509342942.

Nafees, B., Setyawan, J., Lloyd, A., Ali, S., Hearn, S., Sasane, R., et al. (2014). Parent preferences regarding stimulant therapies for ADHD: A comparison across six European countries. *European Child and Adolescent Psychiatry, 23*, 1189–1200. https://doi.org/10.1007/s00787-013-0515-6.

Padela, A. I., Killawi, A., Forman, J., DeMonner, S., & Heisler, M. (2012). American Muslim perceptions of healing: Key agents in healing, and their roles. *Qualitative Health Research, 22*, 846–858. https://doi.org/10.1177/1049732312438969.

Pham, A. (2015). Understanding ADHD from a biopsychosocial-cultural framework: A case study. *Contemporary School Psychology, 19*, 54–62.

Pham, A. V., Carlson, J. S., & Kosciulek, J. F. (2010). Ethnic differences in parental beliefs of Attention-Deficit/Hyperactivity Disorder and treatment. *Journal of Attention Disorders, 13*, 584–591. https://doi.org/10.1177/1087054709332391.

Pham, A. V., Goforth, A. N., Chun, H., Castro-Olivo, S., & Costa, A. (2017). Acculturation and help-seeking behavior in consultation: A sociocultural framework for mental health service. *Journal of Educational and Psychological Consultation*, 1–18. https://doi.org/10.1080/10474412.2017.1287574.

Piacentini, J., Bennett, S., Compton, S. N., Kendall, P. C., Birmaher, B., Albano, A. M., et al. (2014). 24- and 36-week outcomes for the Child/Adolescent Anxiety Multimodal Study (CAMS). *Journal of the American Academy of Child and Adolescent Psychiatry, 53*, 297–310. https://doi.org/10.1016/j.jaac.2013.11.010.

Rhodes, R. L., Ochoa, S. H., & Ortiz, S. O. (2005). *Assessing culturally and linguistically diverse students: A practical guide*. New York: Guilford Press.

Schlosser, A. V., & Ninnemann, K. (2012). Introduction to the special section: The anthropology of psychopharmaceuticals: Cultural and pharmacological efficacies in context. *Culture, Medicine and Psychiatry, 36,* 2–9. https://doi.org/10.1007/s11013-012-9249-z.

Sentell, T., Shumway, M., & Snowden, L. (2007). Access to mental health treatment by English language proficiency and race/ethnicity. *Journal of General Internal Medicine, 22,* 289–293. https://doi.org/10.1007/s11606-007-0345-7.

Sirin, S. R., Ryce, P., Gupta, T., & Rogers-Sirin, L. (2013). The role of acculturative stress on mental health symptoms for immigrant adolescents: A longitudinal investigation. *Developmental Psychology, 49,* 736–748. https://doi.org/10.1037/a0028398.

Smedley, B. D., Stith, A. Y., & Nelson, A. R. (2012). *Unequal treatment: Confronting racial and ethnic disparities in health care*. Washington, DC: The National Academies Press.

Todd-Bazemore, B. (1999). Cultural issues in psychopharmacology: Integrating medication treatment with Lakota Sioux traditions. *Journal of Clinical Psychology in Medical Settings, 6,* 139–150. https://doi.org/10.1023/a:1026211515879.

United States Department of Health and Human Services. (2001). Mental health: Culture, race, and ethnicity—A supplement to mental health: A report of the Surgeon General. Rockville, MD: U.S. Department of Health and Human Services, Substance Abuse and Mental Health Services Administration, Center for Mental Health Services.

Visser, S. N., Danielson, M. L., Bitsko, R. H., Holbrook, J. R., Kogan, M. D., Ghandour, R. M., et al. (2014). Trends in the parent-report of health care provider-diagnosed and medicated Attention-Deficit/Hyperactivity Disorder: United States, 2003–2011. *Journal of the American Academy of Child and Adolescent Psychiatry, 53,* 34–46.e32. https://doi.org/10.1016/j.jaac.2013.09.001.

Yeh, M., McCabe, K., Hough, R. L., Lau, A., Fakhry, F., & Garland, A. (2005). Why bother with beliefs? Examining relationships between race/ethnicity, parental beliefs about causes of child problems, and mental health service use. *Journal of Consulting and Clinical Psychology, 73,* 800–807. https://doi.org/10.1037/0022-006x.73.5.800.

Zong, J., & Batalova, J. (2015). Frequently requested statistics on immigrants and immigration in the United States. Retrieved from http://www.migrationpolicy.org/article/frequently-requested-statistics-immigrants-and-immigration-united-states.

Chapter 12
Integrated Behavioral Health: Coordinating Psychosocial and Pharmacological Interventions Across Family, School, and Health Systems

Thomas J. Power, Jennifer A. Mautone, Nathan J. Blum, Alexander G. Fiks and James P. Guevara

Behavioral Health: Coordinating Psychosocial and Pharmacological Interventions Across Family, School, and Health Systems

Mental health conditions are estimated to occur among at least 20% of children and adolescents (Merikangas et al., 2010), and treatment of mental health concerns among youth is more costly than any other childhood medical condition (Soni, 2015). Less than 30% of children with significant mental health needs receive services (Soni, 2015), and, on average, there is a delay of 8–10 years between symptom onset and engagement in behavioral health intervention (Wang et al., 2005). Families from low-income, urban, culturally diverse communities often face additional barriers to care that make it difficult for them to become engaged in evidence-based treatment and sustain their involvement throughout the duration of intervention (Eiraldi, Mazzuca, Clarke, & Power, 2006). Service use often depends on a combination of individual beliefs (e.g., knowledge and beliefs about mental health conditions, stigma) and access factors (e.g., insurance, transportation, fragmentation of care; Eiraldi et al., 2006). Lack of service use is a significant problem because untreated mental health conditions are associated with poor educational and health outcomes (Institute of Medicine, 2009).

As a response to the challenges children and adolescents experience in accessing mental health care, strategies to deliver mental health services in primary care and schools are being developed and expanded. Primary care providers (PCPs) may

T. J. Power (✉) · J. A. Mautone · N. J. Blum · A. G. Fiks · J. P. Guevara
The Children's Hospital of Philadelphia, Perelman School of Medicine at University of Pennsylvania, Philadelphia, PA, USA
e-mail: power@email.chop.edu

J. S. Carlson and J. A. Barterian (eds.), *School Psychopharmacology*, Pediatric School Psychology, https://doi.org/10.1007/978-3-030-15541-4_12

identify children's mental health needs early in the course of problem development through regular screening, which can facilitate timely diagnosis and improve access to treatment (LaVigne, Feldman, & Meyers, 2016); however, most pediatricians report feeling inadequately trained to address their patient's mental health needs (Horwitz et al., 2015). Additionally, children with emotional and behavioral difficulties receive support from school providers through school-based programming (e.g., Rones & Hoagwood, 2000); however, school-based mental health providers also face challenges with implementation of evidence-based behavioral health interventions (Eiraldi et al., 2014).

Fragmentation of Mental Health Services

When multiple systems (e.g., primary care, school, community mental health) are involved in children's mental health care, which is common when both pharmacological and psychosocial interventions are provided, coordination across these systems is generally poor (Guevara et al., 2005). Fragmentation in service delivery, including poor communication and collaboration across systems, may prevent families from accessing and benefiting from evidence-based interventions, which can preclude children from achieving successful outcomes (Hoagwood, Kelleher, Feil, & Comer, 2000). The failure to collaborate across disciplines and between systems of care is especially problematic for the treatment of mental health conditions because effective treatment often requires integration of psychosocial, educational, and pharmacological treatments that involve multiple disciplines and providers, who are based in different service systems. In these cases, parents or caregivers are typically placed in the untenable situation of having to manage care coordination among the multiple systems and providers involved in a child's care (Power, Blum, Jones, Guevara, & Leslie, 2013).

Potential Benefits of Integrated Behavioral Health

To address some of the challenges inherent in the provision of mental health care across multiple systems, models of integrated behavioral health (IBH) are becoming increasingly common. Integrated behavioral health refers to models of medical service delivery that include medical providers and behavioral health providers (e.g., psychologists, social workers, psychiatrists) working in collaboration to provide coordinated, team-based care (McDaniel et al., 2014). In many cases, the focus is on team-based care in the primary care setting; however, integrated care can be offered in specialty medical services as well (e.g., inpatient hospital programs, outpatient specialty care practices). Models of integrated care exist along a continuum including coordinated, co-located, and integrated based on the level of collaboration between medical and mental health providers (Collins, Hewson, Munger, & Wade,

2010). Coordinated care includes minimal or basic collaboration between providers who are typically based in different settings; co-located care involves basic or close collaboration between providers in shared offices, although the providers often have separate systems (e.g., different health records), and integrated care includes close or full collaboration between providers who operate using the same systems and are members of the same care team (Njoroge, Hostutler, Schwartz, & Mautone, 2016). In this chapter, we extend the meaning of IBH to include integration of care across the medical and educational systems, a connection that is critically important to provide effective services to children with mental health conditions (Power & Bradley-Klug, 2013).

IBH has proliferated over the last several years in response to calls to reduce health care costs while increasing quality and access for patients. Specifically, the Patient Protection and Affordable Care Act prompted the acknowledgement that behavioral health care is an "essential health benefit" and encouraged health systems to develop models of care that supported cost-effective, efficient, multidisciplinary care (Croft & Parish, 2013). These models may be especially beneficial for pediatric populations; early identification and treatment of behavioral health problems among youth has the potential for long-term benefit into adulthood (Asarnow, Rozenman, Wiblin, & Zeltzer, 2015). IBH services offered in pediatric primary care likely increase access to and engagement in behavioral health care (Asarnow & Miranda, 2014). In addition, IBH improves coordination across systems and collaboration between disciplines.

Purposes of Chapter

The purposes of this chapter are to: (a) describe examples of integrated care designed to improve children's educational functioning through the use of pharmacological and psychosocial treatments, (b) describe models of integrated behavioral health involving collaboration between school professionals and primary care providers to implement pharmacological and psychosocial interventions, and (c) describe strategies for coordinating treatment services between schools and health professionals in specialty practices, such as child psychiatry, developmental and behavioral pediatrics, and pediatric neurology. Additionally, the chapter addresses the role of school psychologists in IBH contexts, including implications for training. Given that most of the literature related to IBH focuses on integration of behavioral health and primary care systems, the main focus of this chapter is on models of integrated behavioral health in primary care that foster connections with school professionals. Limitations of current models of integrated care, future directions for research, and implications for training and practice are discussed.

Integrating Medical and Psychosocial Care to Improve Student Success in School

A major venue for the delivery of pharmacological interventions for children with mental health problems is primary care (Stancin & Perrin, 2014). The integration of behavioral health services into primary care can facilitate the coordination of medical and psychosocial care for children and adolescents. Unfortunately, primary care providers and mental health professionals working in primary care generally are limited in their efforts to assist students in school because there is infrequent contact between providers in primary care and those in school (Power et al., 2013). Integrated care to promote student success in school can be enhanced by promoting collaboration between the primary care and school teams. In addition, co-locating school psychologists with training emphasizing integrated behavioral health in primary care practices may be an approach to bridge the health and school systems to promote school success (Adams, Hinojosa, Armstrong, Takagishi, & Dabrow, 2016).

Children with moderate to severe internalizing disorders and those with autism spectrum disorder (ASD) and complex comorbidities often cannot be served adequately in primary care, which may be due to a lack of mental health training among primary care providers and their self-perceived lack of competence in managing the needs of children with these mental health conditions (Power, Mautone, Manz, Frye, & Blum, 2008). In these cases, specialty-level mental health care may be indicated. Children with developmental disabilities, such as ASD and intellectual disabilities, are often treated by subspecialists in developmental and behavioral pediatrics or pediatric neurology and those with internalizing disorders and complex comorbidities are generally treated in child and adolescent psychiatry. The primary focus of specialty care is to provide family-centered care to patients, which often includes pharmacological treatment to improve school performance and may also include brief consultation about how to address school issues. However, collaboration between medical specialists and school professionals is typically highly limited, which may contribute to fragmentation in care (Guevara et al., 2005). Once again, the quality of care may be improved by strategic efforts to link the medical practice with the school system.

Although models of integrated care usually are based in health systems, in some school districts medical providers may be available in schools through school health centers or consultative arrangements with the schools. However, these arrangements are the exception to the rule; the services offered by medical providers in schools generally are limited to diagnostic evaluations for special education placement decisions or consultations to school staff, and may not include medication consultation and monitoring. Given that a majority of students who receive mental health care obtain these services in schools (Merikangas et al., 2010) and that complex mental health problems often require a combination of pharmacological, educational, and behavioral interventions, schools are a compelling setting within which to locate integrated behavioral health services. Although there are clear challenges to basing integrated behavioral health services in school settings, recommendations have been advanced for how to adapt models of integrated care to be feasible and effective in schools (Lyon et al., 2016).

Models of Integrating Services Across Schools and Primary Care Practices

Although research on strategies to link schools and primary care is in its infancy, there is a sufficient knowledge base at this point to propose models for linking these systems. Figure 12.1 depicts a multi-tier model for promoting collaboration between schools and primary care.

Tier 1 (universal approach): Web-based practice supports. Tier 1 supports have generally been implemented in the context of primary care. The Institute of Medicine (now referred to as the National Academies of Science, Engineering, and Medicine) has defined primary care as the "provision of integrated, accessible health care services by clinicians who are accountable for addressing a large majority of personal health care needs, developing a sustained partnership with patients, and practicing in the context of the family and community" (Institute of Medicine, 1996, p. 1). This definition highlights that care integration in the context of a longitudinal relationship is fundamental to primary care. Nonetheless, time and other constraints limit primary care clinicians' ability to achieve this vision for behavioral conditions

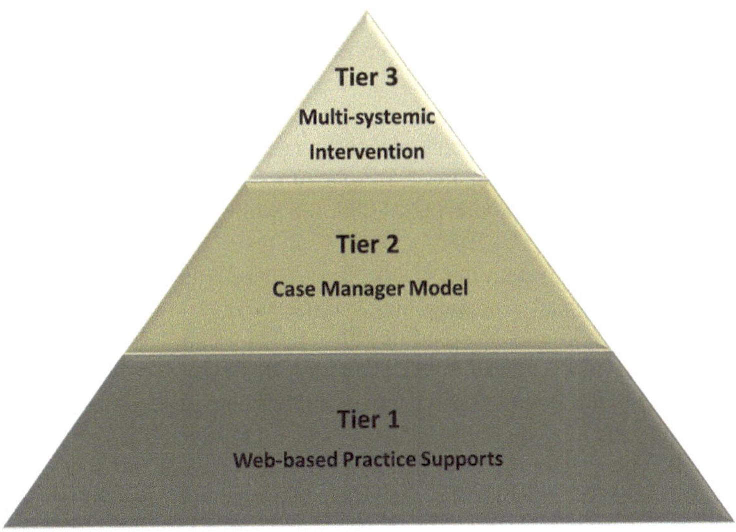

Fig. 12.1 Multi-tier model for promoting cross-system collaboration to coordinate psychosocial and pharmacological interventions

(Fiks, Hughes, Gafen, Guevara, & Barg, 2011). Electronic systems help to overcome these barriers and increasingly are able to promote communication between primary care and schools to assist in assessment, intervention planning, and monitoring of the effectiveness of behavioral health care.

Several web-based systems have been developed to assist in the assessment and intervention monitoring of children with mental health conditions. A system that is used in many primary care practices across the country and is commercially available is the Comprehensive Health and Development Interactive System (CHADIS; http://www.childhealthcare.org/chadis). This system facilitates screening, assessment, and progress monitoring of a wide range of developmental and mental health conditions, including autism, ADHD, disruptive behavior problems, anxiety, and depression, from infancy through late adolescence. CHADIS supports approximately 200 measures, which has enabled it to be highly versatile and useful for clinicians. The system facilitates the collection of data from parents, teachers, and youth; scores the data; and provides guidelines to clinicians for interpretation. The system can be highly useful for monitoring the effects of intervention, in particular medication. In addition, CHADIS offers a wealth of resources about the management of developmental and mental health conditions, which can be downloaded and distributed to families.

Several additional web-based systems have been developed, most of which focus on children with ADHD between the ages of 5 and 12 years. One well-researched system is myADHDportal, developed and evaluated by a team of researchers at Cincinnati Children's Hospital Medical Center (Epstein et al., 2011). This commercially available system collects, scores, and interprets rating scales completed by parents and teachers in assessing ADHD and comorbid conditions. In addition, the system monitors the effects of intervention, particularly medication, over time using rating scales and facilitates communication among health providers, parents, and teachers. Research has documented that training of primary care pediatricians in the use of this system resulted in significant increases in the use of parent and teacher rating scales to assess ADHD and increased use of teacher rating scales to monitor medication effects (Epstein et al., 2011). In addition, these researchers have developed quality improvement strategies to facilitate implementation of rating scales in the diagnostic assessment and treatment monitoring of children with ADHD (Epstein, Langberg, Lichtenstein, Kolb, & Simon, 2013).

Another web-based system that has been developed to promote evidence-based practices for assessing and managing ADHD is the ADHD Care Assistant, developed by researchers at Children's Hospital of Philadelphia where it is exclusively being used (Power et al., 2016). Like myADHDportal, this system collects, scores, and interprets rating scales completed by parents and teachers for initial assessment and ongoing monitoring of intervention effects (i.e., psychosocial and/or psychopharmacological). The system provides detailed information (e.g., handouts) about the effects of treatment on ADHD, disruptive behavior, and internalizing symptoms as well as functional impairments. In addition, the system monitors the occurrence of side effects so that clinicians can determine the benefits and risks of pharmacological treatment. A unique feature of the system is that it facilitates assessment of parents' preferences and helps to monitor goals for treatment, which is highly useful in promoting shared decision-making between clinicians and families (Fiks, Mayne, DeBartolo, Power, & Guevara, 2013). A particularly useful feature of this tool is that it is linked directly to the electronic health record used in the hospital, which facilitates the usability of the system among primary care providers.

Recent iterations of ADHD Care Assistant have included automatic communication of teacher-rated data to parents via email and communication of parent-approved components of data from parent rating scales to teachers. The system has been developed to be fully compliant with the Health Insurance Portability and Accountability Act (HIPAA) regulations regarding the transmission of personal health information through the internet and regarding the necessity of parent consent for the sharing of information with teachers. In addition, the system was built to be responsive to the Family Educational Rights and Privacy Act (FERPA) regulations that require parental consent for the sharing of teacher information with health providers.

Although most web-based systems to facilitate information exchange and communication between health practices and schools focus specifically on ADHD, a system that has been adapted for a range of conditions is TriVox Health, developed by researchers at Boston Children's Hospital (Chan et al., 2016). The system is currently being used to facilitate assessment and intervention monitoring for ADHD, autism, anxiety, depression, epilepsy, and asthma, and it includes information obtained from parents, teachers, and adolescent patients. A feature that contributes to its acceptability and usability to providers is that it is linked with the electronic health record. The system is highly useful for titrating and monitoring the effects and side effects of pharmacological treatments in home and school settings. TriVox Health was initially established as a web-based system, but it has been adapted to be used as a mobile app. System developers anticipate that the mobile app will increase usage of the system among adolescents. Although TriVox Health is currently available in a limited number of hospitals in the Boston area, the developers are working to make the system available in other institutions.

Tier 2 (selective approach): Care manager model. The care manager approach assigns a professional to promote communication among key intervention participants and facilitate coordination of care. The care manager, who may have master- or bachelor-level training in nursing, social work, or a related discipline, provides support to families in addressing the cumbersome process of coordinating communications across systems of care. This approach is a response to the need for cost-effective methods to provide care between medical visits. The care manager model was developed initially to facilitate communication and coordination of care for the treatment of adults with depression and has been shown to be feasible to implement and to improve outcomes with modest effect sizes (Gilbody, Bower, Fletcher, Richards, & Sutton, 2006). Care manager interventions using professionals with mental health training, who were carefully supervised on a regular basis have been shown to achieve better outcomes relative to less rigorous interventions (Katon, Von Korff, Lin, & Simon, 2001). Although research using this strategy with families coping with children's mental health problems is just beginning to emerge (Power et al., 2013), the approach would appear to have substantial promise.

Among the numerous roles of the care manager, this professional meets with families to understand their preferences for treatment (i.e., medication and behavior therapy), identify intervention goals (e.g., academic performance, interpersonal competence, behavior compliance), engage them in treatment decisions, provide education, and refer them for psychosocial services, when indicated. The care manager facilitates shared decision-making among families, health providers, and school professionals to communicate family preferences and goals for treatment, identify emerging problems, and facilitate measurement of outcomes. Through this process, many families are able to resolve concerns they might have about using medication or behavioral treatments to address their child's problems at school and home. The care manager maintains contact with families on at least a quarterly basis by telephone or text message to monitor progress, assist with problem-solving, make referrals when needed, and provide support with the implementation of interventions. Similarly, the care manager maintains contact on at least a quarterly basis with teachers and any external mental health providers to monitor progress, communicate emerging problems, and facilitate sharing of treatment recommendations. The care manager also communicates with primary care providers on an ongoing basis through the electronic health record. In addition, the care manager coordinates the efforts of teachers and mental health providers through ongoing phone and email contact.

A pilot study of this intervention model was tested among children diagnosed with ADHD between 5 and 12 years using a quasi-experimental design based in two urban primary care practices, with 19 children referred from one primary care practice receiving the care manager intervention and 10 children referred from a practice with similar demographic characteristics receiving treatment as usual. Parent ratings of treatment acceptability for the care manager intervention were high, and outcome data demonstrated reductions in ADHD symptoms and related impairments with small to medium effect sizes (Power et al., 2013).

Tier 3 (targeted intervention): Multi-systemic interventions. For many families coping with their children's mental health conditions, facilitated communication and coordination of care is not sufficient to address their concerns. Families may not be able to access culturally effective, evidence-based mental health interventions to address their children's problems. To address the need for evidence-based intervention while promoting coordination of care, multi-systemic intervention approaches have been developed that involve collaboration across systems of care. Multi-systemic interventions are often applied in the context of primary care using an integrated model. For example, a multi-systemic intervention based in primary care was developed and evaluated for the treatment of children with ADHD, disruptive behavior disorders, and anxiety disorders (Kolko et al., 2014). The psychosocial intervention was offered by a supervised master-level clinician who provided evidence-based interventions for ADHD, behavior disorders, and anxiety. The clinician worked collaboratively with the PCP and assisted with the monitoring of medication effects and side effects at home and school, when indicated. In a randomized controlled trial, the intervention was demonstrated to be feasible to implement and generally effective (Kolko et al., 2014). In addition, multi-systemic interventions based in primary care have been used effectively to treat adolescent depression (Richardson et al., 2014). The intervention included an initial session to promote youth engagement and assist the family in determining the optimal approach to treatment, which consisted of cognitive behavior therapy (CBT), medication for depression, or a combined approach. The initial engagement session and CBT were provided by supervised, master-level clinicians, who worked in collaboration with PCPs. The results of a randomized clinical trial demonstrated the feasibility of this approach, its effectiveness in reducing symptoms of depression (Richardson et al., 2014), and its cost-effectiveness (Wright et al. 2016).

Although several collaborative care interventions based in primary care have been found to be feasible and effective, a limitation is that these approaches do not focus on linking with the school system and targeting school performance and behavior. To address these limitations, multi-systemic approaches have been developed that promote coordination among the family, school, and health systems. For example, Partnering to Achieve School Success (PASS) is a multi-systemic intervention approach based in pediatric primary care practices that include behavioral parent training and parent–teacher consultation, in addition to components to improve family engagement in intervention and team-based care (Power et al., 2014).

PASS was designed for families of children with ADHD in the context of practices serving primarily low-income families of minority racial background. PASS infuses three core principles into every session: (a) engagement and motivation, (b) trauma-informed care, and (c) team-based care. Given the challenges low-income families often experience in becoming engaged in mental health services (Power et al., 2010), PASS therapists utilize engagement and motivation strategies to encourage family involvement. Additionally, given the relatively high prevalence of chronic stress and trauma among inner-city families (Marsac et al., 2016), PASS therapists apply trauma-informed care principles to acknowledge parental stress, provide empathy, reinforce coping, and develop a self-care plan with the parent, when necessary.

Given the potential for collaborative care between medical and mental health providers to improve outcomes (Asarnow et al., 2015), PASS places an emphasis on team-based care. Team-based care includes the following elements: (a) supporting PCPs in using a common factors approach to treatment (e.g., listening with empathy, instilling hope, obtaining permission to explore sensitive issues; Wissow et al., 2008); (b) regular communication between the PASS clinician and PCP about family progress toward goals; and (c) collaboration to monitor the effects of pharmacological treatments, when indicated. Initial efforts to evaluate PASS indicated reductions in parent-perceived barriers to care, increases in parental ratings of medication acceptability, reductions in ineffective parenting practices, and reductions in child impairment with modest effect sizes (Power et al., 2014).

Models of Integrating Care Across Schools and Specialty Medical Practices

A high percentage of children with mental health problems have complex needs, which can complicate intervention planning and implementation. Children with complex mental health needs often cannot be addressed adequately through collaboration between families, school professionals, and PCPs (Power et al., 2008). In these cases, specialty care health professionals (e.g., child psychiatrists, developmental and behavioral pediatricians) may be needed.

The multi-tier approaches described above for coordinating care across schools and primary care practices certainly can be adapted for complex cases (e.g., ASD, epilepsy, substance use disorder) in which medical care is provided by a specialist. Indeed, within pediatric hospital settings, a unitary electronic health record is used across the entire system and it may be feasible to adapt web-based systems to promote cross-system communication and coordination of care. In addition, specialty care practices may have a nurse or social worker available to serve the functions of a care manager. Further, in some practices, it may be feasible to offer intensive multi-systemic intervention involving team-based care with the medical clinician, family–school consultation, and family-behavioral interventions.

An example of multi-systemic intervention provided in the context of specialty care practice was provided by a team at University of Nebraska (Sheridan et al., 2009). The integrated behavioral health team included developmental-behavioral pediatricians (DBP) based in a medical center and behavioral health clinicians who worked in the medical clinic as well as the communities in which the students went to school. The behavioral health clinicians were advanced graduate students trained in conjoint (family–school) behavioral consultation (CBC). Team-based care involved collaboration among parents, the DBPs, and the CBC clinicians throughout the course of intervention. DBPs and CBC clinicians collaborated to determine the appropriateness of referral for CBC and behavioral intervention, and DBPs maintained ongoing communication with the CBC clinician and family to coordinate care, which often included initiation and monitoring of medication. About 80% of the children enrolled in the project were diagnosed with ADHD and 77% were treated with stimulants, highlighting the importance of a combined approach to treatment for a relatively large proportion of children with ADHD.

Consultation provided by the CBC clinicians followed the steps of CBC, involving parents and teachers in the process of target behavior identification, behavior analysis, intervention implementation, and evaluation. Consultation typically identified multiple interventions to be applied at school and/or at home. The CBC clinicians provided consultation to teachers and parents to develop specific intervention plans and coach them with implementation. Throughout the process of consultation, CBC clinicians, DBPs, and parents continued to communicate to coordinate intervention efforts. The findings of the project indicated that the intervention process was acceptable to parents and teachers and that outcomes with regard to changes in targeted behaviors were generally favorable (Sheridan et al., 2009).

Limitations of Existing Models and Directions for Future Research

Research focused on developing models to promote communication between health care and school systems is in its infancy. Most of the research to promote coordination between health and school systems has been conducted with individuals who have ADHD; there is very little research on disruptive behavior disorders and internalizing disorders, despite the fact that numerous studies have applied an integrated behavioral health model for targeting behavior and internalizing problems in primary care (e.g., Kolko et al. 2014; Richardson et al., 2014). Although the focus of almost all of the research has been on children between the ages of 5 and 12 years; models for linking systems of care for adolescents are strongly needed. Further, research to this point has emphasized the development of models that can be effective in promoting intersystem communication; there has been a lack of emphasis on how to implement these models in real-world settings and how to sustain the use of these strategies over time.

Several research teams are developing web-based methods to promote the exchange of information among parents, health providers, and school professionals. Although these systems are improving the use of evidence-based practices for assessing child disorders and monitoring medication effects (Epstein et al., 2013), barriers to collecting this information from school providers have been identified (e.g., school official concerns about protecting student privacy and questions about sharing information with health providers and parents without sufficient consideration of the implications for student classification and placement; Power et al., 2016). Additional research is needed to understand and address these barriers, which can have an effect on implementation by teachers. Finally, models being developed to promote system interconnections generally are based in health systems, especially primary care; comparable models based in schools are needed (Lyon et al., 2016). Research is needed to develop the role of a school-based service coordinator, who can work with health providers, parents, and teachers to coordinate communications and promote integrated services.

Implications for Training and Practice

Doctoral-level school psychologists have many of the competencies necessary to be effective in engaging in integrated care that links the health and school systems (Adams et al., 2016). Table 12.1 describes the competencies of health service psychologists (i.e., licensed, doctoral-level providers with internship and supervised experience in a health setting; Health Service Psychology Education Collaborative [HSPEC], 2013), school psychologists (National Association of School Psychologists, 2010), and psychologists working in IBH contexts (Hoffses et al., 2016), School psychology competencies generally are closely aligned with those of health service

Table 12.1 Comparison of professional competencies in health service psychology, school psychology, and pediatric psychology in integrated behavioral health

Health service psychology[a]	School psychology[b]	Psychology in integrated behavioral health[c]
Evidence-based assessment	Data-based decision-making and accountability	Screening, assessment, documentation in medical record
Evidence-based consultation	Consultation and collaboration	Consultation and interdisciplinary collaboration
Evidence-based intervention, prevention, health promotion	Intervention, instructional support, mental health services	Brief intervention, prevention services
Practice in interdisciplinary systems; professional development; advocacy	School-wide practices; preventive services; family–school collaboration services	Systems-oriented practice in pediatric setting; practice management
Individual and cultural diversity	Diversity in development and learning	Cultural competence and adaptation
Scientific knowledge and methods; research and evaluation	Research and program evaluation	Research and evaluation; practice-based research, quality improvement
Professional values; ethical and legal standards; reflective practice, self-care	Legal, ethical, and professional practice	Professional values; ethical and legal standards, reflective practice, self-care
Interpersonal skills and communication; interdisciplinary practice	Communication applicable to individuals, families, groups, and systems	Interpersonal communication; interdisciplinary practice
Teaching and supervision		Teaching and supervision

[a]Health Services Psychology Education Collaborative
[b]National Association of School Psychologists (2010)
[c]Hoffses et al. (2016)

psychologists, who include doctoral-level professionals trained in clinical, counseling, and school psychology (Daly, Doll, Schulte, & Fenning, 2011; HSPEC, 2013). In addition, school psychology's specific focus on cross-system (family–school) collaboration, systems-oriented practice, preventive services, and individual and cultural diversity is closely aligned with competencies required for providers in IBH practices. Although doctoral-level school psychologists have many of the competencies to function effectively as health service providers in IBH contexts, they typically require additional training to be highly effective (Mautone, Booster, and Ridgard, 2019). For example, they might benefit from training related to systems-oriented practice in an IBH context, interdisciplinary collaboration in a health context, care coordination across health and school systems, research informing IBH practice, quality improvement methods using data extracted from the electronic health record, and ethical and legal issues arising in IBH practice. In addition, training may be needed in psychiatric diagnostic evaluation and evidence-based interventions (e.g., cognitive behavioral therapy for anxiety and depression). Models of training at the doctoral level have been incorporated into programs with an emphasis on pediatric school psychology (Power & Bradley-Klug, 2013).

Collaboration across school and health systems typically is very limited. In general, school practitioners engage in a limited amount of communication with health professionals, in particular PCPs, even though they consider this practice to be important for providing effective services to students (Bradley-Klug et al., 2013). School practitioners are advised to form connections with health providers in the community who provide services to children in their school districts (Power & Bradley-Klug, 2013). In some cases, web-based systems may already be in place to promote cross-system collaboration, and school practitioners can learn about these methods. In some districts, there may be concerns about using web-based systems; in these cases, it is important to provide feedback to health providers as there may be an opportunity to improve the system so it is more feasible to use across schools in the region (Power et al., 2016).

Most medical practices do not have care managers and multi-systemic intervention programs that link with the school. However, practices may have nurses or nurse practitioners who have some responsibility for communicating with professionals in the community. It is important for school practitioners to identify these individuals, build strong relationships with them, and coordinate efforts in the care of children with mental health problems.

The sharing of mental health information across medical and school systems raises privacy issues. Privacy regulations present significant challenges when creating web-based systems (Power et al., 2016). School practitioners are strongly encouraged to carefully review privacy regulations and consult with school district attorneys when questions about privacy arise in the course of collaborating with professionals across systems of care.

Conclusions

Access to evidence-based mental health treatment can be challenging, especially for children and adolescents of minority status from low-income communities. When services are available, coordination of care across systems is typically inadequate. Models of integrated care, based mostly in primary care, have proliferated to increase access to care and coordinate medical and psychosocial interventions, but these models typically do not focus on linking with schools to promote student educational success. This chapter proposes a multi-tier model for promoting linkages between primary care and school systems to provide pharmacological and psychosocial interventions. Tier 1 incorporates web-based technologies to promote information exchange between primary care and schools; Tier 2 provides the support of a care manager to promote information exchange and monitor the effects of pharmacological and psychosocial interventions; and Tier 3 provides evidence-based psychosocial and pharmacological treatment in an integrated manner that is linked with the school.

Research on models of service delivery that link the health and school systems to provide pharmacological and psychosocial interventions is in its infancy. Most of the existing research is based on primary care settings, but the link with school systems is extremely limited. Research based on both health and school settings is needed to demonstrate the feasibility and effectiveness of models of service delivery that connect health and school systems to provide pharmacological and psychosocial interventions. Given their competencies as health service providers and researchers, doctoral-level school psychologists are well positioned to conduct this research and develop programs of integrated service delivery that link the family, school, and health systems.

Funding Preparation of this chapter was supported by grants from Pfizer Independent Grants for Learning and Change, the Maternal and Child Health Bureau (R40MC08964, T73MC00012), and the Department of Education, Office of Special Education Programs (H325D100019), as well as a contract from the Patient-Centered Outcomes Research Institute (PCORI, CDI-140820669), In addition, several of the projects described in this chapter were supported by the resources of the Pediatric Research Consortium (PeRC) of Children's Hospital of Philadelphia. The information and conclusions of this chapter are those of the authors and should not be construed as the official position or policy of, nor should any endorsements be inferred by, the funding agencies or the U.S. Government.

Disclosure Alexander Fiks is a co-inventor of the Care Assistant software used to develop the ADHD Care Assistant, described in this chapter.

List of Key Readings

Bradley-Klug, K. L., Jeffries-DeLoatche, K. L., Walsh, A. S., Bateman, L. P., Nadeau, J., Powers, D. J., & Cunningham, J. (2013). School psychologists' perceptions of primary care partnerships: Implications for building the collaborative bridge. *Advances in School Mental Health Promotion, 6,* 51–67. DOI:

This article describes school psychologists' perceptions of their communications with pediatricians in primary care. The findings demonstrated that communication is relatively infrequent despite the recognition of the importance of this collaboration.

Lyon, A. R., Whitaker, K., French, W. P., Richardson, L. P., Wasse, J. K., & McCauley, E. (2016). Collaborative care in schools: Enhancing integration and impact in youth mental health. *Advances in School Mental Health, 9,* 148–168. https://doi.org/10.1080/1754730x.2012.760921

This article describes the effectiveness of collaborative care models for addressing children's mental health problems. In addition, the article proposes a set of recommendations for implementing a collaborative care model in schools.

Power, T. J., Michel, J., Mayne, S., Miller, J., Blum, N. J., Grundmeier, R. W., Guevara, J. P., & Fiks, A. G. (2016). Coordinating systems of care using health information technology: Development of the ADHD Care Assistant. *Advances in School Mental Health Promotion, 9,* 201–218. https://doi.org/10.1080/1754730x.2016.1199283

This article describes the development and initial implementation of an electronic health record portal to facilitate the sharing of information between schools and primary care to facilitate shared decision-making and the monitoring of pharmacological and psychosocial treatments.

List of Websites

The Academy for Integrating Behavioral Health and Primary Care (https://integrationacademy.ahrq.gov/)

The Agency for Healthcare Research and Quality sponsors this website (The Academy for Integrating Behavioral Health and Primary Care). The goal of the academy is to be a resource and coordinating center for professionals interested in integrated care. This resource is not specific to providers working in pediatric practices.

SAMHSA-HRSA Center for Integrated Health Solutions (http://www.integration.samhsa.gov/integrated-care-models/children-and-youth)

This website is sponsored by the SAMHSA-HRSA Center for Integrated Health Solutions and provides updated resources related to integrated behavioral health in pediatric primary care.

Milbank Memorial Fund (Behavioral Health Integration in Pediatric Primary Care) (https://www.milbank.org/publications/behavioral-health-integration-in-pediatric-primary-care-considerations-and-opportunities-for-policymakers-planners-and-providers/)

The mission of the Milbank Memorial Fund is to improve individual and population health by applying research and learning to health policy and practice. This website links to a document that provides an overview of the need for pediatric IBH and suggestions for policy and implementation.

References

Adams, C. D., Hinojosa, S., Armstrong, K., Takagishi, J., & Dabrow, S. (2016). An innovative model of integrated behavioral health: School psychologists in pediatric primary care settings.

Advances in School Mental Health Promotion, 9, 188–200. https://doi.org/10.1080/1754730X.2016.1215927.
Asarnow, J. R., & Miranda, J. (2014). Improving care for depression and suicide risk in adolescents: Innovative strategies for bringing treatments to community settings. *Annual Review of Clinical Psychology, 10,* 275–303. https://doi.org/10.1146/annurev-clinpsy-032813-153742.
Asarnow, J., Rozenman, M., Wiblin, J., & Zeltzer, L. (2015). Integrated medical-behavioral care compared with usual primary care for child and adolescent behavioral health: A meta-analysis. *JAMA Pediatrics, 169*(10), 929–937. https://doi.org/10.1001/jamapediatrics.2015.1141.
Bradley-Klug, K. L., Jeffries-DeLoatche, K. L., Walsh, A. S. J., Bateman, L. P., Nadeau, J., Powers, D. J., et al. (2013). School psychologists' perceptions of primary care partnerships: Implications for building collaborative bridges. *Advances in School Mental Health Promotion, 6,* 51–67. https://doi.org/10.1080/1754730X.2012.760921.
Chan, E., Fleegler, E., Weas, S., Zhang, X., Rhodes, E., Kahn, J., … Loddenkemper, T. (2016). *Implementation of an internet-based patient monitoring system improves families' perception of quality of communication and experience of care.* Paper presented at the Pediatric Academic Societies Annual Meeting, Baltimore, Maryland, United States.
Collins, C., Hewson, D. L., Munger, R., & Wade, T. (2010). Evolving models of behavioral health integration in primary care. In M. M. Fund (Ed.), *The Milbank Quarterly*. New York.
Croft, B., & Parish, S. L. (2013). Care integration in the Patient Protection and Affordable Care Act: Implications for behavioral health. *Administration and Policy in Mental Health, 40*(4), 258–263. https://doi.org/10.1007/s10488-012-0405-0.
Daly, E. J., Doll, B., Schulte, A. C., & Fenning, P. (2011). The competencies initiative in American professional psychology: Implications for school psychology preparation. *Psychology in the Schools, 48*(9), 872–886. https://doi.org/10.1002/pits.20603.
Eiraldi, R. B., McCurdy, B., Khanna, M., Mautone, J. A., Jawad, A. F., Power, T. J., … Sugai, G. (2014). A cluster randomized trial to evaluate external support for the implementation of positive behavioral interventions and supports by school personnel. *Implementation Science, 9*(12). https://doi.org/10.1186/1748-5908-9-12.
Eiraldi, R. B., Mazzuca, L. B., Clarke, A. T., & Power, T. J. (2006). Service utilization among ethnic minority children with ADHD: A model of help-seeking behavior. *Administration and Policy in Mental Health and Mental Health Services Research, 33*(5), 607–622. https://doi.org/10.1007/s10488-006-0063-1.
Epstein, J., Langberg, J., Lichtenstein, P., Kolb, R., Altaye, M., & Simon, J. (2011). Use of an internet portal to improve community-based pediatric ADHD care: A cluster randomized trial. *Pediatrics, 128,* e1201–e1208. https://doi.org/10.1542/peds.2011-0872.
Epstein, J., Langberg, J., Lichtenstein, P., Kolb, R., & Simon, J. (2013). The myADHDportal.com improvement program: An innovative quality improvement intervention for improving the quality of ADHD care among community-based pediatricians. *Clinical Practice in Pediatric Psychology, 1*(1), 55–67. https://doi.org/10.1037/cpp0000004.
Fiks, A. G., Hughes, C. C., Gafen, A., Guevara, J. P., & Barg, F. K. (2011). Contrasting parents' and pediatricians' perspectives on shared decision making in ADHD. *Pediatrics, 127,* e188–e196. https://doi.org/10.1542/peds.2010-1510.
Fiks, A. G., Mayne, S., DeBartolo, E., Power, T. J., & Guevara, J. P. (2013). Preferences, goals, and ADHD treatment initiation. *Pediatrics, 132,* 692–702. https://doi.org/10.1542/peds.2013-0152.
Gilbody, S., Bower, P., Fletcher, J., Richards, D., & Sutton, A. J. (2006). Collaborative care for depression: A cumulative meta-analysis and review of longer-term outcomes. *Archives of Internal Medicine, 166*(21), 2314–2321. https://doi.org/10.1001/archinte.166.21.2314.
Guevara, J. P., Feudtner, C., Romer, D., Power, T., Eiraldi, R., Nihtianova, S., et al. (2005). Fragmented care for inner-city minority children with attention-deficit/hyperactivity disorder. *Pediatrics, 116,* e512–e517. https://doi.org/10.1542/peds.2005-0243.
Health Service Psychology Education Collaborative. (2013). Professional psychology in health care services: A blueprint for education and training *American Psychologist, 68*(6), 411–426. https://doi.org/10.1037/a0033265.

Hoagwood, K., Kelleher, K. J., Feil, M., & Comer, D. M. (2000). Treatment services for children with ADHD: A national perspective. *Journal of the American Academy of Child and Adolescent Psychiatry, 39*(2), 198–206. https://doi.org/10.1097/00004583-200002000-00020.

Hoffses, K. W., Ramirez, L. Y., Berdan, L., Tunick, R., Honaker, S. M., Meadows, T.,…, & Stancin, T. (2016). Topical review: Building competency: Professional skills for pediatric psychologists in integrated primary care settings. *Journal of Pediatric Psychology, 41*(10), 1140–1160. https://doi.org/10.1093/jpepsy/jsw066

Horwitz, S. M., Storfer-Isser, A., Kerker, B. D., … Stein, R. E. K. (2015). Barriers to the identification and management of psychosocial problems: Changes from 2004 to 2013. *Academic Pediatrics, 15*(6), 613–620.

Institute of Medicine. (1996). *Primary care: America's health in a new era*. Washington, DC: National Academy Press.

Institute of Medicine. (2009). Committee on comparative effectiveness research prioritization. In: *Initial national priorities for comparative effectiveness research.* Washington, DC: National Academy Press.

Katon, W., Von Korff, M., Lin, E., & Simon, G. (2001). Rethinking practitioner roles in chronic illness: The specialist, primary care physician, and the practice nurse. *General Hospital Psychiatry, 23*(3), 138–144. https://doi.org/10.1016/S0163-8343(01)00136-0.

Kolko, D. J., Campo, J., Kilbourne, A. M., Hart, J., Sakolsky, D., & Wisniewski, S. (2014). Collaborative care outcomes for pediatric behavioral health problems: A cluster randomized trial. *Pediatrics, 133*(4), e981–e992. https://doi.org/10.1542/peds.2013-2516.

Lavigne, J. V., Feldman, M., & Meyers, K. M. (2016). Screening for mental health problems: Addressing the base rate fallacy for a sustainable screening program in integrated primary care. *Journal of Pediatric Psychology, 41,* 1081–1090. https://doi.org/10.1093/jpepsy/jsw048.

Lyon, A. R., Whitaker, L., French, W. P., Richardson, L. P., Wasse, J. K., & McCauley, E. (2016). Collaborative care in schools: Enhancing integration and impact in youth mental health. *Advances in School Mental Health, 9,* 148–168. https://doi.org/10.1080/1754730X.2012.760921.

Marsac, M. L., Kassam-Adams, N., Hildenbrand, A. K., Nicholls, E., Winston, F. K., Leff, S. S., et al. (2016). Implementing a trauma-informed approach in pediatric health care networks. *JAMA Pediatrics, 170*(1), 70–77. https://doi.org/10.1001/jamapediatrics.2015.2206.

Mautone, J. A., Booster, G., & Ridgard, T. (2019). Current practice: Schools vs. alternative settings. In M. Burns (Ed.), *Introduction to school psychology: Controversies and current practice*. Oxford, United Kingdom: Oxford University Press.

McDaniel, S. H., Grus, C. L., Cubic, B. A., Hunter, C. L., Kearney, L. K., Schuman, C. C., et al. (2014). Competencies for psychology practice in primary care. *American Psychologist, 69*(4), 409–429. https://doi.org/10.1037/a0036072.

Merikangas, K. R., He, J., Burstein, M., Swanson, S. A., Avenevoli, S., Cui, L., et al. (2010). Lifetime prevalence of mental disorders in U.S. adolescents: Results from the national comorbidity survey replication-adolescent supplement (NCS-A). *Journal of the American Academy of Child and Adolescent Psychiatry, 49,* 980–989. https://doi.org/10.1016/j.jaac.2010.05.017.

National Association of School Psychologists. (2010). Model for comprehensive and integrated school psychological services: NASP practice model overview. In National Association of School Psychologists. (Ed.), (Vol. 4, pp. 1–6). Bethesda, MD: National Association of School Psychologists.

Njoroge, W. F. M., Hostutler, C. D., Schwartz, B. S., & Mautone, J. A. (2016). Integrated behavioral health in pediatric primary care. *Current Psychiatry Reports, 18*(106), 1–8. https://doi.org/10.1007/s11920-016-0745-7.

Power, T. J., Mautone, J. A., Marshall, S. A., Jones, H. A., Cacia, J., Tresco, K., et al. (2014). Feasibility and potential effectiveness of integrated services for children with ADHD in urban primary care practices. *Clinical Practice in Pediatric Psychology, 2*(4), 412–426. https://doi.org/10.1037/cpp0000056.

Power, T. J., Michel, J., Mayne, S., Miller, J., Blum, N. J., Grundmeier, R. W., et al. (2016). Coordinating systems of care using health information technology: Development of the ADHD

Care Assistant. *Advances in School Mental Health Promotion, 9,* 201–218. https://doi.org/10.1080/1754730X.2016.1199283.
Power, T. J., Blum, N. J., Guevara, J. P., Jones, H. A., & Leslie, L. K. (2013). Coordinating mental health care across primary care and schools: ADHD as a case example. *Advances in School Mental Health Promotion, 6,* 68–80. https://doi.org/10.1080/1754730X.2013.749089.
Power, T. J., & Bradley-Klug, K. (2013). *Pediatric school psychology: Conceptualization, applications, and strategies for leadership development.* New York: Routledge.
Power, T. J., Hughes, C. L., Helwig, J. R., Nissley-Tsiopinis, J., Mautone, J. A., & Lavin, H. J. (2010). Getting to first base: Promoting engagement in family–school intervention for children with ADHD in urban, primary care practice. *School Mental Health, 2*(2), 52–61. https://doi.org/10.1007/s12310-010-9029-2.
Power, T. J., Mautone, J. A., Manz, P. H., Frye, L., & Blum, N. J. (2008). Managing ADHD in primary care: A systematic analysis of roles and challenges. *Pediatrics, 121,* e65–e72. https://doi.org/10.1542/peds.2007-0383.
Richardson, L. P., Ludman, E., McCauley, E., Lindenbaum, J., Larison, C., Zhou, C., et al. (2014). Collaborative care for adolescents with depression: A randomized clinical trial. *Journal of the American Medical Association, 312*(8), 809–816. https://doi.org/10.1001/jama.2014.9259.
Rones, M., & Hoagwood, K. (2000). School-based mental health services: A research review. *Clinical Child Family Psychology Rev, 3*(4), 223–241. https://doi.org/10.1023/A:1026425104386.
Sheridan, S. M., Warnes, E. D., Woods, K. E., Blevins, C. A., Magee, K. L., & Ellis, C. (2009). An exploratory evaluation of conjoint behavioral consultation to promote collaboration among family, school, and pediatric systems: A role for pediatric school psychologists. *Journal of Education and Psychological Consultation, 19,* 106–129. https://doi.org/10.1080/10474410902888566.
Soni, A. (2015). Top five most costly conditions among children, ages 0–17, 2012: Estimates for the U.S. civilian noninstitutionalized population. In Agency for Healthcare Research and Quality (Ed.), *Medical expenditure panel survey* (Statistical Brief #472.).
Stancin, T., & Perrin, E. C. (2014). Opportunities for collaboration in Primary care. *American Psychologist, 69*(4), 332–343. https://doi.org/10.1037/a0036046.
Wang, P. S., Berglund, P., Olfson, M., Pincus, H. A., Wells, K. B., & Kessler, R. C. (2005). Failure and delay in initial treatment contact after first onset of mental disorders in the national comorbidity survey replication. *Archives of General Psychiatry, 62*(6), 603–613. https://doi.org/10.1001/archpsyc.62.6.603.
Wissow, L., Anthony, B., Brown, J., DosReis, S., Gadomski, A., Ginsburg, G., et al. (2008). A common factors approach to improving mental health capacity in pediatric primary care. *Administration and Policy In Mental Health, 35,* 305–318. https://doi.org/10.1007/s10488-008-0178-7.
Wright, D. R., Haaland, W. L., Ludman, E., McCauley, E., Lindenbaum, J., & Richardson, L. P. (2016). The costs and cost-effectiveness of collaborative care for adolescents with depression in primary care settings: A randomized clinical trial. *JAMA Pediatrics, 170*(11), 1048–1054. https://doi.org/10.1001/jamapediatrics.2016.1721.

Chapter 13
School-Based Medication Evaluations: Implications for School Personnel and Physicians

Robert J. Volpe, Brian Daniels and Christina Sakai

Introduction

Approximately, 10–20% of school-age children and adolescents are affected by psychiatric disorders (Kieling et al., 2011), and the number of children and adolescents receiving psychotropic medication (e.g., stimulants, antidepressants, and antipsychotics) has consistently increased over the past 20 years (Olfson, Druss, & Marcus, 2015). Estimates indicate that, on average, 7.5% of school-aged children and adolescents (6–17 years old) use at least one psychotropic medications for social–emotional difficulties; however, rates vary based on medication type and child age and gender (Howie, Pastor, & Lukacs, 2014; Jonas, Gu, & Albertorio-Diaz, 2013). Overall, more school-aged males (9.7%) are prescribed psychotropic medication than school-aged females (5.2%), with more male (10.2%) and female (6.2%) adolescents (12–17 years old) receiving prescriptions than male (9.2%) and female (4.0%) children (6–11 years old). The six most commonly prescribed classes of medication for children and adolescents include anxiolytics/sedatives/hypnotics, Central Nervous System (CNS) stimulants, antidepressants, antipsychotics, antiadrenergic agents, and mood stabilizers (Chirdkiatgumchai et al., 2013). CNS stimulants are the most frequently used medications, with 5.1% (1.5 million) of children (6–12 years old) and 4.9% (1.3 million) of adolescents (13–18 years old) taking stimulants (Zuvekas & Vitiello, 2012). Use of stimulants is consistently higher among males (5.3%) than females (1.6%; Zuvekas & Vitiello, 2012). Estimated use of antidepressants, antipsychotics,

R. J. Volpe (✉)
Northeastern University, Boston, MA, USA
e-mail: r.volpe@northeastern.edu

B. Daniels
University of Massachusetts, Boston, Boston, MA, USA

C. Sakai
Floating Hospital for Children at Tufts Medical Center, Boston, MA, USA

J. S. Carlson and J. A. Barterian (eds.), *School Psychopharmacology*,
Pediatric School Psychology, https://doi.org/10.1007/978-3-030-15541-4_13

and anxiolytics/sedatives/hypnotics is lower at 3.2%, 1.0%, and 0.5%, respectively (Jonas et al., 2013).

Positive impacts have been demonstrated across social, behavioral, and academic domains for all three of the most frequently prescribed classes of psychotropic medications (stimulants, antidepressants, and antipsychotics); however, side effects are commonly associated with their use (Baweja et al., 2016; Harvey, James, & Shields, 2016; Walkup, 2017).

What Types of Assessments Are Needed to Evaluate Psychotropic Medication?

Despite the potential benefits of medical treatments, there are important differences in the way individuals respond (or fail to respond) to psychotropic medication. Careful monitoring of trials of psychotropic medication is important for several reasons including: (a) the identification of appropriate doses of medication, (b) monitoring of potential side effects, and (c) monitoring of the integrity of administration procedures. Evaluation of psychotropic medication for individual cases can be divided into two essential assessment tasks: (a) medication titration and (b) ongoing monitoring of medication effectiveness.

Medication titration. Medication titration is a procedure to identify the most appropriate dose of medication for a given client (hereafter referred to as "student"). Medication titration involves comparing student functioning between a non-medication condition and conditions where a student is prescribed one or more doses of medication, although if there is inadequate response to a particular medication, different medications may be substituted and evaluated. Non-medication conditions may simply be business as usual or might involve a placebo control (more on this later). Our definition of medication titration above begs the question as to what we mean by "appropriate dose of medication." One might argue that given a student's response to multiple doses of medication, the *appropriate* dose would be the one associated with the best overall response. Let us call this the "optimal dose" approach. Others may argue that it would be better that children and adolescents are prescribed less psychoactive medication if a lower dose offers significant therapeutic benefits. In this case, the *appropriate* dose would be the lowest dose offering the desired benefit. Let us call this the "minimally effective dose" approach.

In group design studies examining the efficacy of stimulant medication on (attention-deficit/hyperactivity disorder ADHD) symptoms, a linear dose response is typical. That is, higher doses of medication are associated with greater benefits (Stein et al., 2003). Although some individual children will exhibit a linear response to higher doses of medication, a significant proportion of students will not respond to one or more different stimulants and many more show nonlinear dose responses (see Fig. 13.1).

Specifically, some children exhibit a threshold response wherein an initial benefit is observed at lower doses of medication; however, gains plateau at higher

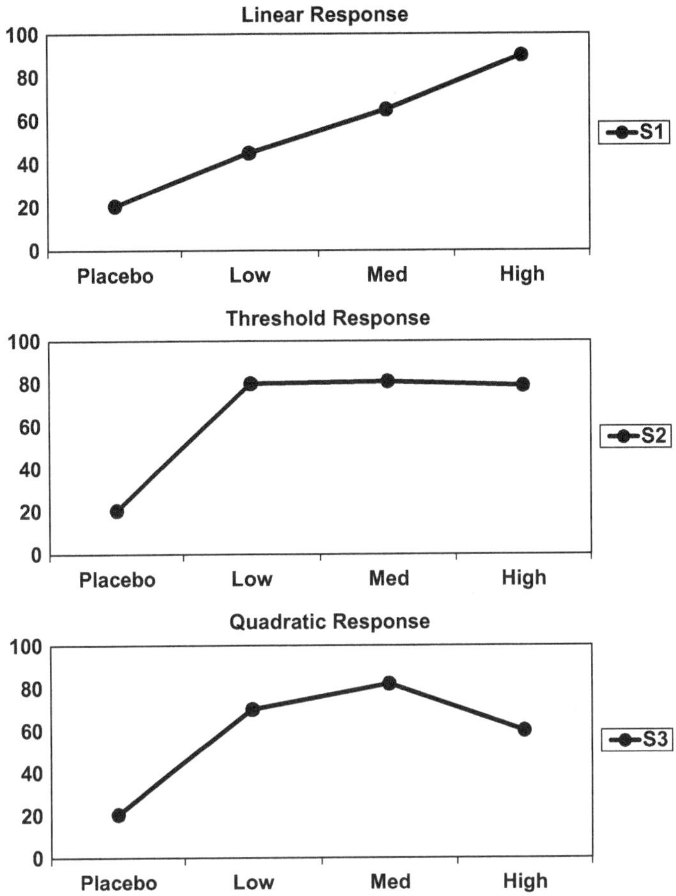

Fig. 13.1 Hypothetical response curves to low, medium, and high doses of stimulant medication. Student 1 (S1) exhibits a linear response, Student 2 (S2) exhibits a threshold response, and Student 3 (S3) exhibits a quadratic response

doses. In addition, some children will exhibit a quadratic response wherein initial improvements are evident as dose increases, but there is a decline in performance at higher doses (Rapport, DuPaul, & Kelly, 1989). Moreover, children may demonstrate idiosyncratic responses to medication across different domains of functioning including math and reading performance, disruptive behavior, and social engagement (Northup, Gulley, Edwards, & Fountain, 2001). To be clear, for a given student, the most therapeutic dose of medication in one domain (e.g., disruptive behavior) may offer little benefit in another domain (e.g., oral reading fluency).

Ongoing monitoring of medication effectiveness. Once medication has been appropriately titrated, it is important to conduct ongoing monitoring of medication effectiveness. Monitoring procedures may involve weekly or biweekly assessments across key domains (e.g., symptomatology, social behavior, academic performance, and side effects). This is important for several reasons. First, although careful medication titration can identify effective maintenance doses for most students, subsequent dose adjustments are necessary (Vitiello et al., 2001). Ongoing monitoring of medication effectiveness and potential side effects is helpful in determining if dose adjustments are necessary. Moreover, particularly as students age, adherence to medication administration is problematic (e.g., Hougue, Lichvar, & Bobek, 2016), and thus ongoing monitoring can help to identify problems with dosage and adherence.

Why Evaluate Psychotropic Medication in the School Setting?

Schools are an ideal place for monitoring the effects of medication for several reasons. First, children spend many of their waking hours in school. Second, schools are an optimal place to assess key areas of student functioning because adults are in the position to witness and supervise students' (a) performance on a range of academic tasks and (b) social interactions. Third, schools are staffed by professionals with expertise in areas relevant to treatment evaluation. For example, school psychologists, teachers, and school nurses have extensive knowledge of the biological, cultural, developmental, and social factors affecting learning and behavior. School psychologists have a variety of skills that can be applied to the evaluation of medication effectiveness including training in single-case research design, behavioral assessment, and behavioral consultation (c.f., DuPaul & Stoner, 2014). In addition, school psychologists have experience collaborating with professionals from other disciplines (Power & Bradley-Klug, 2013). Two studies have indicated that between 55 and 63% of school psychologists surveyed were involved in school-based medication evaluation procedures (Carlson & Demaray, 2001; Gureasko-Moore, DuPaul, & Power, 2005).

Although there are numerous classes of medications that may require school-based monitoring, we will focus most of our discussion on school-based medication evaluation of stimulant medication for two reasons. First, stimulants are the most frequently prescribed medications for school-age children and adolescents (Sultan & Olfson, 2016). Stimulant medication has a rapid onset of action and short half-life, which affords a variety of options for evaluation. Second, many of the methods used to evaluate the effects of stimulant medication may be adapted to the evaluation of other classes of medication with more delayed onsets of action and half-lives. These adaptations involve longer phases in medication conditions to allow time for medication effects to be observed and require washout phases when evaluating return to non-medicated conditions or before a different medication is administered.

The importance of medication titration and ongoing monitoring and management cannot be overstated. Results of large-scale studies have shown that medication is more effective when it is carefully titrated and monitored. Findings from the Multimodal Treatment Study of ADHD (MTA) conducted by the National Institute of Mental Health indicated children who received ongoing (i.e., monthly) monitoring of stimulant medication following initial titration (i.e., "optimal medication management") showed greater improvement with regard to (a) inattentive and hyperactive impulsive symptoms, (b) oppositional/aggressive symptoms, (c) social skills, (d) internalizing symptoms, and (e) academic achievement than children who received less frequent follow-up without initial titration (i.e., "community care"; Jensen et al., 2001). Furthermore, when optimal monthly medication management was discontinued and subjects reverted to care from their community providers after the initial 14-month period, initial differences between the groups regarding the symptoms were no longer evident 3 years later (American Academy of Pediatrics, 2011).

Despite the rationale for monitoring the effects of medications, current procedures often fall short of recommended practices. For example, only about one half (53.3%) of adolescents (12–19 years old) who reported using any psychotropic medication had seen a mental health professional within the past year, and the percentage was slightly lower for adolescents using only one psychotropic medication (42.8%; Jonas et al., 2013). It is important to note that follow-up may in part depend on the type of medication. Reviews of electronic medical records in a large national database indicated that only 38% of 66,719 children in the database diagnosed with ADHD (1995–2010) had a follow-up visit within 30 days of receiving a prescription for ADHD medication (Patel et al., 2017). Within these follow-up appointments, use of information provided by schools is even more infrequent. For example, teacher-completed rating scales were used to monitor medication response for only 7.5% of children with ADHD based on a survey of pediatricians (Epstein et al., 2014).

Medication Evaluation Procedures

It is important to note that medication represents only one method of available treatment, and it may not be appropriate for every student. Several circumstances should be considered before deciding on whether medication is an appropriate treatment option including the severity of the child's symptoms, the parents' and child's attitudes toward medication, and the extent to which other treatments have been implemented (Connor, 2015; DuPaul & Stoner, 2014). If behavioral interventions have not been attempted or adequately adjusted, it may be prudent to delay medication until behavioral interventions have been implemented, modified (if necessary), and accurately evaluated (DuPaul & Stoner, 2014; Fabiano et al., 2007). Numerous components need to be coordinated for school-based medication evaluation to be feasible and valid. The first step in any school-based medication evaluation is to secure written parental consent for school personnel to share information with the prescribing clinician and vice versa. The limits of confidentiality should also be discussed with the parents at the beginning of the process.

In the next section, we will describe the primary stages involved in school-based medication evaluation. Roles of key stakeholders who may lend their expertise to each stage will be examined.

Evaluation Design and Dosage Schedule

Double-blind, placebo-controlled crossover trials have long been considered the "gold standard" for clinical medication evaluation, and several authors extended this methodology to school-based evaluation. For example, Gadow (1993) proposed a model of school-based medication evaluation which employed a double-blind, placebo-controlled design to evaluate student response to two standard doses of stimulant medication. The order of the 2-week dose conditions was randomized and student response during each dose condition was assessed using (a) three different parent and teacher behavior rating scales and (b) systematic direct observation of the student in the classroom, in the lunchroom, and on the playground. Side effects were also monitored via anecdotal caregiver reports and a 13-item checklist completed by both parents and teachers. Similarly, Pelham, Bender, Cadell, Booth, and Moorer (1985) used a double-blind, placebo-controlled design to evaluate student response to three different doses of stimulant medication. The order of 1-week dose conditions was randomized and student response during each dose condition was evaluated on academic performance (e.g., reading comprehension workbooks, math worksheets, and spelling tests) and classroom behavior during daily 30-min observations. Although the designs of these models enhance the internal validity of medication evaluation, the time and resources needed to complete many of the procedures (e.g., daily classroom observations, multiple behavior rating scales) are prohibitive. As a result, stakeholders are left to choose between devoting large amounts of time to technically sound medication evaluation procedures or reverting to an informal, and likely unreliable, process of anecdotal reporting. Consequently, comprehensive medication evaluation procedures have not been widely adopted in school settings and the impact of medication has been systematically assessed for only small percentages of children using psychotropic medication (Shahidullah & Carlson, 2014).

To balance technical rigor with feasibility, Volpe, Heick, and Guerasko-Moore (2005) developed the Agile Consultative Model for Medication Evaluation (ACMME), which utilizes a behavioral consultation process to identify targets for intervention, set specific goals, and devise the treatment evaluation plan. A major advantage of the ACMME is that evaluation procedures can be individualized for different cases and settings based on an evaluation of the feasibility of each evaluation component. Tailoring the assessment in this way is likely to increase the use of and fidelity to medication evaluation procedures. Volpe et al. (2005) cited four advantages of placing school-based medication evaluation in a behavioral consultation framework. First, it places decision-making in a problem-solving framework, which focuses on observable changes in functioning rather than attempting to "cure" underlying pathology. Second, it is a collaborative process involving multiple stakeholders, which is likely to increase social validity. Third, it allows for the prioritization of target behaviors which aids in decision-making. Finally, the model is commonly used for designing and evaluating school-based interventions and facilitates multimodal approaches to intervention, which can be individualized for each student. Stages of the ACMME are outlined in the following paragraphs and in Fig. 13.2.

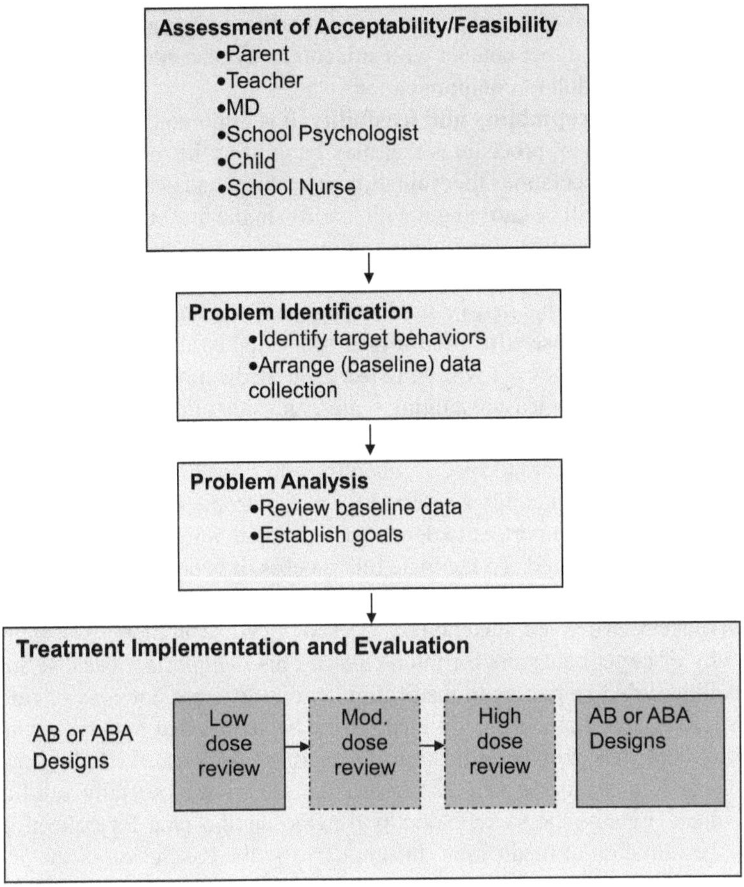

Fig. 13.2 The *Agile Consultative Model of Medication Evaluation* (ACMME; adapted from Volpe, Heick, & Guerasko-Moore, 2005). Boxes in the vertical progression represent stages in the consultative model. Boxes in the horizontal progression within treatment evaluation represent stages in stimulant medication titration

Because there are numerous stakeholders involved in school-based medication evaluation, the ACMME involves a multidisciplinary team approach to leverage the expertise of each member in the evaluation and decision-making process. Although the exact team composition may vary, the stakeholders most commonly involved in school-based medication evaluation include prescribing clinicians, school nurses, teachers, parents, and mental and behavioral health professionals, such as the school psychologist. We have found it helpful to identify one member of the team (hereafter referred to as the "evaluation coordinator") who can facilitate and streamline communication across home, school, and clinical settings. Owing to their expertise in behavioral consultation, assessment, and single-case designs, school psychologists make an ideal team leader who can coordinate the overall process of school-based medication evaluation. Although, as mentioned earlier, school nurses, owing to their medical training and direct contact with students, may also adopt the role of being the cross-setting conduit of communication.

Assessment of acceptability and feasibility. It is important to assess the acceptability and feasibility of procedures that may be used in the medication evaluation because it sets the expectations for evaluation procedures and increases the likelihood that the procedures will be carried out with fidelity. In the first stage of the ACMME, the school-based evaluation coordinator communicates with stakeholders (e.g., parent, teacher, and prescribing physician) to determine the acceptability and feasibility of potential procedures that may be used during the treatment evaluation phase. Parents and teachers may use structured forms (see Volpe et al., 2005) to indicate the frequency with which they are willing to use each medication evaluation procedure (e.g., curriculum-based measures, rating scales, and side effect checklists).

Problem identification. As in a behavioral consultation model, goals of the problem identification phase are to specify, quantify, and prioritize problem(s) exhibited by the student. Although children referred for psychotropic medication may exhibit several problems, it is important to define each problem in observable terms so that it can be reliably measured. To facilitate this process, it is helpful to clarify the discrepancy between the student's current performance and expected performance. Once problems have been defined, stakeholders work to prioritize problems by establishing a hierarchy of target behaviors for intervention. This is important because students often exhibit varied responses to medication across different domains of functioning. Therefore, stakeholders should identify the behaviors that may be sensitive to medication and thus provide indication of treatment response. Including multiple stakeholders in this process will also ensure the selection of socially valid targets for treatment. Finally, the stakeholders will agree upon a plan for collecting data prior to the initiation of medication. In summary, by the conclusion of the problem identification phase, target behaviors should be clearly and objectively defined and a timeline for collecting pretreatment (baseline) data from all relevant stakeholders should be established.

Problem analysis. The two primary tasks to accomplish in the problem analysis phase are to (a) review baseline data and (b) establish goals for intervention. Clearly defined goals will allow the evaluation team to accurately identify the minimally effective dose. Medication can continue at the dose associated with the student's goal achievement. Once the evaluation team has agreed upon goals, they will have a clearer direction to develop the stimulant medication treatment plan.

In addition to medication, the evaluation team should discuss other factors that may be contributing to the problem, including environmental variables or potential skill deficits. Based on these considerations, the evaluation team may decide to implement other components in addition to medication including environmental accommodations, more intensive academic instruction, or a behavioral intervention plan.

Treatment implementation and evaluation. The structure of the treatment evaluation phase in part depends on the medication used, target behaviors identified, and measures deemed to be feasible and acceptable. With short-acting medication, such as stimulants, rigorous single-case research designs (e.g., alternating treatments) have traditionally been employed; however, these designs require rapid changes in dose (i.e., frequent alternating and counterbalanced dose administration) and daily assessment of outcomes, which are likely not feasible in typical public school settings. For this reason, we recommend an evaluation design that is easier to manage and includes a stepwise increase in dose over time (e.g., AB, ABC). When the evaluation team uses some form of an AB design, team members should meet at the end of each dose phase to review implementation fidelity and outcomes. In cases in which side effects increase dramatically, the evaluation team may meet sooner, as needed, to discontinue the medication trial or reduce the dose.

There are four main goals of the treatment evaluation phase. First, the evaluation team must determine the extent to which medication was dispensed and used as intended. To aid in this endeavor, it is helpful for parents and school nurses to keep a log of the student's medication use. Second, the team should determine whether treatment goals were met at a specific dose. Measures agreed upon in the earlier ACMME phases will be used to evaluate the impact of medication on target outcomes and side effects. Third, the evaluation team should determine whether a particular dose should be reduced (or discontinued), continued, or increased. The evaluation team may decide to discontinue the medication trial or reduce the dose of medication if side effects reach a level of concern. The dose may also be reduced if no clear benefit has been observed on target outcomes in comparison to lower doses and side effects become intolerable. Conversely, the team may decide to continue medication if improvement on target outcomes is evident and side effects are tolerable, although monitoring procedures should also continue. The team may increase the dose if the student has not yet achieved treatment goals specified in the ACMME problem analysis phase.

The final goal of the treatment evaluation phase is to plan for continued medication evaluation; however, the exact procedures will depend on whether medication is still being titrated. If the evaluation team decides to increase the dose (i.e., the minimally effective dose has not yet been identified), the evaluation team should continue frequent evaluation procedures as part of the titration process. However, if the minimally effective dose has been identified, a monitoring plan should be developed and agreed upon.

Dispensing Medication

Effective school-based medication evaluation requires systematic, tightly controlled manipulation of dose. Therefore, it is important for the school-based evaluation team to agree upon the evaluation plan (e.g., AB design, alternating treatments design) in the ACMME prior to beginning the medication trial. When medication is administered at home, it is important for parents to accurately record administration and ingestion of medication and inform school personnel of lapses, incorrect dosage, or other problems dispensing the medication. Parents may need training to accurately and consistently determine whether their child ingested the medication; therefore, the school-based team must coordinate this training with the prescribing physician. When medication is administered at school, it is important for the school nurse to administer the medication according to the treatment plan and accurately record whether the child ingested the medication. The school nurse may also serve as the primary contact for the parents when problems dispensing medication at home arise. School nurses serve an important role in promoting treatment adherence. They can check in with students in the morning as to whether they received their morning dose of medication, can provide reminders to parents about administration and refilling prescriptions, and can administer medication in the school setting.

Best Practices in Measuring School Outcomes

Behavior, symptomatology, and problem behaviors. Table 13.1 summarizes the advantages and limitations of common measures in school-based medication evaluation. The most frequently used measures of behavior are Systematic Direct Observation (SDO), behavior rating scales such as the IOWA Conners Teacher Rating Scale, and daily behavior report cards (see Fabiano et al., 2007). Although SDO has the advantage of being an objective measure that is sensitive to small changes in behavior, training requirements, and time demands are barriers to its broad use in evaluation procedures (see Briesch, Volpe, & Floyd, in press). Rating scales can be useful in the assessment of behavioral response to medical interventions, but many common rating scales are too lengthy to be appropriate for frequent assessment. Investigators have examined abbreviating such measures to create shorter scales that are individualized for each student (e.g., Hyman et al., 1998; Volpe & Gadow, 2010). Likewise, investigators have advocated for the use of daily report cards as individualized measures of student classroom functioning (Pelham, 1993; Fabiano et al., 2007; Volpe & Fabiano, 2013). Over the last decade, increasing attention has been focused on Direct Behavior Ratings (DBR; see Briesch, Chafouleas, & Tillman, 2016). DBR are a hybrid assessment method involving characteristics of both SDO (real-time observation) and rating scales (e.g., rating the frequency of a behavior or the proportion of time it was present). Both single-item scales and multiple-item scales have been investigated (see Volpe & Briesch, 2012, 2015). Although DBR are not as well studied in the context of school-based medication evaluation as the other methods described here, given their feasibility and flexibility, they show much promise in this regard.

Academic performance. Assessment tools used to measure changes in academic performance during medication titration need to be capable of detecting changes in the short term. Curriculum-Based Measures (CBM) are useful in this regard because initial research has shown math computation and oral reading fluency CBM to be sensitive to the effects of stimulant medication (Northup & Gulley, 2001; Stoner, Carey, Ikeda, & Shinn, 1994).

Table 13.1 Advantages and limitations of methods commonly used to assess response to psychotropic medication

Domain/measures	Advantages	Limitations	Source
Behavior and symptomatology			
Systematic direct observation	• Objective • Sensitive to short-term changes	• Time intensive • Requires training	School Psychologist
Behavior rating scales	• Strong technical characteristics (e.g., reliability validity)	• Time intensive • Not sensitive to short-term changes	Teacher Parent
Daily behavior report cards	• Individualized • Sensitive to treatment	• Lack evidence of traditional reliability	Teacher Parent
Direct behavior rating	• Feasible • Flexible	• Has not been evaluated in the context of medication evaluation	Teacher
Academic performance			
Curriculum-based measures	• Sensitive to short-term changes in academic skills	• Requires training • Requires frequent and repeated administration	Teacher
Side effects			
Anecdotal student reports	• Specific • Qualitative	• Highly subjective	School Nurse
Structured side effect rating scales	• Focused	• High ratings may reflect symptoms of the disorder itself and not medication side effects	Student Parent

Monitoring Side Effects

To effectively monitor the side effects of medication, the evaluation team must first understand what potential side effects are associated with a specific medication. Additionally, it is important to collect information about pretreatment side effects for comparison during treatment because behaviors reported as medication side effects have also been reported while children receive placebo (Barkley, McMurray, Edelbrock, & Robbins, 1990). Anecdotally, the school nurse is often the first person a student interacts with when he or she is experiencing discomfort including headaches, stomachaches, loss of appetite, or insomnia, and given that the aforementioned symptoms are common side effects associated with psychotropic medication, the school nurse is indispensable in monitoring side effects. Furthermore, school nurses are trained to look for adverse changes in physiology, mood, or behavior in the assessment of overall health.

In addition to providing anecdotal reports to adults, students may be asked to complete standardized self-report measures of medication side effects, such as the Stimulant Drug Side Effects Rating Scale (SDERS; Barkley & Murphy, 2006). The SDERS is a 17-item rating scale designed to assess the most common adverse reactions to stimulant medication, which may be completed by teachers, parents, and/or students; each item is rated on a 10-point scale ranging from *Absent* (0) to *Serious* (9). Students are likely the most accurate reporters of certain side effects during treatment with methylphenidate, including internalizing symptoms, drowsiness, and insomnia (DuPaul & Stoner, 2014).

Teachers may be useful in monitoring medication side effects because they spend the most time with children of anyone in the school; however, caution should be exercised. Some studies have shown that the severity of teacher-reported side effects is actually higher during placebo than during treatment with methylphenidate (Barkley et al., 1990; DuPaul et al., 1996). The hypothesized reason for this is that teachers and parents may misperceive some symptoms of the disorder as side effects (Rapport & Moffitt, 2002). Similar patterns have been demonstrated with regard to parent ratings of side effects; however, parents may be in the best position to monitor some side effects such as insomnia and reduced appetite (Barkley et al., 1990), although school nurses also can provide valuable information in this regard owing to their training in communicating with children about how they feel. Together, these results suggest multiple informants, including the students themselves, should be included in monitoring medication side effects.

Physician/School Communication

The school psychologist's role in medication evaluation is rooted in the concept of "pediatric school psychology" first advanced by Power, DuPaul, Shapiro, and Parrish (1995), who highlighted the need for school psychologists to develop expertise in the provision of services to children with medical conditions. Specifically, Power and colleagues (1995) defined the roles of a pediatric school psychologist as "(a) advocacy for the educational needs of children with medical conditions; (b) evaluation of the efficacy of interventions designed to improve the ability of children with medical conditions to adapt in educational settings; (c) promotion of more effective communication between pediatric and educational professionals; and (d) collaboration with educational professionals to design programs to promote health among all children and adolescents" (p. 248).

As such, the school psychologist serves as a bidirectional link between pediatricians and educators with regard to evaluating the effects of medication. In one direction, the school psychologist educates pediatricians about single-case research design, behavioral assessment methods, and the unique culture and features of school settings (e.g., available personnel; Power et al., 1995). In the other direction, the school psychologist helps educators to understand the medical treatment model and the culture of clinical settings, as well as to effectively evaluate the impact and side effects of medication (Power et al., 1995).

The need for the school psychologist to serve as a link between school and clinical settings is even more imperative when one considers the fact that children taking psychotropic medication are also likely to receive other interventions and supports in school that need to be integrated with the psychopharmacological intervention (DuPaul & Carlson, 2005). Ideally, targets for school-based academic, social–emotional, and behavioral interventions should be aligned with targets for psychopharmacological intervention (DuPaul & Carlson, 2005). Furthermore, when social–emotional and behavioral interventions are used in conjunction with medication, the intensity or duration of the intervention, as well as the dose of medication may be reduced, thus the potential for side effects is also reduced (Fabiano et al., 2007).

Implications for Psychologists and Physicians

Given the role school psychologists play in medication evaluation, it is important that they continue to develop advanced skills. Power, Shapiro, and DuPaul (2003) outlined key competency domains necessary for school psychologists to serve as an effective link between pediatric and school settings. First, psychologists must have knowledge of *interventions for chronic illnesses*, including methods to assess the needs of children with chronic illness and interventions to support their families. Specific knowledge of (a) child development, (b) the impact of specific classes of medication on children's cognitive, social, and emotional functioning, and (c) side effects associated with commonly prescribed medications all fall within this domain. Second, psychologists must develop competency in *prevention programming*, including understanding risk and protective factors related to chronic health problems, as well as skills to implement core components of wellness programs. Third, psychologists must develop competency in *program evaluation*, including the use of single-case research design and quasi-experimental research methods to determine whether interventions are effective for helping children achieve desired outcomes. Finally, psychologists must develop competency in *intersystem collaboration*, including interdisciplinary collaboration skills to facilitate communication and intervention across pediatric, home, and school settings.

One important consideration in communicating across home, school, and clinical settings is understanding that stakeholders in these settings have different perspectives and foci regarding the medication regimen. Communication across settings must take into consideration differences in perspective, training, and constraints on time. When communicating across settings, the content and format of information should be: (a) accessible, (b) concise, and (c) usable. By this, we mean that the liaison should use language that is easily understood by the recipient, that it be in a format that does not overwhelm the recipient, and that when thinking about communication, the liaison should start by thinking about why he/she is communicating the information and provide the information in that context. School psychologists are used to communicating findings with single-case design charts, but these may be overwhelming to a parent (or a prescribing physician for that matter). Effective communication across settings may involve synthesizing this information for these stakeholders. For example, when titrating medication, the prescribing physician wants to know if there has been an improvement in symptoms and functional impairment (e.g., academic functioning) from baseline to a particular dose of medication or between two doses of medication. A 10-minute office visit does not afford much time to critically examine several different single-case design charts. A better start might be to have a one-page summary sheet that includes all the domains assessed across two or more conditions (e.g., symptom counts, academic performance scores, points earned on daily behavior report cards, and side effects). If stakeholders are interested in gaining more information, it can be provided, but working closely with these stakeholders will help ensure that the data are actionable to the end user.

Summary

Millions of schoolchildren in the United States are being prescribed psychotropic medication. However, despite the clear importance of careful titration and ongoing monitoring of the effectiveness of medication and potential side effects, such assessments are the exception rather than typical practice. Although prescribing physicians would appreciate receiving information from school regarding student response to medication (Haile-Mariam, Bradley-Johnson, & Johnson, 2002), there are several barriers to conducting assessments and communicating findings across settings including time, clear role assignments, and accessibility to prescribing physicians.

In this chapter, we have summarized the ACMME, which is a flexible approach to evaluating medication in the school setting. Although the model was developed to address challenges in assessing the effects of stimulant medication for children and adolescents with ADHD, the model can be adapted to the evaluation of longer acting psychotropic medications. In summarizing the model, we discussed the roles different stakeholders can play in applying the model. Key considerations in the success of carrying out such evaluations are to clearly delineate roles, design procedures that are acceptable and feasible, and establish a structure to facilitate frequent communication.

Acknowledgements The authors would like to thank Wanda Visnick for sharing her expertise in the delivery of school-based mental health services.

Readings

American Academy of Child and Adolescent Psychiatry. (2009). Practice parameter on the use of psychotropic medication in children and adolescents. *Journal of the American Academy of Child and Adolescent Psychiatry, 48,* 961–973.

The American Academy of Child and Adolescent Psychiatry (AACAP) is an organization of psychiatrists whose mission is to promote the healthy development of children, adolescents, and families and the safe use of psychotropic medication in children and adolescents with mental health needs. AACAP guidelines recommend that medications should be used for the minimal duration possible; therefore, frequent and continuous monitoring can identify clinical response in children and adolescents and facilitate efficient and effective use of psychotropic medication.

DuPaul, G. J., & Stoner, G. (2014). *ADHD in the schools: Assessment and intervention strategies* (3rd edn.). New York: Guilford.

This book serves as a comprehensive guidebook for assessing and intervening with students with ADHD. It offers guidelines for evaluating the effects of medical interventions in the school setting including a detailed review of measures that might be used to evaluate the effects (and side effects) of medical interventions. In the Appendix of the book, the authors provide several exemplars of communication between a school psychologist and a prescribing physician including an initial referral letter, a referral for a possible medication trial, a description of a school-based medication procedure, and a letter summarizing the results of a school-based medication trial.

Websites

https://ccf.fiu.edu/about/resources/index.html

The Center for Children and Families at Florida International University provides (a) information on ADHD medication and (b) behavioral intervention resources for improving classroom management practices and implementing daily behavior report card interventions. The website also provides tools for assessing the extent of students' impairment with regard to ADHD and teachers' classroom management practices.

http://www.chadd.org/

Children and Adults with Attention-Deficit/Hyperactivity Disorder (CHADD), is a national non-profit organization whose mission is to "improve the lives of people affected by ADHD." The National Resource Center on ADHD (a program of CHADD) provides up-to-date evidence-based information about assessment, diagnosis, and treatment of ADHD (including medication).

http://parentsmedguide.org/

The website provides extensive information regarding medication for treating ADHD, Bipolar Disorder, and Depression, including medication guides that were developed by the American Psychiatric Association and the American Academy of Child and Adolescent Psychiatry. Although the intended audience is parents, the information is relevant for anyone working in childcare systems (e.g., teachers, school psychologists).

References

American Academy of Pediatrics, Committee on Quality Improvement, & Subcommittee on Attention-Deficit/Hyperactivity Disorder. (2011). ADHD: Clinical practice guideline for the diagnosis, evaluation, and treatment of attention-deficit/hyperactivity disorder in children and adolescents. *Pediatrics, 128,* 1–16.

Baweja, R., Belin, P. J., Humphrey, H. H., Babocsai, L., Pariseau, M. E., Waschbusch, D. A., … Waxmonsky, J. G. (2016). The effectiveness and tolerability of central nervous system stimulants in school-age children with attention-deficit/hyperactivity disorder and disruptive mood dysregulation disorder across home and school. *Journal of Child and Adolescent Psychopharmacology, 26,* 154–163.

Barkley, R. A., McMurray, M. B., Edelbrock, C. S., & Robbins, K. (1990). Side effects of methylphenidate in children with attention deficit hyperactivity disorder: A systemic, placebo-controlled evaluation. *Pediatrics, 86,* 184–192.

Barkley, R. A., & Murphy, K. R. (2006). *Attention-deficit hyperactivity disorder: A clinical workbook.* New York: Guilford Press.

Briesch, A. M., Chafouleas, S. M., & Riley-Tillman, T. C. (2016). *Direct behavior rating (DBR): Linking assessment, communication, and intervention.* New York, NY: Guilford Press.

Briesch, A. M., Volpe, R. J., & Floyd, R. G. (in press). *A practical guide to classroom observation.* New York: Guilford Press.

Carlson, J. S., & Demaray, M. K. (2001, February). *A survey of knowledge and training in school psychopharamacology.* Poster presented at the annual National Association of School Psychologists Convention, Washington, DC.

Chirdkiatgumchai, V., Xiao, H., Fredstrom, B. K., Adams, R. E., Epstein, J. N., Shah, S. S., … Froehlich, T. E. (2013). National trends in psychotropic medication use in young children: 1994–2009. *Pediatrics, 132,* 615–623.

Connor, D. F. (2015). Stimulant and nonstimulant medications for children with ADHD. In R. A. Barkley (Ed.), *Attention-deficit hyperactivity disorder: A handbook for diagnosis and treatment* (pp. 666–685). New York: Guildford Press.

DuPaul, G. J., Anastopoulos, A. D., Kwasnik, D., Barkley, R. A., & McMurray, M. B. (1996). Methylphenidate effects on children with attention deficit hyperactivity disorder: Self-report of symptoms, side-effects, and self-esteem. *Journal of Attention Disorders, 1,* 3–15.

DuPaul, G. J., & Carlson, J. S. (2005). Child psychopharmacology: How school psychologists can contribute to effective outcomes. *School Psychology Quarterly, 20,* 206–221.

DuPaul, G. J., & Stoner, G. (2014). *ADHD in the schools: Assessment and intervention strategies.* New York: Guilford Press.

Epstein, J. N., Kelleher, K. J., Baum, R., Brinkman, W. B., Peugh, J., Gardner, W., … Langberg, J. (2014). Variability in ADHD care in community-based pediatrics. *Pediatrics, 134,* 1136–1143.

Fabiano, G. A., Pelham, W. E., Jr., Gnagy, E. M., Burrows-MacLean, L., Coles, E. K., Chacko, A., et al. (2007). The single and combined effects of multiple intensities of behavior modification and methylphenidate for children with attention deficit hyperactivity disorder. *School Psychology Review, 36,* 195–216.

Gadow, K. D. (1993). A school-based medication evaluation program. In J. L. Matson (Ed.), *Handbook of hyperactivity in children* (pp. 186–219).

Gureasko-Moore, D. P., DuPaul, G. J., & Power, T. J. (2005). Stimulant treatment for attention-deficit/hyperactivity disorder: Medication monitoring practices of school psychologists. *School Psychology Review, 34,* 232–245.

Haile-Mariam, A., Bradley-Johnson, S., & Johnson, C. M. (2002). Pediatricians' preferences for ADHD information from schools. *School Psychology Review, 31,* 94–105.

Harvey, R. C., James, A. C., & Shields, G. E. (2016). A systematic review and network meta-analysis to assess the relative efficacy of antipsychotics for the treatment of positive and negative symptoms in early-onset schizophrenia. *CNS Drugs, 30,* 27–39.

Hogue, A., Lichvar, E., & Bobek, M. (2016). Pilot evaluation of the medication integration protocol for adolescents with ADHD in behavioral care: Treatment fidelity and medication uptake. *Journal of Emotional and Behavioral Disorders, 24,* 223–234.

Howie, L. D., Pastor, P. N., & Lukacs, S. (2014). *Use of medication prescribed for emotional or behavioral difficulties among children aged 6–17 years in the United States, 2011–2012.* US Department of Health and Human Services, Centers for Disease Control and Prevention, National Center for Health Statistics.

Hyman, I. A., Wojtowicz, A., Lee, K. D., Haffner, M. E., Fiorello, C. A., Storlazzi, J. J., & Rosenfeld, J. (1998). School-based methylphenidate placebo protocols: Methodological and practical issues. *Journal of Learning Disabilities, 31,* 581–594.

Jonas, B. S., Gu, Q., & Albertorio-Diaz, J. R. (2013). Psychotropic medication use among adolescents: United States, 2005–2010. *NCHS Data Brief, 135,* 1–8.

Jensen, P. S., Hinshaw, S. P., Swanson, J. M., Greenhill, L. L., Conners, C. K., Arnold, L. E., … March, J. S. (2001). Findings from the NIMH multimodal treatment study of ADHD (MTA): Implications and applications for primary care providers. *Journal of Developmental & Behavioral Pediatrics, 22,* 60–73.

Kieling, C., Baker-Henningham, H., Belfer, M., Conti, G., Ertem, I., Omigbodun, O., … Rahman, A. (2011). Child and adolescent mental health worldwide: Evidence for action. *The Lancet, 378,* 1515–1525.

Northup, J., & Gulley, V. (2001). Some contributions of functional analysis to the assessment of behaviors associated with attention deficit hyperactivity disorder and the effects of stimulant medication. *School Psychology Review, 30,* 227–238.

Northup, J., Gulley, V., Edwards, S., & Fountain, L. (2001). The effects of methylphenidate in the classroom: What dosage, for which children, for what problems? *School Psychology Quarterly, 16,* 303–323.

Olfson, M., Druss, B. G., & Marcus, S. C. (2015). Trends in mental health care among children and adolescents. *New England Journal of Medicine, 372,* 2029–2038.

Patel, A., Medhekar, R., Ochoa-Perez, M., Aparasu, R. R., Chan, W., Sherer, J. T., … Chen, H. (2017). Care provision and prescribing practices of physicians treating children and adolescents with ADHD. *Psychiatric Services.* Advance online publication. https://doi.org/10.1176/appi.ps.201600130.

Pelham, W. E. (1993). Pharmacotherapy for children with attention-deficit hyperactivity disorder. *School Psychology Review, 22,* 199–227.

Pelham, W. E., Bender, M. E., Caddell, J., Booth, S., & Moorer, S. H. (1985). Methylphenidate and children with attention deficit disorder: Dose effects on classroom academic and social behavior. *Archives of General Psychiatry, 42,* 948–952.

Power, T. J., & Bradley-Klug, K. (2013). *Pediatric school psychology: Conceptualization, applications, and strategies for leadership development.* New York: Routledge.

Power, T. J., DuPaul, G. J., Shapiro, E. S., & Parrish, J. M. (1995). Pediatric school psychology: The emergence of a subspecialty. *School Psychology Review, 24,* 244–257.

Power, T. J., Shapiro, E. S., & DuPaul, G. J. (2003). Preparing psychologists to link systems of care in managing and preventing children's health problems. *Journal of Pediatric Psychology, 28,* 147–156.
Rapport, M. D., DuPaul, G. J., & Kelly, K. L. (1989). Attention-deficit hyperactivity disorder and methylphenidate: The relationship between gross body weight and drug response in children. *Psychopharmacology Bulletin, 25,* 285–290.
Rapport, M. D., & Moffitt, C. (2002). Attention deficit/hyperactivity disorder and methylphenidate: A review of height/weight, cardiovascular, and somatic complaint side effects. *Clinical Psychology Review, 22,* 1107–1131.
Shahidullah, J. D., & Carlson, J. S. (2014). Survey of nationally certified school psychologists' roles and training in psychopharmacology. *Psychology in the Schools, 51,* 705–721.
Stein, M. A., Sarampote, C. S., Waldman, I. D., Robb, A. S., Conlon, C., Pearl, P. L., ... Newcorn, J. H. (2003). A dose-response study of OROS methylphenidate in children with attention-deficit/hyperactivity disorder. *Pediatrics, 112,* e404–e404.
Stoner, G., Carey, S. P., Ikeda, M. J., & Shinn, M. R. (1994). The utility of curriculum-based measurement for evaluating the effects of methylphenidate on academic performance. *Journal of Applied Behavior Analysis, 27,* 101–113.
Sultan, R. S., & Olfson, M. (2016). National rates of psychotropic medication use in pediatric populations. *Journal of the American Academy of Child and Adolescent Psychiatry, 55,* S166.
Vitiello, B., Severe, J. B., Greenhill, L. L., Arnold, L. E., Abikoff, H. B., Bukstein, O. G., ... March, J. S. (2001). Methylphenidate dosage for children with ADHD over time under controlled conditions: Lessons from the MTA. *Journal of the American Academy of Child and Adolescent Psychiatry, 40,* 188–196.
Volpe, R. J., & Briesch, A. M. (2012). Generalizability and dependability of single-item and multiple-item direct behavior rating scales for engagement and disruptive behavior. *School Psychology Review, 41,* 246–261.
Volpe, R. J., & Briesch, A. M. (2015). Multi-item direct behavior ratings: Dependability of two levels of assessment specificity. *School Psychology Quarterly, 30,* 431–442.
Volpe, R. J., & Fabiano, G. A. (2013). *Daily behavior report cards: An evidence-based system of assessment and intervention.* New York: Guilford Press.
Volpe, R. J., & Gadow, K. D. (2010). Creating abbreviated rating scales to monitor classroom inattention-overactivity, aggression, and peer conflict: Reliability, validity, and treatment sensitivity. *School Psychology Review, 39,* 350–363.
Volpe, R. J., Heick, P. F., & Guerasko-Moore, D. (2005). An agile behavioral model for monitoring the effects of stimulant medication in school settings. *Psychology in the Schools, 42,* 509–523.
Walkup, J. T. (2017). Antidepressant efficacy for depression in children and adolescents: Industry- and NIMH-funded studies. *American Journal of Psychiatry, 174,* 430–437.
Zuvekas, S. H., & Vitiello, B. (2012). Stimulant medication use in children: A 12-year perspective. *American Journal of Psychiatry, 169,* 160–166.

Chapter 14
Clinical Case Studies: Evaluating Medication Outcomes in Schools

Sally Askar, Danielle Haggerty, Justina Yohannan, Courtney Darr, Allison Siroky, Rachel Korest and Adrianna Crossing

The purpose of this chapter is to provide a follow-up to the series of cases presented in Chap. 3. Those case studies highlighted difficult situations when children fail to respond to psychosocial treatment approaches in schools/at home and an emergent need for a psychiatric consultation develops in an effort to attempt to improve mental health functioning. Case studies (Attention Deficit Hyperactivity Disorder, Conduct Disorder, Depression, Social Anxiety Disorder, Autism Spectrum Disorder, Bipolar Disorder, Psychosis) related to each of the mental health conditions reviewed in the prior chapters of this book are presented.

Each case study provides a brief summary of the reason for the psychiatric consultation. Then a summary of the findings of the consultation is provided including the diagnostic criteria met and the psychiatrist's recommendation for treatment. The rationale for the psychotropic medication(s) prescribed for each case is provided in the context of the treatment side effects that may emerge. An overview of the methods used to gather the data necessary to further examine the costs and benefits of the treatment selected is provided. Specific attention in each case study is given to the data collection methods and procedures to be employed. Finally, each case ends with a summary of the treatment cost-benefit analysis based on the progress monitoring data collected at home and school.

The purpose of each case study is to provide readers with a sense of the importance of a data-based approach to progress monitoring when psychotropic medication treatments are used to improve the mental health functioning of school-aged youth. The costs (e.g., side effects) and benefits (e.g., intended effects) of psychotropic medications in these cases are reviewed.

S. Askar (✉) · D. Haggerty · J. Yohannan · A. Siroky · R. Korest · A. Crossing
Michigan State University, East Lansing, MI, USA
e-mail: askarsal@msu.edu

C. Darr
East Lansing, MI, USA
e-mail: courtneyldarr@gmail.com

J. S. Carlson and J. A. Barterian (eds.), *School Psychopharmacology*,
Pediatric School Psychology, https://doi.org/10.1007/978-3-030-15541-4_14

Attention Deficit Hyperactive Disorder

Sally Askar

Reason for Referral

Jim is a 10-year-old male who was referred by his parents for a psychiatric consultation because his externalizing behaviors have become more severe in recent weeks despite implementing a series of interventions targeting his behavior at school and home. Symptoms of inattention, hyperactivity, and impulsivity are more pervasively affecting his school and home life. In addition, Jim has become more aggressive toward his parents, increasingly engaged in negative self-talk at school, and showing an increased level of frustration with his schoolwork.

Results of Psychiatric Consultation

The psychiatric consultation consisted of a review of Jim's medical/family history and a collection of information about Jim's symptoms across home and school. Jim, his parents, and his homeroom teacher all completed both broadband (i.e., internalizing and externalizing symptoms) and narrow-band (i.e., impulsivity, hyperactivity, inattention) behavioral rating scales. Data gathering efforts resulted in a diagnosis of ADHD-combined presentation type because of consistent and severe symptoms of hyperactivity, inattention, and impulsivity that are impairing multiple areas of Jim's functioning. The psychiatrist prescribed methylphenidate, a psychostimulant medication, as an adjunctive treatment to his current school-based interventions to help reduce his behavioral symptoms of impulsivity and inattention. A close examination of stimulant side effects (e.g., appetite and sleep difficulties) was recommended. In addition, Jim's parents were encouraged to closely monitor his behavior for any additional signs of depression and conduct problems as an alternative or additional treatments may be warranted to address any co-occurring emotional or behavioral symptoms.

Rationale for Psychotropic Medication Treatment

Jim has struggled with symptoms of ADHD since he was a young child and he has a family history of ADHD as both his father and brother present with the disorder. His symptoms (e.g., fidgeting, inattention, disorganization, talking excessively to peers, difficulties with self-regulation) have become more severe in the past couple of months. Recently, aggressive behaviors toward his parents have emerged. Jim's symptoms are negatively impacting his work in school and his ability to make and keep friends. Jim has gone through multiple psychosocial treatments that have failed to help him manage his symptoms. Methylphenidate, a psychostimulant, was selected for treatment given its impact on the core features of ADHD (i.e., reductions in hyperactivity/impulsivity, improvements in attention) and its relatively minimal side effect profile. Implementing psychotropic medication treatment along with psychosocial treatments has the potential to bring about the most positive outcomes for Jim at the lowest possible dosage (i.e., less potential for negative side effects). Medication treatments combined with psychostimulant treatments have also been found to allow for improvements in social and academic behaviors.

Evaluation Methods

Before beginning the evaluation of psychotropic medication treatment, Jim's parents provided consent to release information about his treatment to both school personnel and his physician. The school psychologist worked closely with Jim's doctor, teacher, and parents to discuss and create a plan on how Jim's psychotropic medication treatment would be evaluated. The specific plan involved the completion of daily behavior ratings from his teacher related to hyperactivity, impulsivity, and inattention. It was expected that these symptoms would improve within the first couple of weeks after the onset of methylphenidate treatment. Jim's physician recommended that data collection occurs at school and home to help determine if any dosage changes were necessary. In addition to daily behavior ratings, his mother and homeroom teacher were asked to complete an ADHD behavior rating form once a week. Jim and his parents were also asked to complete a daily five-item questionnaire aimed at identifying any changes in appetite, sleep, irritability, somatic concerns, and depressive symptoms. A structured classroom observation was completed once a week to determine if Jim's classroom behavior more closely approximated that of his teacher's expectations (i.e., comparison to a peer). Jim was also involved in the evaluation of his psychotropic medication treatment to help better understand his perception of change. The school psychologist also asked Jim to complete a behavioral rating scale once a week to examine changes in his attention and behavior.

Cost-Benefit Analysis/Treatment Response

Jim and his parents met with his doctor to review the results of the data collected at home and school after 4 weeks of treatment. A two-page summary document was created by the school psychologist with attention to the medication target behaviors and potential side effects. A reduction in Jim's appetite was reported by his parents and his physician recommended that he increase his caloric intake. Jim also experienced sleep difficulties (i.e., trouble falling asleep) initially but his sleep improved in the past 2 weeks. No other side effects were reported. According to multiple sources of information, Jim's behaviors are now more consistent with others his age. Jim's parents reported that he has been more cooperative at home and has been completing his homework without being told. Additionally, his parents noticed that when they ask Jim to do chores around the house he actively listens and responds. Jim's teacher noted that he has not been walking around disturbing others during his independent work time. Further, he pays closer attention to his seat work and does not daydream as often. His teacher indicated that when she is lecturing the class, she now notices that Jim is attending to the presentation and consistently raising his hand to answer questions. Improvements have also been noticed with respect to his grades and school personnel have now backed away from their prior recommendation to retain Jim in the fourth grade. According to school-based observations, Jim displays more positive interactions with his peers and he has begun to sit with the same group of friends at lunch. Jim's parents were especially happy to see his irritability decline and he has been much more respectful of them at home.

Conduct Disorder

Danielle Haggerty

Reason for Referral

Brian is a 15-year-old male who was referred by his mother for a psychiatric consultation due to worsening conduct problems. Brian and his friends were suspended from school after being caught drinking in the school bathroom. That same day, Brian was arrested for shoplifting. School personnel and Brian's mother believed the school-based interventions were not reducing problem behaviors to an acceptable level. A psychiatric consultation, including a substance use assessment, was completed to try and more effectively treat his emotional and behavioral challenges.

Results of Psychiatric Consultation

The psychiatric consultation involved an in-depth interview with Brian and his mother. Specific attention was given to the behaviors that were impairing his functioning at school, home, and in the community. Brian, his mother, and one of his teachers provided their behavioral ratings on a set of broad-band and narrow-band measures. The school also provided the psychiatrist with progress monitoring data from Brian's check and connect intervention. A write-up of the incident at school and a copy of the police report were also reviewed by Brian's physician. Brian's lack of remorse for stealing, his aggression toward others, and his pervasive engagement in oppositional behaviors and conduct problems were found to be particularly concerning. Brian was diagnosed with Conduct Disorder. A trial of the antipsychotic medication, risperidone, was recommended as an adjunct to his current school-based interventions. Additionally, it was recommended that Brian see a substance abuse counselor once a week. Brian was responsible for monitoring antipsychotic side effects (e.g., tiredness, weight gain, somatic complaints) and any other physical or cognitive changes.

Rationale for Psychotropic Medication Treatment

Brian has struggled with academic and conduct problems since early in elementary school. His behaviors have become more severe and he is at risk for being sent to juvenile detention. A series of school-based interventions had limited impact on improving Brian's conduct problems. His association with a deviant peer group combined with recent substance use are particularly worrisome. Brian's recent legal troubles at school and in the community indicated his behaviors have worsened in recent weeks. Risperidone, an atypical antipsychotic, was selected for treatment given its potential impact on reducing his aggressive and impulsive behaviors. Additionally, the psychiatric consultation highlighted that not treating Brian's current symptoms with a psychotropic medication could result in additional harm to himself or others. Brian's recognition of the negative path that he is on resulted in an openness to a trial of risperidone. A combination of substance use counseling, school-based psychosocial interventions, and medication treatment were agreed to by Brian (i.e., assent) and his mother given their realization of the need to quickly reduce problem behaviors.

Evaluation Methods

Brian's mother provided consent for the release of information pertaining to his treatment across all parties involved, including school personnel. Brian's response to a trial of risperidone was closely monitored by his psychiatrist through daily text messages from Brian about his treatment response and any emergent side effects. Brian, his mother, and the school psychologist shared responsibility for gathering and summarizing behavioral data to help to determine if risperidone was effective. First, Brian's mother was responsible for ensuring that he was taking the prescribed dosage of risperidone at the correct times. She was responsible for summarizing treatment adherence data. Brian kept a daily journal about how he was feeling physically (e.g., headache, stomachache) and psychologically (e.g., irritability, anger). The school psychologist was responsible for gathering data about the impact of the in-school psychosocial interventions (i.e., multisystemic therapy, parent/teacher management training, check and connect) and produced a brief monthly summary of his progress (i.e., attendance, behavior, office referrals). Finally, his substance abuse counselor was responsible for monitoring his abstinence from alcohol and other drugs given the potential impact these medications would have when combined with risperidone. The information gathered across time was used to help the psychiatrist weigh potential costs and benefits of the medication trial. Brian was responsible for bringing all this data with him to his 4-week follow-up appointment.

Cost-Benefit Analysis/Treatment Response

There were costs and benefits associated with Brian's risperidone trial. Costs included emergence of common side effects (lethargy, weight gain) associated with risperidone. During the 4-week trial, Brian was excused from class three times to take a short nap in the nurse's office. Additionally, Brian's mother noted that he was hungry late into the night and ate more than before he started taking risperidone. Brian was unhappy that he had gained ten pounds over the past month but overall indicated feeling less angry and irritable, especially after stopping his substance use. Brian reported improvements that resulted from taking risperidone in combination with his school-based interventions. First, he had not engaged in any illegal activity in the past month which was especially important given that he was put on probation for his prior shoplifting arrest. Second, he was only absent two days during the medication trial and sent to the principal's office once. Brian's teachers reported improvements in Brian's behavior during class and were encouraged by the progress he appeared to be making. They noted that his outbursts were less severe and more manageable than in the past. Teachers were beginning to feel more comfortable addressing Brian's classroom misbehavior, compared to before when they would immediately send him to the office. Ultimately, the decision was made between Brian's psychiatrist, school psychologist, mother, and Brian that the benefits of taking risperidone appeared to outweigh the costs though close monitoring was necessary over the next month. Brian's psychiatrist offered him resources to help combat his side effects of sleepiness and weight gain (i.e., a food and exercise log). Brian's psychiatrist will continue to monitor his behavior and adjust his dosage of medication as needed.

Depression

Justina Yohannan

Reason for Referral

Chris is a 13-year-old male who was referred for a psychiatric consultation by his parents because his internalizing symptoms have become more severe in recent weeks despite implementing a series of interventions targeting his behavior at home and school. Both Chris's teachers and parents have raised numerous concerns about his emotional well-being. Specifically, his depressed mood, irritability, and a recent increase in talk reflecting potential self-harm led to the need for additional treatment to improve his functioning at home and school.

Results of Psychiatric Consultation

The psychiatric consultation consisted of a review of Chris's medical/family history, a clinical interview, and a collection of information about his symptoms across home and school. Chris, his parents, and one of his teachers completed both broad-band (i.e., internalizing and externalizing symptoms) and narrow-band (i.e., depression) behavioral rating scales. Due to reports of depressed mood, diminished interest, and pleasure in most activities, withdrawal, and recent concerns regarding suicidal ideation, Chris was diagnosed with Major Depressive Disorder (MDD). Due to the lack of success with psychosocial evidence-based interventions, the psychiatrist prescribed fluoxetine as an adjunctive treatment. A close examination of side effects (e.g., gastrointestinal issues, headaches) associated with fluoxetine treatment was recommended to be undertaken by both Chris and his parents. A safety plan was developed, and suicidal ideation was closely monitored. School personnel were included in the consultation to ensure that the three school-based interventions were maintained with additional progress monitoring data collected.

Rationale for Psychotropic Medication Treatment

Chris has struggled with anxiety and depressive symptoms for years. A family history of depression and suicidal behavior were particularly concerning. This prior family history combined with an increase in Chris's irritability, withdrawal, and negative self-talk (i.e., "make all this sadness go away") warranted immediate attention via the use of an adjunctive psychotropic medication. While a relatively limited number of studies support the efficacy of selective serotonin reuptake inhibitor (SSRI) with children and adolescents, fluoxetine has been approved by the Food and Drug Administration (FDA) for youth up to 18 who have been diagnosed with MDD or obsessive-compulsive disorder. Given the pervasiveness of Chris's depressive symptoms and the emergence of potential self-harm, prescribing fluoxetine to Chris appeared to outweigh the costs of not providing him additional treatment. The intended target behaviors of medication treatment included depressed mood, irritability, and feelings of worthlessness. Implementing fluoxetine treatment in combination with his school-based psychosocial treatments has the potential to bring about the most positive outcomes for Chris at the lowest possible dosage (i.e., less potential for side effects).

Evaluation Methods

Chris's parents provided a release of information between home–school–physician's office to facilitate communication regarding treatment progress monitoring information. Chris's physician recommended that data collection be completed across settings to assist with any dosage change decisions and to closely monitor the intended and unintended effects of fluoxetine treatment. Chris's mother kept a chart recording the consistency of medication intake (e.g., days and times) and she provided this to the clinic during follow-up visits to ensure treatment compliance. She also sent weekly brief reports via text to the psychiatrist's office regarding the emergence of side effects (e.g., changes in sleep, appetite, impulsivity). Chris's school psychologist scheduled weekly meetings to continue cognitive-behavior therapy. During these meetings, Chris completed brief ratings on his depressed mood. Rating increases and decreases were summarized monthly and provided to his parents. Chris, his mother, and one of his teachers each completed weekly behavior ratings pertaining to depression symptoms and a summary table of results was also shared. Chris's symptoms were expected to improve within four to 6 weeks following treatment onset. A structured classroom behavioral observation was scheduled 4 weeks after treatment began to explore whether his behavior more closely approximated his teachers' expectations. A summary of all the progress monitoring data was provided to Chris's physician at the 6-month follow-up.

Cost-Benefit Analysis/Treatment Response

Chris and his parents met with the psychiatrist 6 weeks after treatment began to review the information collected at home and at school. A reanalysis of treatment costs and benefits was conducted to determine if modifications to his treatment were warranted. Chris lost five pounds over the span of 6 weeks of treatment, as he experienced daily stomachaches, nausea approximately twice a week, and overall reduced appetite.

Positively, Chris's sleeping behaviors were reported to be substantially improved. Multiple sources of information indicated a substantial decrease in depressive symptoms, an increase in academic motivation, and no ideation of self-harm. Improvements in Chris's irritability were associated with more positive social interactions with peers and adults. In the past week, Chris initiated a meeting with the wrestling club coach and received approval to resume workouts with the team. Improvements in Chris's school attendance and grades were also observed. Teacher reports and a classroom observation indicated substantially improved attention to task, completion of seatwork, and a calm demeanor. School personnel too reported that Chris was actively and positively engaged in his self-monitoring for homework completion, cognitive-behavioral therapy, and activity planning. Chris's parents reported substantial improvements at home especially related to his mood and his regular sleep patterns. Chris has been helping with chores and has been keeping his room clean. While concerned with Chris's weight loss, his parents are pleased with the improvements they have seen and are very supportive of continued fluoxetine treatment as an adjunct to current school-based interventions.

Social Anxiety Disorder

Courtney Darr

Reason for Referral

Kate is a 16-year-old female who was referred for a psychiatric consultation due to her withdrawn and socially anxious behaviors (i.e., cognitive distortions, somatic complaints, avoidance, poor coping strategies). She has previously participated in several evidence-based interventions at her high school to reduce her social anxiety symptoms. However, due to increased avoidance of psychosocial interventions, Kate was referred for psychiatric consultation.

Results of Psychiatric Consultation

The consultation consisted of a review of medical history, a clinical interview, and a series of rating scales completed by Kate and her mother. A review of Kate's medical history determined that Kate has exhibited symptoms of anxiety (e.g., marked fear of social activities, avoidance of feared activities, enduring social situations with intense anxiety) persistently for at least the past year. Her family history of anxiety and depression too was concerning. Kate and her mother completed both broad-band (i.e., internalizing, externalizing) and narrow-band measures (i.e., social phobia, generalized anxiety, obsessive-compulsive behaviors). A summary of rating scale data combined with other information indicated Kate's behaviors were consistent with a diagnosis of Social Anxiety Disorder (SAD). To reduce her anxiety toward social situations, Kate was prescribed sertraline, a selective serotonin reuptake inhibitor commonly prescribed for adolescents with anxiety disorders. A follow-up appointment was scheduled 6 weeks after the initial appointment to determine how Kate responded to treatment and if the dosage should be adjusted.

Rationale for Psychotropic Medication Treatment

Kate has struggled with symptoms of social anxiety (e.g., cognitive distortions, avoidance, somatic complaints) most of her life. Recently, Kate's symptoms worsened, and her social avoidance has become more entrenched. Concerns about self-medicating (i.e., alcohol) have emerged. Her family history of internalizing disorders highlights a potential biological component to her social anxiety. Kate's current behaviors and symptoms are substantially impairing her functioning at home and at school. Given Kate's avoidance of school-based interventions, psychotropic medication (i.e., sertraline) was recommended as an adjunctive treatment. Sertraline was selected due to its prior use in effectively treating youth with social phobia and other anxiety disorders. Treatment plans that incorporate both cognitive-behavioral therapy and psychotropic medication can often be more effective at improving social anxiety symptoms. Ideally, sertraline treatment would help reduce Kate's physiological symptoms that influence her avoidance of select social situations and may increase the likelihood of her benefiting from the school-based interventions being implemented.

Evaluation Methods

The school counselor worked closely with Kate, her mother, and Kate's doctor to ensure that progress monitoring data provided the necessary information to determine if her sertraline treatment was having the expected impact on her symptoms (i.e., improvements expected after 4–6 weeks of treatment). Several pieces of data were collected across time as Kate's doctor wanted to be able to determine if any dosage changes may be needed. Kate completed weekly ratings related to her comfort in social situations and the coping strategies she was using to reduce her anxiety. Specific attention was given to whether Kate was engaging in any self-medication efforts to cope with her discomfort. Kate also completed daily ratings related to common side effects associated with sertraline (e.g., stomachaches, headaches). Kate's mother recorded daily data pertaining to her daughter's treatment compliance. Kate, her mother, and one of her teachers completed a brief measure of social anxiety after 4 weeks of treatment. Structured classroom observation was completed 3 weeks after treatment onset to closely examine changes in Kate's participation and interactions with peers within class. Kate's school counselor summarized data from the cognitive-behavior therapy group sessions and the self-monitoring intervention aimed at attendance and class participation. Kate and her mother were responsible for bringing the summary reports to their follow-up doctor's appointment.

Cost-Benefit Analysis/Treatment Response

At her 6-week follow-up appointment, Kate reported that she generally "felt calmer" when taking the sertraline, though she did not feel like she was having many benefits related to her social anxiety and still reported anxious thoughts. Kate also experienced insomnia and gastrointestinal issues (e.g., nausea, diarrhea) during the first week of treatment. Rating scale data indicated a slight decrease in Kate's overall anxious behaviors. Information from her school indicated improved participation and slight benefits from the psychosocial interventions being implemented. Kate's physician recommended a slight increase in sertraline dosage given the overall perceptions that side effects were minimal and small improvements had been evident.

After an additional 4 weeks of sertraline treatment, Kate no longer rated herself as experiencing school avoidance as she reported reductions in her anxious thoughts and feelings related to social situations. Teacher reports also suggested an improvement in Kate's behavior in class following the increased dose. Specifically, they reported that she increased how often she was participating in class. Teachers also report that Kate has not left the classroom for extended time periods for the past 2 weeks. Based on Kate's progress, it was determined that the benefits of the increased sertraline dose were outweighing any prior (i.e., stomach issues) or newly emergent side effects (e.g., headaches). While Kate did experience some side effects on the increased sertraline dose, those side effects did not substantially impact her daily functioning. Based on these results, it was determined that Kate should continue the medication treatment in combination with school-based cognitive-behavioral therapy interventions to continue to improve her social anxiety.

Autism Spectrum Disorder

Allison Siroky

Reason for Referral

Danny is a 12-year-old male with a history of ASD who was referred by his mother for psychiatric consultation. After 9 weeks of school-based interventions with adequate adherence, Danny continued to present with difficulty managing his repetitive, stereotyped behaviors in the classroom (i.e., frequently requesting to check the news, rocking back and forth when unable to access the news) and occasional aggression toward peers and school staff members. Possible medication treatment for Danny's aggressive and stereotyped behaviors was considered.

Results of Psychiatric Consultation

After a careful review of the school-based intervention report, the consulting psychiatrist gathered additional information about Danny's behaviors. She administered a standardized behavior rating scale to both Danny and his mother. On both forms, scores on the withdrawal and social skills subscales fell within the clinical range. In addition, scores on the hyperactivity, anxiety, aggression, and adaptability subscales were within the clinical range on the parent rating form. These results were consistent with recent observations and brief interviews, which informed the earlier intervention process at school. Based on the school-based report and the psychiatrist's supplemental assessment, a polypharmacological treatment approach (i.e., use of multiple medications; fluoxetine and risperidone) was recommended to address Danny's obsessive-compulsive symptoms and his aggressive behaviors. Potential risks and benefits of both medications, as well as considerations for combining the two medications, were discussed. The consulting psychiatrist recommended a team-based approach to monitor treatment effects at home and school.

Rationale for Psychotropic Medication Treatment

While Danny didn't endorse items related to anxiety within his self-ratings, youth with ASD tend to express anxiety differently and they typically are unable to verbalize their anxious feelings. Danny's psychiatrist believed that his concern for current events may reflect anxiety caused by the persistent influx of stories depicting unrest, violence, or danger. Selective serotonin reuptake inhibitors (SSRIs) can be prescribed to reduce anxious symptoms, but they have also been shown to help individuals with ASD manage restrictive repetitive behaviors. Danny's psychiatrist recommended fluoxetine treatment. Given Danny's lack of response to the video self-modeling intervention to reduce his aggressive behaviors toward peers and teachers, Danny's psychiatrist also recommended a small dose of risperidone for short-term treatment. Risperidone is one of two medications approved by the United States Food and Drug Administration (FDA) to treat irritability or aggression in individuals with ASD. Danny's psychiatrist recommended a 4-week titration plan with brief weekly appointments to slowly work up to the full dose for both medications. With these considerations in mind, a school- and home-based evaluation plan was also essential to this effort.

Evaluation Methods

Following Danny's appointment with his psychiatrist, he, his mother, his teacher, and the school psychologist met to initiate a medication evaluation plan. The school psychologist spoke directly with the psychiatrist, who noted that both target behaviors and potential adverse effects should be monitored over time. The school psychologist decided to track three target behaviors (e.g., the frequency of requests to check the news, rocking back and forth in the seat after a denied request, instances of physical or verbal aggression) and four potential adverse effects (e.g., hyperactivity, distractibility, impulsivity, sedation). The school psychologist developed a Direct Behavior Rating (DBR) form with one item for each of these seven behaviors. Danny's teacher agreed to complete the form each day. Danny was also asked to use a daily symptom tracker to mark any somatic symptoms associated with his medications. The tracker prompted him to mark whether he experienced nausea, difficulty sleeping, difficulty paying attention, increased appetite, fatigue, or dizziness. Danny's mother reviewed the symptom tracker each week and was asked to note any other changes in his mood or behavior. The psychiatrist arranged to meet with Danny and his mother for a lengthy appointment after 10 weeks of treatment (i.e., 6 weeks after the titration phase was complete) to review the progress monitoring data.

Cost-Benefit Analysis/Treatment Response

After 10 weeks of treatment, noticeable decreases in Danny's requests to check the news during class were reported by his teacher. DBR ratings also demonstrated a steady decline in requests, starting 2 weeks after reaching the maximum prescribed dose for both medications. Danny now asks to check the news only "once or twice each class" but does not tend to ask again after being denied a request. DBR ratings across 10 weeks, including 4 weeks of titration, also showed some improvement over time in Danny's repetitive rocking behavior while in his seat. No incidents of aggression were noted at home or in school. His teacher's ratings of potential adverse effects on the DBR suggests that Danny has become slightly more hyperactive and inattentive than when prior to beginning medication. A review of Danny's daily symptom tracker suggests that Danny experienced a short period (i.e., 11 days) of insomnia shortly after reaching the full dose of both medications. Danny did not self-report any change in his attention but did note a persistently increased appetite, 5 weeks into the treatment plan. Danny's parents chose to start weighing Danny weekly after also noticing his change in appetite. Danny has gained approximately six pounds. Despite these side effects, Danny's mother reported a decrease in his interest in current events at home. She and his siblings noticed an unanticipated response, too, noting that Danny also became much less resistant when asked to complete tasks he previously avoided such as cleaning his room, getting ready for bed, or going to visit family friends. Danny had little comment on his overall response to his treatment but explained that he did enjoy going to school more now that he was getting along better with his classmates and teachers.

Psychosis

Rachel Korest

Reason for Referral

April is a 15-year-old female who was referred for a psychiatric consultation by her parents due to her recent engagement in self-harm (i.e., cutting her forearms). After 8 weeks of school-based psychosocial interventions, concerns also remained about April's poor school attendance, her increased isolation from her friends and family, poor hygiene habits, and her hostility toward others. April's beliefs that her friends and teachers were plotting against her have also worsened in the past week.

Results of Psychiatric Consultation

April's psychiatrist used an evidence-based comprehensive diagnostic assessment that included a general screening measure of psychosis, structured interviews with April, her mother, and school personnel, as well as a review of past records (e.g., medical history, family history of mental illness, school records). The psychiatrist asked about April's behavior, thinking, and perceptions (e.g., "Does your mind ever play tricks on you?" "Do you hear voices talking to you when no one is there?"). April confided that she has been hearing voices (i.e., "No one likes you April") in the past week which has led her to engage in cutting behavior. The psychiatrist also collected information from April's parents, and the school social worker related to April's history of mental health issues and observations of April's behavior at school. Through the assessments and data collected, it was determined that April meets diagnostic criteria for Major Depressive Disorder (MDD), with psychotic features. A prescription of fluoxetine, an SSRI, to treat her depressive symptoms along with a dose of risperidone to help treat April's delusions and auditory hallucinations were recommended.

Rationale for Psychotropic Medication Treatment

Fluoxetine has been approved by the FDA to treat MDD and risperidone has been approved to treat schizophrenia and bipolar disorder in youth. Prescribing April with a combination of fluoxetine (e.g., potential for increased suicidal thinking and behavior), and risperidone (e.g., potential for metabolic disturbance) was particularly worrisome to her parents. The family met at length with the psychiatrist to discuss the potential costs and benefits of this treatment combination. A chart of the benefits and potential risks of the current treatment plan was created. April's lack of response to multiple psychosocial interventions was closely reviewed. Considerable attention was given to the possible harmful effects of April's current untreated symptoms (i.e., delusions, hallucinations, depression). Working closely with school personnel, a trial of adjunctive medication treatment to the current school-based psychosocial interventions, in addition, to intensive therapy with a community-based psychologist was agreed to by all parties to try and improve April's mental health functioning. A plan to closely monitor April's behavior and symptoms for signs of improvement or adverse effects were developed.

Evaluation Methods

Before beginning treatment, April's parents signed a release of information form to allow the school to collect and communicate (i.e., to them and April's psychiatrist) information pertaining to April's behavior before and after starting medication. April's social withdrawal, delusions and hallucinations, and academic performance/attendance were tracked at school. A behavioral rating scale was used to progress monitor April's behaviors weekly by her mother and one of her teachers. The data was summarized monthly by the school psychologist and provided to April for her to bring to her doctor's visits. Before April began taking medication, her psychiatrist described to April and April's parents the potential mild to severe side effects of the medication and symptoms to look for. Some of the mild to moderate symptoms include weight gain, motor impairments, and memory difficulties that commonly occur with risperidone as well as drowsiness, stomachache, nervousness, and impulsivity that can occur with fluoxetine. Less frequent but more severe side effects (e.g., metabolic issues, suicidal thoughts/behaviors) were also discussed. To evaluate for the emergence of any side effects, April was asked to create a daily journal of any side effects she experienced and to review those nightly with her mother. April's psychiatrist also recommended she visit her general practitioner to monitor her weight and physical health at least twice prior to her follow-up appointment when possible dosage changes would be considered.

Cost-Benefit Analysis/Treatment Response

After 6 weeks of treatment, a follow-up was conducted by April's psychiatrist to closely review the costs and benefits associated with the combined fluoxetine/risperidone treatment plan. Data were encouraging as April demonstrated no hallucinations since treatment began and her delusions had decreased significantly since the start of medication treatment. April reported feeling much more comfortable at school and around her friends. She also reported hanging out with her best friend more frequently than she had been prior to medication treatment. April's mother reported that April's sleep, eating, and self-hygiene have all improved. Her interactions at home have been considerably more pleasant and she has been doing more with the family in the past 2 weeks. Data collected by the school psychologist showed an improvement in daily functioning and social withdrawal as well as decreased delusions. While April has experienced an increase in stomachaches and headaches, she has been able to treat those with over-the-counter medications. April expressed some frustration with her weight gain and reported that her appetite has increased considerably since treatment began. From April's experience, using medication to treat her symptoms in combination with psychosocial interventions has outweighed the risks. She reports that a substantial improvement in her psychological well-being and her self-esteem. April also indicated that she is not obsessing over others' feelings toward her and that her urge to cut herself has gone away. A decision was made by April's psychiatrist to taper off the risperidone treatment with the belief that fluoxetine treatment, combined with her current psychosocial interventions, may help to further treat her depressive symptoms and maintain her improved functioning at home and school.

Bipolar Disorder

Adrianna Crossing

Reason for Referral

Dylan is a 14-year-old male who was referred for psychiatric consultation by his parents and pediatrician due to his recent engagement in cutting behavior and his acknowledgement of suicidal ideation. Dylan presents with numerous mental health challenges (e.g., impulsivity, defiance, irritability, depression) that have failed to respond as expected to a series of school-based interventions and medication trials. Dylan has a history of being unsuccessfully treated with methylphenidate and is currently taking atomoxetine.

Results of Psychiatric Consultation

An assessment of the nature, severity, and duration of Dylan's symptoms was completed. Dylan's psychiatrist noted an unusual pattern with his mood, including one extended period of increased risk-taking behavior, inflated self-esteem, and irritability. Following that perceived manic episode, Dylan presented as lethargic, disengaged at school, and experiencing an increased need for sleep. The severity of Dylan's current symptoms combined with his developmental, behavioral, and family history, led to a diagnosis of Bipolar Disorder, Not Otherwise Specified (BP-NOS). The diagnosis was based on a history of at least one prior manic or hypomanic episode and a major depressive episode, and the current presentation of a possible mixed episode. Dylan's psychiatrist also noted, from a review of records, what appeared to be a manic reaction to stimulant medication and a decision to terminate atomoxetine treatment was advised. Dylan's psychiatrist recommended that he instead be prescribed divalproex sodium, a mood stabilizer, to reduce his current symptoms and reduce the chance of other mood swings in the immediate future. A decision was made to initiate a trial of an atypical antipsychotic (e.g., risperidone) if improvements were not evident within the first 6 weeks.

Rationale for Psychotropic Medication Treatment

Dylan has struggled with numerous mental health challenges over the past few years with little reprieve from prior treatments. His current endorsement of suicidal ideation and cutting behavior warrants the need for an alternative or adjunctive treatment. Due to several manic episodes, a current suspicion of a mixed episode, and present thoughts of suicide and self-injurious behavior, Dylan's psychiatrist recommended beginning a trial of a mood stabilizer to be added to his current school-based interventions. Divalproex sodium has been approved by the FDA for the treatment of bipolar disorder in youth. A close examination of the risks and benefits of treating or not treating Dylan's current symptoms was completed with Dylan and his parents. A chart detailing the costs and benefits of divalproex treatment was created and was to be reexamined in 6 weeks during a follow-up appointment. It was recommended that intensive monitoring of treatment effects be undertaken at home and in school.

Evaluation Methods

Dylan's parents signed a release of information form to allow for close communication across home, school, and the psychiatrist's office regarding his response to divalproex sodium. Dylan's manic and depressive symptoms, along with his behavior at home and school were tracked across time. Dylan worked with the school psychologist as a part of his check and connect meetings to complete daily behavior ratings regarding his mood, irritability, suicidal ideation, impulsivity, and attention. He reviewed those ratings with his mother nightly. Dylan also completed a daily journal of any side effects (e.g., headaches, lethargy, stomach issues, tremors) he experienced which he was to share with his parents on a regular basis. Dylan's mother and one of his teachers completed a brief standardized behavior rating form on a weekly basis to gather information on improvements in his social, emotional, and behavioral functioning. The school social worker provided a one-page summary of the weekly progress observed during her conjoint behavioral consultation sessions with Dylan's mother and teachers. The school counselor also created a summary of her social skills intervention work with Dylan. Each of these summaries were gathered by Dylan's mother. Finally, Dylan's psychiatrist also recommended that he visit with his nursing staff to monitor his weight, have his blood drawn to test liver functioning, and examine his physical health at least once prior to the follow-up appointment when possible dosage changes would be considered.

Cost-Benefit Analysis/Treatment Response

After 6 weeks of treatment, a follow-up appointment was conducted to closely review the costs and benefits of Dylan's divalproex sodium treatment. Dylan's liver functioning and physical health were reviewed and determined to be normal. Data summaries from school personnel and from home indicated improvements in Dylan's mood, impulsivity, and irritability. School personnel were particularly pleased to see that Dylan appeared to be more open and receptive to his school-based interventions. As a result, he had been engaging more appropriately with peers during class time. He has also been regularly eating lunch and going over to his friends to play video games. During the visit, Dylan reported feeling more calm and comfortable at school and with friends. Dylan denied any feelings or thoughts of suicide and reported feeling much more hopeful about the future. While Dylan noted that he experienced some headaches and nausea during the first week of treatment, he had not recently noted any side effects in his daily log. Dylan's parents reported improved compliance with their requests and a dramatic decline in his irritability and hostility at home. The decision to continue his current dose of divalproex sodium, as opposed to switching to an atypical antipsychotic medication, was made. Continued involvement in his school-based interventions was recommended along with further monitoring of the intended and potential side effects of his mood stabilizer medication. A 2-month follow-up visit to review progress monitoring data across home and school was scheduled.

Index

J. S. Carlson and J. A. Barterian (eds.), *School Psychopharmacology*, Pediatric School Psychology, https://doi.org/10.1007/978-3-030-15541-4

Kolibri 360 GmbH
Ferdinand-Jühlke-Straße 7
99095 Erfurt, Deutschland
produktsicherheit@kolibri360.de